Acupressure and Acupuncture during Birth

of related interest

Acupuncture for Babies, Children and Teenagers
Treating Both the Illness and the Child
Rebecca Avern
Illustrated by Sarah Hoyle
ISBN 978 1 84819 322 2
eISBN 978 0 85701 275 3

Treating Emotional Trauma with Chinese Medicine
Integrated Diagnostic and Treatment Strategies
CT Holman, M.S., L.Ac.
ISBN 978 1 84819 318 5
eISBN 978 0 85701 271 5

Complementary Therapies in Maternity Care
An Evidence-Based Approach
Denise Tiran
ISBN 978 1 84819 328 4
eISBN 978 0 85701 284 5

Chinese Medical Gynaecology
A Self-Help Guide to Women's Health
Eddie Dowd
ISBN 978 1 84819 382 6
eISBN 978 0 85701 340 8

ACUPRESSURE AND ACUPUNCTURE DURING BIRTH

An Integrative Guide for Acupuncturists and Birth Professionals

CLAUDIA CITKOVITZ

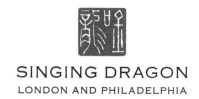

SINGING DRAGON
LONDON AND PHILADELPHIA

First published in 2020
by Jessica Kingsley Publishers
73 Collier Street
London N1 9BE, UK
and
400 Market Street, Suite 400
Philadelphia, PA 19106, USA

www.jkp.com

Library of Congress Cataloging in Publication Data
A CIP catalog record for this book is available from the Library of Congress

British Library Cataloguing in Publication Data
A CIP catalogue record for this book is available from the British Library

ISBN 978 1 84819 358 1
eISBN 978 0 85701 317 0

Printed and bound by CPI Group (UK) Ltd, Croydon, CR0 4YY

For my very own Mom,
who has taught me so much.

Contents

Foreword

It was a joy meeting Claudia in 2006 when we lectured together in New York. It was obvious Claudia had built on my earlier acupressure pamphlet and textbook on using acupuncture in pregnancy to develop her own unique and practical applications. As the director of the acupuncture program at NYU Langone Hospital–Brooklyn, her experiences teaching students and supporting women in a busy US hospital have resulted in a practical approach that can be used by health professionals, acupuncturists and support people to assist women prior to and during labor.

In 1992, as an acupuncturist working with midwives in New Zealand, it seemed logical to teach support people and midwives how to use pressure on the points acupuncturists needle to provide pain relief in labor. I could not have foreseen that positive feedback from this simple approach would have resulted in an acupressure booklet that has now been translated into nine different languages, a textbook on using acupuncture in pregnancy, and the opportunity to run workshops with acupuncturists and midwives around the world. It is a great pleasure to see these initial ideas on using acupressure expanded to provide a more detailed East Asian medicine toolkit of hands-on techniques.

My textbook focused on using acupuncture for pregnancy, with midwives sharing their experiences of using acupressure and acupuncture during birth. Claudia takes East Asian medicine during childbirth to a deeper level, providing an integrative guide for health professionals, acupuncturists and support people on assisting women during their labor. The layout is particularly useful, with Chapter 1 giving specific acupressure and other tools that can be used immediately. Chapter 2 introduces East Asian medical principles for Western birth practitioners, while Chapter 3 provides a readable introduction for acupuncturists interested in understanding the birth process. Chapter 4 provides deeper insight into physical and emotional challenges encountered by differing patient types during birth, as well as which Eastern and Western interventions may be beneficial and for whom.

Chapters 5 and 6 provide detailed hand and acupuncture toolkits of interventions that can be used by anyone interested in supporting a woman during labor, while Chapter 7 is a systematic guide to differential problem-solving throughout the labor course. The Appendices that complete this book are particularly valuable, giving information about how East Asian medicine can be used for birth preparation, breech, postpartum and recovery post-Cesarean section.

I am grateful Claudia has taken the time and care to share her expertise through this publication. *Acupressure and Acupuncture during Birth* stands out as a leading text in this field, providing the information health professionals, acupuncturists and support people need to bring East Asian medicine into the birthing room. I can only hope it stimulates further interest in the potential East Asian medicine has to offer women during this crucial time of their lives. Having read this book, I have no hesitation in recommending it as an essential text for any practitioner working in childbirth.

Debra Betts
Author – *The Essential Guide to Acupuncture in Pregnancy and Childbirth*
Wellington, New Zealand, 2019

Acknowledgments

"Birth work is not for lone wolves," I often say in class. Nowhere in my life has this been more true than in conceiving, gestating and delivering this book. Everything in it was learned from somebody's hard work writing or teaching it, and any mistakes in transmission are mine alone. Throughout every cycle of learning, practice, teaching and reevaluating, I have been sustained by the support and constructive criticism of several extraordinary tribes of people, each improving the world in her own way and helping others to do the same. I am grateful to all of them more than I can say, and will mention only a fraction by name.

My beloved mentors in the world of birth include Debra Betts, Sarah Budd, Raven Lang, Debra Pascali-Bonaro and Zena Kocher. I am also deeply indebted to my teachers and role models in East Asian medicine: Tom Bisio, Sharon Weizenbaum, Maryanne Travaglione, Kathy Taromina, Frank Butler and Caroline Radice. Jill Blakeway changed my life when she nurtured me into the world of hospital care, and has continued to inspire me and many others with her work and vision. Other guardian angels – without whose wings I might never have gotten off the ground in the hospital – include Kell Julliard, Jenny Kakleas, Salman Azhar, Elena Klimenko, Vincent Cavallaro and Khadijah Matin. In the world of Labor and Delivery, I am particularly grateful to Irene Scully, Lisa Eng, Iffath Hoskins, D'Arby Toledano, Marie Versaggi, George Aglioloro, Ralph Ruggiero, Meera Kesavan, Emad Al-Janabi, Siongpan So, Barbara Gordon and Barbara Delgado, Gail Besson, Shira Samet Patricia Wuensch, Monique DeFour Jones, Jacqueline Ford, Rosemary Ruggiero-Decarlo, Amanda Francis, Xin Guan, Elissa Marsh, Maureen Liberth, Sam Shahem, Susan Rodriguez, Amy Spurling, and Jacqueline Marecheau; also Asmaa, Masha, Irina, Agatha, Karolina, Bang, Maffel, Kadijah, Maryam, Terry, Jackie, Celina, Edie, Yonina, and so many others for their many kindnesses great and small over the years.

Among Labor and Delivery acupuncturists, my deepest, most precious gratitude is to the program's preceptor, Tzivya Kraus. Without her partnership practicing, teaching and administrating as well as discussing cases and working out new treatment ideas, neither the Labor and Delivery program nor I could not have survived the past decade. I am also deeply grateful to Melani Bolyai for her vision and drive in the early years of the program, as well as the Master's thesis and clinical work that got our first study going. Other members of the Acuteam over the years to whom I am most grateful include Holly Nochimson, Cristina Terre, Tuesday Hoffman, SooHee Straub Kristen Manges, Melanie Clemons, Brittany Harris, Robin Maza, Yael Sverdlik, Mona Elhadry, Paul Ryan, Patricia Cassidy, Sally Rappeport, Sarah Gamble, Elizabeth Shiah, Carla Kreft, Maryanne Travaglione, Moshe Heller, and Debra Barbiere.

In putting this book together, I would have been lost without the inspirational companionship of the Medicine Women gathering. Tireless and endlessly kind readers include Suzanne Connole, Marnae Ergil, Maureen Larkin, Jenn Schwartz, Jeremy Lehrer, Kate Levett, Anna Dix, Margaret Sikowitz – and a star turn by my sweet partner John Barnard (John also deserves a medal of honor for never once saying "I told you so" – out loud at least). At Singing Dragon, I deeply appreciate Claire Wilson's vision and encouragement, and Emma Holak's precise work throughout. Fred Hatt's cover photo and beautiful life drawings are a magnificent and ongoing gift to the world, as is his website and weekly(ish) blog, "Antimony". My sincerest thanks also to his body painting model: I know nothing about her other than that she has a PhD and kindly agreed to let us reproduce her magnificent image. I am extremely grateful to Tiffany Davanzo for her radiant medical illustrations, and for her patience with the endless detail of the acupuncture world. Special appreciation also to Sarah Berube for her very kind help with illustrations, and Michael Miller and Karen O'Neil for additional graphic work.

My profoundest debt is to all of the moms over the years, who have given me the sacred gift of their trust at this most private and vulnerable time.

Chapter 1

INTRODUCTION

I offer this book to acupuncturists, midwives, doulas, physicians and physician assistants, obstetrical nurses and residents, shiatsu practitioners, massage therapists, and anyone else who works or wants to work in the glorious, messy, occasionally terrifying and eternally inspiring world of birth. My purpose in writing is twofold. First, I see the principles of Yin and Yang as powerful lenses that can shed much-needed light on how the birth experience unfolds differently for different body and emotional types, helping birth team members to anticipate challenges and provide optimal support. And second, using those principles, I want to share the powerful tools I have learned for identifying and addressing the specific physical and emotional challenges that arise in difficult labors.

The insights and technical approaches in this book grew out of my experience practicing, teaching and conducting research in acupuncture and associated techniques during labor and delivery over the past 15 years. In 2003 I started teaching acupuncture students at Lutheran Medical Center in Brooklyn, New York. Now called NYU Langone Hospital-Brooklyn, it is a so-called "safety net" hospital treating a diverse and underserved population that includes many recent immigrants from China and Mexico. With a minimal budget supplemented by various educational programs and occasional grants, the team size has fluctuated over the years from just me to seven experienced acupuncture practitioners. This "Acuteam" provided prenatal care in the hospital's women's health clinic for some of that time, and in the early days I also codirected an "AcuDoula" service, attending home and hospital births throughout New York City.

In 2006 the Acuteam produced the country's first study on acupuncture during labor and delivery. We treated 45 patients with acupuncture during labor, and only three of them (7%) went to Cesarean section, versus 20 percent in 127 previous cases taken from the hospital's records. We systematically matched the two groups on characteristics that might affect labor progress such as age and number of previous births.[1] The study had been planned to explore whether acupuncture was effective for pain in American labor and delivery settings, as a series of studies in Scandinavia had shown reductions in mothers' experience of pain and use of epidural. There was some thought at that time that acupuncture might shorten the duration of labor, but seeing our study results was the first time I thought about presenting labor progress as a primary goal of acupuncture treatment. If a 7 percent Cesarean section rate was the result of treating for pain, what would we see if we treated for progress?

Circumstances have not been right to do a follow-up clinical trial, but in continuing to host acupuncture students in the years since, the program's preceptor Tzivya Kraus and I saw a number of cases where it seemed quite clear that the acupuncture had greatly accelerated labor progress, in many cases making the difference between vaginal and Cesarean birth. "I was going to cut her open," I remember one doctor saying with mixed gratitude and sadness, when a patient scheduled for C-section due to lack of progress delivered vaginally. We had done a mere 20 minutes of acupuncture, acupressure and gentle rocking of the hips – a treatment opportunity we only had because the patient was held in queue for an available operating room as we started our shift.

What struck me most about this case was how difficult the situation had looked when we started, and how easy it had been to get back on track. The mom – we'll call her Leticia – was young and strong but had a dry, pinched look to her face; likely some combination of a difficult labor and long hours at her work as a house cleaner. The labor was being induced due to low levels of amniotic fluid, and had stalled with the cervix dilated to 7–8 cm; at the time we met her there had been no change for over 4 hours, other than the cervix swelling slightly. Our analysis of the case had been that the cervix was just like the mom – strong, but with a dry, tight quality that could not easily relax and yield during painful contractions. The first element of our treatment was targeted labor support to help her system relax: turning down the lights, rocking her hips, and rubbing her feet and inner ankles. The second element was a set of specific acupressure and electro-acupuncture techniques to reduce the cervical swelling and help the tissue to soften and dilate.[2] There was a near-immediate shift in Leticia's manner

---

1   Citkovitz, C., Klimenko, E., Bolyai, M., Applewhite, L., Julliard, K., & Weiner, Z. (2009). Effects of acupuncture during labor and delivery in a US hospital setting: A case–control pilot study. *The Journal of Alternative and Complementary Medicine*, 15(5), 501–505.

2   These included "dredging" with strong thumb pressure along the inside of the shin bone to soften the cervix (discussed in Chapter 5), and electrical stimulation between the points Liver-2 and Liver-5 to reduce cervical swelling (discussed in Chapter 6).

during the contractions – from agitated to purposeful – and over the next 15 minutes her bump moved visibly downward. Her reflexive pushes, which had been spasmodic now seemed inexorable. It took some convincing for the doctor to come in and recheck her progress, as the last exam had been at shift change perhaps 30 minutes before. But indeed the previously swollen cervix had reduced to only a slight lip, which the doctor was able to push out of the way. "I was going to cut her open, like a flounder," the doctor said repeatedly, shaking her head – thankfully out of earshot of the patient.

Not all difficult labors resolve that easily, but many can, or can at least proceed much more smoothly – it's slow work though, one birth at a time. I am therefore strongly motivated to teach these conceptual and technical approaches as widely as possible. To date some 160 acupuncturists and students have trained in clinical intensives or internships on the Labor and Delivery Unit. Additionally I've taught my "Birth Basics" class, constructed on those principles, to some 400 acupuncturists from 14 countries (that I know of), and more have taken it online. My hope is that this book carries the powerful principles and techniques of East Asian medicine (EAM), as I've learned to apply them to birth, beyond the circle I would normally reach through teaching. I have therefore set out background information, basic principles and advanced techniques in stages throughout the book, so that acupuncturists, midwives, doulas, nurses, physicians and anyone else reading the book can find their own path through the material. For anyone who works in birth, a basic grasp of Yin, Yang and related concepts – as described in Chapters 2 and 4 – can provide important new tools for understanding the lived experience and anticipating possible challenges for a given birth, based on Mom's physical and emotional presence beforehand. Subsequent chapters introduce methods for supporting labor using these principles, then technical and analytical approaches to problem-solving. It is my hope that readers will find and assimilate what works for them.

1.1 For Busy Birth Professionals

Ever since I started work in a hospital I have always respected the high volume of precise work that medical professionals do – but the obstetrical nurses, attending physicians, residents and midwives I have worked with seem to me to top the charts for doing a huge number of tasks quickly and accurately in a day, few of which ever get noticed unless there is a problem. So, my valued colleagues: out of respect for your scarce time, I have compiled the list below of "low-hanging fruit." These are acupressure and other EAM techniques that can easily be applied in the moment, or taught to birth team members, without having to read the whole book. Some techniques may be familiar already and some are self-explanatory; section numbers are also provided for reference to subsequent chapters if needed.

It is my belief that the more these techniques are used, the greater the effect will be in shorter labors, fewer and more efficient inductions, fewer Cesarean sections and less blood lost. It is also my hope that, once you see how well they work, you will find the time to read at least Chapters 2, 4 and 5. The techniques are as follows:

- **"Liver Gummies," for cervical ripening and dilatation.** This is a type of acupressure conducted by rubbing upwards along the posterior/medial edge of the tibia with the side of the thumb (see Section 5.1.1.3). This technique strongly promotes cervical ripening and dilatation, particularly when the cervix is tough or edematous, but stimulation can be intense, and needs to be kept within Mom's copability zone to work.

- **Tapping at Bladder-67, to stimulate fetal movement.** A few sharp taps at the same point, with a fingernail or fingertip, nearly always stimulates fetal movements, together with about a five-beat-per-minute acceleration in the heart rate. Lack of response does not always indicate fetal distress, but immediate responsiveness can be reassuring in the context of decreased fetal movements or a flat tracing.

- **Moxibustion at Bladder-67, for breech presentation (see Section 5.4).** Familiar to some from the evidence basis, moxibustion is the practice of heating body points or regions with smoldering cigar-shaped poles of a particular Chinese herb. The technique is easily taught to family members and has several important perinatal uses. For breech presentation, it is used to warm the point Bladder-67 (the posterior/lateral corner of the pinky toenail), 15–20 minutes daily for 10 days, ideally before week 35.

- **Moxibustion on Stomach-36, as supportive care for oligohydramnios or intrauterine growth restriction.** Stomach-36 is at the top of the depression between the tibialis anterior and tibia. I have seldom seen this technique fail to raise fluid levels within a day; over a week or more it does also seem to improve weight in small-for-dates babies. Dosage is 15–20 minutes daily or as often as possible, until resolution or delivery.

- **Acupressure for pain management and labor progress:** familiar to many, the points Large Intestine-4 (on the base of the thumb) and Spleen-6 (a hand's breadth above the medial ankle) can reduce discomfort and shorten labor. Locations and stimulation instructions are found in Section 5.1.1.1, or in obstetrical acupuncturist Debra Betts' excellent app, "Acupressure for Natural Pain Relief in Labor," available via the Apple Store.

- **The Femur Shake.** I learned this technique for the treatment of sacroiliac pain, but it excels at encouraging asynclitic babies to reconsider their approach. Grasping Mom's calf right below the knee, I place my thumbs in the depressions at either side of the patellar tendon and jiggle the femur gently along its long axis, pushing and pulling it toward and away from the pelvis. Thirty seconds, starting quite gently and increasing in amplitude as tolerated without changing Mom's facial expression, is usually sufficient to encourage meaningful change.

- **Liver-14, for retained placenta.** Liver-14 is located in the sixth intercostal space, at the bra line directly below where the nipple would be on a flat chest. Pressed strongly inward and downward, I have never seen it fail to stimulate nearly immediate delivery of the placenta. I therefore press it routinely at 15 minutes postpartum if the placenta has not yet delivered.

- **Spleen-1 for postpartum hemorrhage (Section 5.2.2.1).** In the long moments before uterotonics are administered, and in conjunction with nipple stimulation or other methods to stimulate contractions, it is my experience that strong pressure with a fingernail on Spleen-1, located at the posterior/medial corner of the toenail of the big toe, visibly slows the flow of blood.

- **Moxibustion on the lower back and lower abdomen for postpartum recovery.** Use of moxa to warm the entire area daily for a week or two (or until it stops feeling great) seems to hasten postpartum recovery, increasing blood flow and helping the stretched uterus, muscles and ligaments to recover structural integrity. The effect is particularly strong after Cesarean section (in which case the scar should be thoroughly warmed, well within the bounds of comfort). Other warming methods such as two heating pads can be substituted in a pinch, but are not as useful for Cesarean section recovery.

- **To promote lactation: strong pressure at Gallbladder-21, or, moxibustion at UB-17.** Alone among these introductory techniques, promoting lactation requires some adjustment of the treatment method to Mom's body type and circumstances.

  - Young, strong moms – or stressed-out professionals who worked right up to their due dates – often have plenty of milk, but have trouble relaxing to let it out. For them, strong pressure downward at Gallbladder-21 (the midpoint of the shoulder, right in the belly of the trapezius) can open up the whole chest and shoulder, producing immediate results.

– **Moms who are older, slender, pale, anemic or otherwise lacking in vitality do not benefit from the strong pressure:** the milk is not there to be released; something needs to be added to the system in order to support milk production. Moxibustion at the point Bladder-17 seems to be extremely effective for this; it is located on the back between the spine and the bottoms of the shoulder blades, approximately 1.5 in. (4 cm) lateral to the lower border of the seventh thoracic vertebra). My colleague Debra Betts teaches this technique to New Zealand midwives, who report that milk becomes not only more abundant, but creamier.

1.2 How to Read This Book

A section of my PhD thesis was on how to make practice guidelines for acupuncture in complex conditions. My conclusion was that successful transmission of clinical practice is largely about conveying what the therapeutic goals are and why. From that basis, techniques can be swapped in and out like tools or kitchen implements: if you understand why a slotted spoon is called for in a given recipe and you don't have one, it's not hard to figure out something with two spoons or a large fork. That said, if you poach a lot of eggs, you really want a slotted spoon. This book is constructed first to explain what's needed and supply general tools, then later to provide specific ones – allowing readers to pace themselves in relation to their own needs and experience. Bullet point and tabular summaries at the end of each chapter are also provided to support readers of various learning styles.

Chapters 2 and 3 provide background information for those who need it. Chapter 2 introduces the main principles of EAM as they apply to reproductive health in general and birth in particular. Chapter 3 provides basic background on the three stages of labor, along with clinically relevant anatomy and physiology. It can be skipped by anybody already familiar with this material.

Chapter 4 describes the interface between East Asian medical concepts – Yang activity and Yin stillness – and the differing physical and emotional experience of each person's birth. In particular, this chapter identifies five main pathologies, along with their combinations, variations, and most easily recognized clinical signs and symptoms. Each constitutional tendency has its characteristic challenges in labor; for example, impaired Yin function tends to impede initial cervical ripening, while insufficient Yang often leads to slow, irregular contractions. Lecturing to midwives and doulas in the past, I have found that, once described, the basic constitutional types are very familiar to experienced practitioners and that just having a conceptual framework for these common clinical presentations can sharpen even Western clinical choices going forward. For example, oligohydramnios is often a sign of deficient Yin. Yin-deficient people generally do best in dark, quiet rooms with gentle foot massages, and tend to hyperstimulation or fetal heart rate changes with even low doses of oxytocin. By contrast, Yang-deficient patients tolerate oxytocin relatively well, but tend to require escalating doses if left in the dark without external stimulus.

Chapter 5 is designed as the "starter toolkit" for labor support; that is, helping a labor to proceed as comfortably and smoothly as possible. The chapter introduces acupressure and other non-needling therapeutic methods commonly used in labor, and presents 25 versatile, easy-to-learn techniques that anyone can use to assist labor comfort and progress. These include:

- acupressure and birth bodywork (using elements of Tuina or Chinese medical massage)

- moxibustion (this is the warming technique that helps breech babies turn)

- movement and breathing.

If Chapter 5 is the starter toolkit, Chapter 6 is the large, wheeled toolbox seen in auto repair shops, filled with specialist tools for making specific repairs on a wide range of cars. It organizes the techniques at a higher level of specificity by therapeutic goal. For each goal, a range of therapeutic methods is presented, including acupressure and bodywork as well as a few that require specific training. These include:

- ear acupressure (small herbal pellets on sticky tape applied to specific points on the ears)

- acupuncture, with specific discussion of needle size and stimulation method

- electrical stimulation of acupuncture needles.

Chapter 7 proceeds step by step through the differential analysis of what could be going wrong in dysfunctional labor. It's all very well to know that Yin-deficient patients tend to have difficulty dilating, but what if progress has stopped and there are no signs of Yin deficiency? From labor initiation to delivery, readers learn to probe each potential bottleneck for signs of constitutional pathology, as well as indications that the head and pelvis may be interfacing poorly, or that strong emotions are involved. Suggestions for assistance are also provided for each possibility, using the techniques described in Chapters 5 and 6.

Chapter 8 concludes the book with big-picture advice on implementation. The first section on safety is required reading, then subsequent sections on malpractice insurance and managing a birth practice are useful mostly for acupuncturists new to labor. An annotated list of recommended print and online resources may be of interest to all readers.

- Appendix A is a brief reference for point names and locations. It contains illustrations for all of the acupressure points used in this book.

- Appendix B describes how to perform moxibustion for breech presentation.

- Appendix C describes a non-invasive but powerful moxibustion technique for patients with threatened miscarriage.

- Appendix D provides in-depth instructions for labor preparation treatments. These are broken down both by gestational age and also through differential analysis of Mom's individual physical and emotional challenges.

- Appendix E provides a brief introduction to postpartum care, including post-Cesarean section care, afterpains, constipation, tearing and hemorrhoids, milk supply, mastitis, fatigue and postpartum depression.

- Appendix F is a glossary of East Asian medicine and Western terms that may be unfamiliar to readers.

The commonly requested topics of moxa for breech presentation, labor preparation and immediate postpartum care are covered in the Appendices. A full discussion of prenatal and postpartum care unfortunately can't fit into this book, and will have to wait for another.

1.3 Notes on Terminology

A number of Chinese medical terms do not have good English translations. These include Yin and Yang as well as Qi (pronounced "chee"). Although foreign terms are often rendered in italics, I have chosen to capitalize them instead. Also capitalized are a number of organ names and other words, close enough to the English usage to be used as translations, but with clinical implications that need to be differentiated. Therefore the Chinese Liver promotes emotional resilience, while the Western liver clears toxins.

Readers will notice that the term East Asian medicine is used more often than the more familiar term, Chinese medicine. "East Asian medicine" is preferred by many historians and scholars of the medicine, and is more accurate to use when describing acupuncture and other practices that were developed and used across the shifting boundaries of countries including Korea, Japan and Vietnam, as well as China. Nomenclature for the acupuncture points follows contemporary Western conventions, identifying points by the organ with which they are associated, plus a unique number identifying a particular point's place in line among that organ's points – e.g. Stomach-36, which in writing is generally abbreviated as ST-36. All of the point names and locations used in this book can be found at the end of Chapter 2.

In writing this book, several choices needed to be made regarding how to talk about everybody involved in the birth process. I have worked through these terms in several stages, looking for language that affirms both the diversity and the shared humanity of all involved.

- Not all new parents are married, not all partners are male, and not everybody having a baby has a partner; also some labors are attended by doctors and nurses, some by midwives and doulas. I therefore refer to everybody supporting the birth as "birth team," whether they are family, friends or birth professionals.

- Not everybody having a baby identifies as female. After considerable discussion, reading and unsuccessful experimentation with alternatives such as "birthing person," I have settled on "Mom" as the preferred pronoun for specific individuals and "moms" as the collective noun for birthing people. I hope that the word's utilitarian brevity will allow space for readers to bring their unique embodied human experience to the language – and also that language will continue to evolve in tandem with culture so that we have better choices in the future.

- I sometimes use the word "patient" to describe a pregnant person in the care of an acupuncturist, though this is not preferred, as labor is not a disease.

- Until the moment of delivery, the small creature making his or her way through the pelvis is technically not a baby, but a fetus. In order to emphasize the fetus' active role in the birth process, and also to keep the narrative human and readable, I have in many cases used "Baby," capitalized as though it were a proper name, more or less alternating male and female gender.

Terms that may be unfamiliar to readers are underlined on their first usage to show that they are included in the Glossary. Some abbreviations are used for lengthy terms that recur, such as **occiput posterior** (OP) and East Asian Medicine (EAM). These will be reintroduced in each new chapter.

1.4 Collaborative Worldviews

In working with EAM concepts of physiology and pathology, it is important to understand that they do not conflict with contemporary understandings of biochemistry and tissue function. Rather, they are complementary insights into how things tend to happen in our bodies and minds. The EAM principles in this book can be thought of a transit or traffic map, providing information about the terrain that is different from what is shown on a conventional map, but not aiming to replace it. In some mammals, stereoscopic three-dimensional vision is the result of two eyes viewing the same landscape from slightly different places, with the brain processing and integrating the information. The eyes don't agree, but we would not choose to rectify the discrepancies as they are used to form a more useful total picture than would be possible with only one view.

In writing this book on what I have learned to do in my particular place and time, I am acutely aware that many others are doing wonderful birth work that I either don't feel qualified to speak about in this book, or don't know at all: comprehensive birth education, meditative approaches, hypnobirthing, yoga, belly dancing, Rebozo work and so many others. I have mentioned a scant few, but it is my assumption that every birth worker will build their own repertory of approaches. It has also come to my attention that the approaches here tend to be somewhat problem-based, rather than positive and expansive as birth work would ideally be. This no doubt reflects both my medically oriented training, and also my work in an urban hospital where a lot of problems do indeed arise. Most important to me is that these East Asian medicine ideas and techniques be available for integration and combination with other approaches, at times when they are called for.

When I attended my first doula training with Debra Pascali-Bonaro in 2007, I was already an experienced birth worker; yet her revolutionary assertion that we could make the world a more joyful and peaceful place through joyful and peaceful birth showed me a whole new perspective. In our current fractious times, it is my fervent wish to contribute to this effort with these low-tech, preventatively oriented techniques. Originating as they did millennia ago in a faraway region of considerable conflict, may they now help to plant seeds of peace with every new life.

Chapter 2

A BRIEF INTRODUCTION TO EAM

Vital Substances and Pathological Processes

Chapter Outline

East Asian medicine (EAM) is a large field of study. Professional programs typically take 3–4 years, with an expectation of considerable continuing education thereafter.[1] That said, EAM's core principles are relatively straightforward, and make intuitive sense. They have been applied for comfort and disease prevention in kitchens and bedrooms across the ages and around the world. If there's one thing I would wish for Western-trained providers of perinatal care to take away from this book, it's that *Yin*, *Yang* and other EAM ideas are not brand new concepts to learn, but just new words for experiences that are already quite familiar – clinically and in daily life.

---

1   In some countries, abbreviated training programs are available for medical professionals including midwives.

Case 2.1 Alice, Yang-deficient and borderline hypothyroid.

Alice was 33 years old, seen in a home birth at 41 weeks and 5 days' gestational age.

She was pale and a little bit heavy, with soft flesh that was cool and slightly moist to the touch (even when she was not in the birth pool, which is where I first met her).

Alice's pulse was generally slow although she did not exercise; her blood pressure was also on the low side.

Alice and her husband had struggled with fertility, though with no specific diagnosis other than being borderline hypothyroid. Her menstrual cycles were historically long (31–35 days), with painful cramps that improved with a heating pad or hot bath.

First-trimester fatigue was severe, and her ankles were very swollen for the last month.

I was called by the midwife to help out at the birth because contractions had stalled, about 20 hours after they first became uncomfortable. Initially, the contractions were 5–7 minutes apart, less than a minute in duration and quite painful. Alice got in the birth pool at that point and the discomfort decreased, but so did the contractions. By the time I came she felt waterlogged when in the pool and chilled when out of it, with contractions intermittent, brief and mildly uncomfortable.

My assessment was that Alice's capacity for Yang action, already weak, was being further sapped by the water. I suggested drying off and warming up, using a hair dryer on her head and also the lower back until both were nice and warm. She and her husband then did activating movements such as supported squats and Cat/Cow with strong abdominal breathing, and I taught him to chafe her inner ankles and tap on her pinky toenails to encourage regular contractions. After less than an hour contractions became stronger and more regular, and I left. The midwife reported that Alice progressed rapidly from then on. She got back in the tub at transition with no loss of momentum, and within 6 hours of our visit she pushed out a beautiful baby boy.

Consider the case of Alice: her presentation was nearly opposite to that of Leticia, seen in Chapter 1. Leticia's body suffered from overwork and lacked moisture, and her cervix was reluctant to dilate despite strong contractions. By contrast Alice tended not to move enough; she was cool and moist, with late initiation of labor and sluggish contractions, but she had no trouble dilating once the labor was underway. Birth professionals will likely find both of these patient presentations quite familiar, along with their very different challenges in labor. Western medicine lacks a framework for talking about these differences, however – as though it can't assess the forest for the trees. The blood tests that determine Alice's hormone levels are extraordinary technical achievements, but without EAM interpretation do not offer insight into how her birth may proceed and what may be of help. EAM is more oriented to the basic physical conditions that speed up or slow down chemical reactions. Specifically:

- Heat is activation: it makes everything move faster, including molecules. In EAM, Yang is the force that "warms and activates."

- Cold slows and solidifies things, turning water to ice and making butter hard to spread. When a fire is blazing out of control, Yin water stills the frenetic activity – in EAM terms, cooling and calming.

In birth, Yang drives contractions and labor initiation, while Yin governs relaxation and dilatation. Alice's body was weak on Yang and already had plenty of Yin so relaxing in the birth pool didn't help her, but warming, activating movements did. By contrast, Leticia's Yin was in short supply due to overwork, so acupressure to promote cervical dilatation was actually more helpful in promoting her labor than intravenous oxytocin, which makes contractions stronger but has no direct effect on the cervix.

This chapter explains EAM's basic terms. The first section introduces Yin and Yang plus two other *"vital substances"* (*Qi* and *Blood*), describing their actions in the body, and what happens when there is too little or too much of them. The second and third sections discuss the three *pathological processes* that may disrupt them. The fourth section introduces the main ways in which EAM practitioners assess and work with imbalance and obstructed flow – two basic *therapeutic methods* with a number of variations. Section 5 introduces the acupuncture "meridians" or *channels*, and their associated *acupoints*, as a powerful system for targeting and delivering those therapeutic methods. Section 6 briefly discusses how all of these general principles apply to the specific challenges of birth, while the final section summarizes key information in table and bullet point formats for easy reference.

2.1 The Four Vital Substances

Taken together, these four "substances" broadly delineate EAM ideas on how the body works – much like listing the Western medical systems – digestive, endocrine, circulatory, etc. They are not quite substances *per se*, but can be thought of that way. For working in birth, it's most important to focus on their functions – the jobs they perform in a healthy body – and also their essential qualities, vividly illustrated in the contrast between Alice and Leticia's births. The qualities may be most clearly defined by their absence: nobody finds it remarkable when the garbage is taken out regularly, but once it starts piling up, complaints become very clear and specific. For that reason, this section includes both descriptions of what functions each substance is supposed to accomplish in the body, and also what kind of trash accumulates when the substance is weak or doesn't do its various jobs.

2.1.1 Yin and Yang

Yin and Yang describe contrasting qualities such as black and white, water and fire, moon and sun or night and day. Any phenomenon can be better understood by identifying within it the Yang forces tending toward action, movement and dominance, and the Yin properties of stillness and receptivity. Culturally, these principles are central to such landmark texts as the *I Ching* and *The Art of War*. In human health, there are five main applications:

- temperature

- management of fluids in the body

- digestion and other metabolic activity

- muscle strength and activity level

- mood, cognition and energy level.

Table 2.1 Yin and Yang qualities.

	Yin qualities	Yang qualities
Time	Night, winter	Day, summer
Weather	Cool, damp	Hot, dry
Movement	Stillness, inertia	Action, change
Conflict	Defense, withdrawal Negotiation/compromise	Direct confrontation, attack, dominance
Food	Bland, steamed	Spicy, roasted
Emotions	Grief, concern	Joy, anger
Illness	Chronic, lingering	Acute, changeable
Pain	Low-grade, nagging	Severe, excruciating
Metabolism	Slow; inhibits reactions in muscles, brain, gut	Fast; initiates and catalyzes reactions
Patient presentation	Lethargic, heavy, cold, wet (chills, edema)	Restless, hot, dry, energetic, slender
Complexion and tongue	Pale	Red
Role in birth	Governs dilatation, acceptance, self-soothing	Governs contractions, energy, hormonal activity

As seen in Table 2.1, the faces of Yin and Yang can be found in various aspects of life. Yin is at its peak during winter and the dead of night, while high noon and summer see Yang at its strongest. In movement, action and change belong to Yang, while Yin resists both movement and change. In conflict or war, Yang confronts directly and seeks dominance, while Yin withdraws, placates and seeks compromise. Even foods and food preparation have Yin and Yang polarities, with meat, spices and barbecue on the Yang side, and bland foods, boiled foods, fish and vegetables more Yin.

In the human body, Yang's functions are to warm and activate. Warmth and activation drives all bodily and metabolic activity such as muscle function, cognition, immune response, digestion of food, and processing of fluids into sweat and urine. Yang energy abounds in youth, particularly teenagers and young men: it shows in high energy, high resilience to cold (even with inadequate clothing) and low tolerance for boredom or sitting still. When Yang heat is excessive, symptoms may include fever, sweating, red face, restlessness and agitation, or constipation. Heat may also be localized to a particular area, as with a red swollen infection, joint inflammation or burning urination with a urinary tract infection.

Patients with insufficient Yang may present as cold, overweight and slow-moving, complaining of fatigue or lassitude, loose stools, edema or even congestive heart failure as the Yang activity fails to adequately warm, and Yin fluids and power appropriate metabolic activity. In birth, Yang activity drives contractions, and also the inflammatory hormonal activity of cervical ripening and labor initiation.

Yin functions include cooling and relaxing the body, as well as appropriate inhibition of functions or processes that Yang has begun. Yang promotes inflammation, while Yin quells it. Acceptance (of events and people) and absorption (of nourishment, fluids and life lessons) are also Yin functions. People with abundant Yin tend to be patient and placid to a degree that Yang types may find annoying. Excessive Yin in the body may present as accumulated fluid – including polyhydramnios and severe ankle edema. When muscles retain excess cold, they become tight and painful – like a stiff neck in winter. Excess cold retained in the uterus is a leading cause of painful periods, and resolves remarkably well with EAM therapy.

When Yin is deficient, insomnia, impatience, physical and emotional restlessness, and chronic inflammation are possible signs and symptoms. Yin is particularly important in women's health, as pregnancy's accumulation of flesh and fluid is by nature a Yin phenomenon. During birth, Yin is in charge of cervical softening and dilatation, as well as the relaxation and acceptance that allow labor to progress.

If the signs of deficient Yang seem similar to excess Yin and vice versa, this is because the two principles balance each other in their functions, so that a deficiency of one results in a relative excess of the other and vice versa. In the case of Alice above, her weakened Yang was unable to fully metabolize her Yin fluids, leading to a local excess in her ankles. Conversely, many women experience flashes of excessive heat in their 50s as their bodies have less Yin on hand to balance Yang's warmth.

Case 2.2 Qi deficiency – Lan.

Lan is 27 years old, with a medium build, soft flesh tone and a slouched posture. She seems tired and slightly withdrawn. Her pulse is deep and weak, 72 beats per minute, and her tongue is pale with scalloped edges. As a child she suffered frequent ear infections treated with antibiotics, and has been a picky eater ever since she was adopted from China, where circumstances of her birth and early nutrition are unknown. Lan says that when she eats too much she experiences bloating and loose stools, and when she eats too little, she suffers constipation and occasional hemorrhoids. She has seasonal allergies and exercise-induced asthma; also foot pain and occasional sciatica exacerbated by her work as a nurse.

Lan has been trying to get pregnant for 10 months, and her doctor says there is nothing to worry about; she should just keep trying. Her normal cycle is 22–24 days with 4–5 days of bleeding that starts pale and watery and gets embarrassingly heavy by days 2–3. Some months ago she had a 29-day cycle that ended with extra heavy bleeding; she now thinks it might have been an early miscarriage.

2.1.2 Qi

Qi (pronounced "chee") is a commonplace word in Chinese. Often paired with other words, it defies exact definition on its own, connoting entities as diverse as air, steam and gasoline. Medically, Qi can be thought of as Yang's "boots on the ground." Qi represents Yang energy that is bound up with the body's Yin and Blood in order to implement Yang's agenda of movement and activation. If Yang is leadership, Qi is hands-on management of the other substances doing work in the body. Qi's overarching responsibilities are to flow smoothly, and to keep the other substances in place and functioning appropriately, so that the body is strong and robust. Qi's specific functions are:

- to distribute Yang warmth

- to protect the body

- to raise and hold (this mainly refers to keeping blood and fluids in circulation, rather than leaking out or pooling in the ankles)

- to transform and transport other substances (this includes circulating the blood to carry oxygen and nutrients to the body, as well as digesting food and fluids to produce more Qi and Blood).

Qi's functions are numerous, and they are mission-critical. When Qi is in short supply due to overwork or poor nutrition, all of the body's functions suffer: there is fatigue, shortness of breath and sweating with minimal exercise, and brain fog; over time, muscle tissue gets soft and excess weight may develop. From a Western perspective, it is as though all the mitochondria went on strike and worked at only half capacity. From an EAM perspective, the system first affected by lack of Qi is often the digestion, with gas, bloating, fatigue after eating. This inefficient digestion then does a poor job of extracting nourishment from the food, which only worsens the Qi shortage and leads to a vicious cycle of low energy, sugar cravings and poor nutrition.

Because Qi is responsible for holding blood and fluids up and in, Qi-deficient women often urinate frequently or suffer heavy, frequent menses. During pregnancy, miscarriage and early cervical shortening may occur if deficiency is severe. In birth, Qi is directly responsible for the strength and effectiveness of contractions, as well as Mom's energy, strength and focus overall.

Case 2.3 Blood deficiency – Sierra.

Sierra is a strikingly beautiful 32-year-old African-American woman, slender and graceful. Beneath moderately dark pigmentation, there is a notable pale quality; on closer examination her inner lips, tongue and eyelids are quite pale. A gymnast and dancer since childhood, she became anorexic as a teenager. She now eats a strict organic vegan diet. She works long hours as a highly successful marketing executive, popping awake at 5am. She says that 5 hours' sleep seems to be plenty for her, as long as she does her yoga in the morning; otherwise fatigue and anxiety set in. Sierra has been diagnosed as anemic, but iron supplements give her both indigestion and ferocious constipation; she does better with herbal preparations such as Floradix. Sierra's periods have always been scanty and intermittent, and she has not had a period for 2 years. She has historically avoided treatment, as she figured she was safe from getting pregnant. When the periods come, they last only 2–3 days; the blood is thick and brownish with clots. Cramping is severe the last few days, and she often gets a migraine headache behind her eyes or at the top of her head. She now wants to get pregnant and prefers to start with a more natural approach before seeing Western specialists.

2.1.3 Blood in EAM

Blood seems more straightforward than Qi: it is the red stuff that flows in our arteries and veins. In terms of birth, however, there are a few things that Blood accomplishes in Chinese medicine over and above its Western responsibilities.

Blood's first EAM function is nourishment, which does correspond closely to blood's Western role of carrying oxygen and nutrients to all the tissues. Although there is not a one-to-one relationship between Western anemia and compromised Blood function, there is considerable overlap in signs of pallor, fatigue, dizziness, difficulty concentrating, headaches worse with fatigue, insomnia and leg cramps, as well as tachycardia or palpitations.

Blood's second EAM function is to carry Yin moisture to the tissues. In particular, when blood fails to moisten tissues adequately, athletes suffer injuries and tendinitis due to tight, dry muscles and ligaments. In birth, a tight cervix that does not ripen or dilate adequately may be suffering inadequate nourishment by the blood, or the whole body may be dry, indicating a lack of Yin moisture overall. Blood also stabilizes the body temperature, like water in a car radiator: Yin-deficient patients dislike summer heat, Yang-deficient patients dislike winter cold and Blood-deficient patients dislike them both.

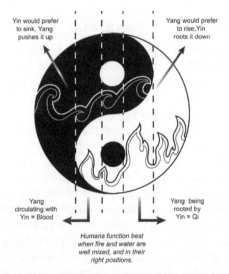

Figure 2.1 Relationships of Yin and Yang, Qi and Blood. Figure 2.1 shows the relationship among the vital substances: Yang is most purely warm and bright, while Yin is most purely cool, dark and moist. Between them, Qi can be seen as pure Yang transforming and transporting Yin, while Blood can be seen as Yin rooting Yang in order to make use of its vitality. Left to their own devices, Yang heat (the white "fish" in the diagram) would rise, while Yin water (the black "fish") would flow downwards. It is only the human metabolism that keeps Yin and Yang productively engaged in this classic picture of health.

Blood has a third responsibility, which is to "house the mind," rooting and stabilizing the flow of Qi so that attention can be steady. Just as blood stabilizes the body temperature, it also stabilizes the perceptions and emotions, providing emotional resilience. Breakdown of this stabilizing function is seen in the anemia symptoms of poor concentration and anxiety: instead of being "rooted" in the present moment, attention flickers nervously between past regrets and future fears.

Common physical signs of blood insufficiency in everyday life include poor night vision and/or floaters, brittle and/or ridged nails and a pale, sallow facial color (in severe cases there may be a yellowish or withered appearance). During birth, Blood-deficient moms tend to experience contractions as disproportionately painful, with low emotional resilience. They may also present as dissociated or "checked out," and are particularly prone to postpartum depression, constipation and difficult lactation.

Table 2.2 summarizes the qualities and functions of the four vital substances.

Table 2.2 Qualities and functions of the four vital substances.

Vital Substance	Qi	Yang	Yin	Blood
Touchstone quality	Vitality/ function	Warmth, activation	Quiescence, moisture	Nourishment, stability
Functions	• Raises & holds • Transforms & transports • Distributes Yang warmth • Protects	Warms Activates	Moistens Settles Cools	• Nourishes & moistens • Houses the mind • Flows with Qi • Determines menstruation
Temperature	Neutral to warm	Warms	Cools	Stabilizes temperature
Water functions	Moves water, holds it in & up	Warms & transforms excess water	Moistens tissues, skin, cervix	
Movement functions	Powers movement	Initiates movement	Slows/stops movement and activity (as appropriate)	Stabilizes, grounds movement
Qualities seen in deficiency	Fatigue, reduced function	Qi deficiency plus cold, wet	Hot, dry, restless, sleepless, irritable	Needy, insecure, unsteady

Vital Substance	Qi	Yang	Yin	Blood
Menstrual cycle in deficiency	Short cycle with prolonged heavy bleeding (e.g. 22 days/ 7 days)	Long cycle with severe cramps	Short or absent cycle with scant, thick, brown blood; possible perimenstrual headaches	Fluid is absent, scanty, or pale and watery; cramps late in cycle
Qualities seen in excess accumulation	Pain, anger, frustration, depression, drama	Heat	Cold Excess fluids	Fixed, stabbing pain; Masses (e.g. cancer); Menstrual clots

2.2 Balance and Flow

A healthy body keeps Yin and Yang in a state of overall balance, despite minor fluctuations. For example, Yang exercise creates excess heat, which the body discharges by boiling off Yin fluids into sweat. The body is then low on Yin water, which it will replenish by getting thirsty and drinking. If the excess heat source were to persist long-term – training for a marathon in a hot country, perhaps, or working as a fry cook – then the physical impact could become more than transitory.

In the given example, Yin can become deficient or *insufficient* when a person's exercise chronically exceeds the body's ability to replace the water lost to sweat. Blood can become deficient through excessive or prolonged menstrual bleeding. Yang can become deficient through prolonged exposure to cold and/or damp, while Qi most commonly becomes deficient through poor diet or lack of exercise. Whichever substance is deficient or insufficient, the overall Qi and vitality of the person is reduced. Indeed, acupuncturists often know that *something* is deficient in a new patient, before they are quite sure which substance or substances. It is as though the *whole* Yin–Yang "picture of health" (Figure 2.1) is reduced in size because one or more of its components is depleted.

It is also possible for the body to get stuck in a state of imbalance that is excess rather than deficient in nature – let's call this accumulation. Accumulation tends to be acute and transitory, and is seen most often in young, strong people. For example, a child with a cold or flu virus may accumulate extraordinary amounts of Yang heat as well as Yin fluid in the respiratory tract, while an older person with the same virus may suffer mainly fatigue and mild congestion. Long-term heat accumulation is sometimes seen in hot, energetic red-faced people. Excess Yin water – generally called damp or dampness – is often seen as excess fluid in the tissues, excess body weight or a constant gurgling of water in the intestine. In most cases, it presents together with Qi and/or Yang deficiency, reflecting the inability of those substances to keep the water moving healthfully through the system – a breakdown of flow.

Flow is the circulation of Qi and the other substances in our bodies, which allows them to rebalance minor fluctuations as described above. In the ocean, we can see the water moving simultaneously in tides, waves within the tides and ripples on the waves. Similarly, the body's Qi flow is experienced in a number of ways. The rhythms of the heartbeat and respiration are relatively short. Longer periods of flow include daily, weekly, and yearly alternations of Yang activity and Yin stillness. Another important form of Qi flow is the emotions, which EAM interprets as body sensations connected to life events. Think of the upward flush of anger, the sinking feeling of fear or the long, slow punch in the chest of grief. From an EAM perspective it is no coincidence that we feel more sociable in summer: our Qi moves outward when we are hot, and also when we are joyful. In winter, when the Qi pulls the blood inwards to keep the organs warm, we similarly pull in to ourselves – this is a normal manifestation of seasonal Qi flow.

2.3 The Pathological Processes

There are three main pathological processes relevant to birth: insufficiency and accumulation – which have been introduced above – and obstruction, meaning any friction or breakdown in the flow of Qi. At its simplest, obstructed Qi is the feeling you might get when you are in a crowded train station, trying to walk through the gate to your train – and the gate shuts abruptly, stopping you in your tracks. Imagine the scene for a moment: the physical sensation of being stopped short, and the feelings of annoyance and frustration that move quickly toward anger if the situation does not quickly resolve. From an EAM perspective, all of those experiences are Qi forms of stuck Qi – and indeed, if you walked into the closed gate and banged yourself painfully, that would be Qi obstruction as well. Our Qi likes, wants and needs to move – and when movement is blocked, we feel some degree of physical or emotional discomfort.

2.3.1 Disrupted Qi flow: Obstruction, stagnation and counterflow

We all experience mild friction or stagnation of our Qi on a daily basis. Qi stagnation is the physical sensation of pressure we feel in our chest, neck or shoulders when angry or frustrated. This feeling is particularly noticeable in situations of sudden change – looking for lost keys, being spoken to rudely or cut off on the highway. In an optimal health situation, we experience the emotion and take action if appropriate, or let the matter go if it's trivial; the Qi moves on and our emotions regain their normal rhythms. When someone cuts in line at the grocery store, if we already have an accumulation of stuck Qi built up from previous annoyances, we may make the mistake of bellowing at them, a welcome release that lasts only until repercussions begin. We could also say nothing and fume inwardly, which from an EAM perspective is a leading cause of emotional depression as well as physical discomfort. Musculoskeletal pain, digestive disturbances and hypertension are all frequently associated with habitual suppression of emotional responses. In Chinese medicine, your emotional life *is* the flow of Qi through your body: the feeling of expansion when joyful; contraction when sad; and tying up in a knot when worried. Many medical problems – including problems in fertility, pregnancy and birth – can be understood and resolved as chronic and acute disruptions of the normal flow of breath and emotions.

During birth, the physical tension of Qi stagnation can prevent the pelvic floor from relaxing and the cervix from dilating. We can think of this as pain causing Qi stagnation (when I stub my toe, the flow of Qi is abruptly blocked), or as Qi stagnation causing pain (after a long day in front of the computer, my shoulders and head may hurt). In EAM, both are true, particularly during birth: pain tends to make us clench, and clenching increases pain. Stagnant Qi can still move; it's just impeded in its flow, causing physical and/or emotional discomfort. The worse the stagnation, the worse the pain: moms who are able to relax and let the contractions stretch the cervix suffer less than those who reflexively clench, fighting progress and increasing stagnation.[2] I generally save the term "obstruction" for when the Qi can't move at all, such as when Baby's head is wedged in the pelvis. The less formal term "stuck Qi" includes both stagnation and obstruction.

One other perturbation of Qi's movement is counterflow, when the Qi moves in the wrong direction. The most obvious example of counterflow is belching or vomiting: the Qi of the Stomach should normally move downward, but may redirect upward if its downward flow is blocked (acupressure at the wrist point Pericardium-6, or needling on the Stomach channel can be very effective in redirecting it downward again). Another important cause of Qi counterflow is when Blood or Yin fails to root Qi and Yang in the flesh where it belongs. The upward-flushing heat of menopause

---

2   If a contraction monitor is in use, this clenching is usually visible as spiky lines radiating up from the smooth curve of the contraction itself. One of the reasons the labor and delivery nurses were so welcoming to the Acuteam from the start, is that they saw how quickly these spikes often resolved with our acupressure and needling.

is often successfully treated using this principle, as are many cases of hypertension. I have also seen symptoms of *preeclampsia* greatly improved with acupuncture and/or Chinese herbs using this principle.

2.3.2 The triad of evils: Stagnation, accumulation and insufficiency

In a healthy body, the smooth flow of Qi ensures a smooth flow of Blood and Yin fluids, while sufficiency and balance of the vital substances is needed for Qi to flow smoothly. The clearest illustration of how balance and flow interact is the menstrual cycle, where imbalance and lack of flow easily engender and complicate each other:

- When the vital substances are abundant and flow freely, the cycle is regular with small if any clots, and minimal or no cramps.

- When Qi is insufficient, it fails to hold the Blood in, so that the cycle is short while bleeding is prolonged and heavy (e.g. a 22-day cycle with 7 days of bleeding). This heavy bleeding easily depletes the Blood.

- When Blood is insufficient, it cannot flow smoothly and also causes the flow of Qi to stagnate. Menstrual fluid may be pale and watery, or scanty with cramps and clots that increase toward the end of the cycle as the flow gets weaker and stagnation increases.

- When stagnant Blood accumulates (in the form of endometriosis, fibroids or other growths) it may obstruct the Qi causing severe pain, or prevent the Qi from holding the blood in place, causing bleeding.

- When Qi is stagnant, the Blood does not flow smoothly: the cycle is irregular, with large clots, cramps and/or premenstrual symptoms of breast tenderness, headache, irascibility, etc.

- When Yin is insufficient, the cycle is short and menses are scanty, thick and brown as though dried up. Toward the end of the cycle there may be headaches as depleted Yin fails to root the Yang and Qi.

- When Yang is deficient, the cycle is long, as the Yang function of initiation is weak. Cramps may be severe with large clots, as slow-moving cold congeals the blood and impedes the flow of Qi.

In many cases, disease combines elements of deficiency, accumulation and stagnation; indeed, over time they tend to encourage each other in vicious cycles. For example, a Yang-deficient person may accumulate extra water in her tissues, making her legs feel extra heavy, which further reduces her desire to exercise and strengthen her Yang and Qi. This all-too-common cycle can begin a downward spiral towards obesity, joint pain, surgery and cardiovascular disease; I see it commonly in stroke and joint replacement patients on the rehabilitation unit. One of EAM's greatest strengths as a medical system is that it can intervene in those vicious cycles early on, spotting and addressing individual pathological processes as they arise. People can be born with constitutional tendencies to a particular insufficiency or accumulation; they may get pushed in a cold, hot, damp or dry direction by weather, diet and life activities; or their Qi flow may be disrupted by emotional challenges. EAM therapeutic methods are simply a repertoire of techniques for nourishing insufficiency, reducing accumulation and restoring flow, so that the body can rebalance itself.

2.4 Overview of EAM Therapeutic Principles and Modalities for Birth

In the West, perception of EAM is sometimes flattened to just the practice of acupuncture. In truth it comprises a large additional range of modalities, including herbal medicine, dietary therapy, Qigong exercises and Chinese medical massage or *Tuina*, each with its own separate history and traditions. What holds these treatment modalities together in contemporary practice is the theoretical system described above, where human suffering is analyzed in terms of the vital substances – what's insufficient, what's accumulating and where flow is stuck.

2.4.1 Therapeutic principles

Broadly speaking, if substances are insufficient, they need to be nourished or replenished, and if there is stagnation and/or accumulation, then Qi needs to be moved in a direction that will carry the accumulation away. In clinical practice, the topping off of insufficient substances tends to be differentiated by what functions are most affected – both because the methods used will differ slightly, and also because there is some sharing of functions between Yang and Qi, as well as Yin and Blood. General principles used in pregnancy, birth and the rest of EAM health care, include:

- **Warming Yang.** Anytime somebody is acutely or chronically cold, Yang is missing in action or blocked by excess cold, so heat needs to be added to the system. For example, soaking the feet in hot water at night can be miraculously effective in turning up a chilly person's inner thermostat.

- **Boosting Qi.** Qi's many functions in the body include driving muscular strength and metabolic function. When they are weak – with symptoms including fatigue, shortness of breath and poor digestion – the principle of "boosting" Qi best encapsulates helping Qi move, hold and carry all the substances. Moderate cardiovascular exercise is actually the best Qi booster over time, but acupressure and other techniques described below can support Qi's actions when needed.

- **Activating Yang and/or Qi.** People may be sluggish due to some combination of insufficient Yang failing in its activating function, and insufficient Qi failing to respond to the call to action. Excess Yin damp also tends to block the flow of *Yang Qi*. Sluggish people often self-medicate with caffeine or other stimulants; healthier methods include martial arts, yoga's "breath of fire," and a "chafing" technique of bodywork, described in Chapter 5.

- **Nourishing Blood.** Healthy Blood is made over time, from good Qi and good food. Stimulating certain acupoints can help to accelerate the process, as can Chinese herbal medicine. As will be seen in later chapters, however, during labor it is more useful to manage acute symptoms of Blood deficiency than to increase production.

- **Nourishing Yin.** Nature's most potent Yin tonics are rest and sleep – both of which can be hard to find during labor and the days before birth – especially for Yin-deficient people who are poor sleepers anyway. Acupressure on Yin points of the feet and ankles can be very helpful in reminding the body to relax, accept the labor process and allow the cervix to dilate. Dimming the lights, reducing screen time and banishing inflammatory personalities can all "calm the spirit," helping the body to shift out of Yang adrenal mode and restore Yin balance, whether during labor or before bedtime.

- **Moving Qi (and other substances).** As discussed above, when Qi flow is impaired by life events, damp, cold or other factors, then symptoms of Qi stagnation may include pain, disrupted menstrual cycle or digestion, and feelings of anger, frustration or depression. Qi stagnation may be caused by accumulation of other substances, or the impaired flow may lead to such accumulation; in either case the accumulation needs to be reduced through moving Qi. Vigorous exercise, strong massage and acupuncture are healthy ways to move Qi; less healthy approaches include temper tantrums and drinking binges. During labor, stagnation is inevitably a large part of the picture:

the contractions are trying to push Baby out, while the cervix and pelvis are holding her in. Most techniques of movement, breathing and acupressure used during labor have a primary purpose of moving Qi to relieve pain, with other secondary purposes. Other uses of the moving principle during labor include:

– **Softening.** Imagine that your shoulders are tight and hard as a rock from long hours of work at the computer. The pain and tightness is indeed a manifestation of stuck Qi, but a vigorous massage or strong acupressure would likely just cause more pain. "Softening" is the principle of gently moving Qi though a stagnant area (in labor, usually the pelvic floor or cervix) to loosen tightness, without causing further pain or exacerbating the Yin or Blood deficiency that often underlie muscular tightness.

– **Clearing heat.** Trapped Yang Qi easily heats up; strong acupressure or acupuncture on certain points can be very effective in restoring flow to help the body to cool itself. I have seen intrapartum fever reduce by a degree and elevated fetal heart rate return to baseline within minutes of acupuncture treatment.

– **Redirecting Qi downwards.** As discussed in Section 2.3.1, Qi may rise due to stagnation, or insufficient rooting by Yin or Blood. Pressure or needling on certain acupoints can be extremely powerful to correct the aberrant flow, often resolving or reducing hypertension, vomiting, or headaches on the spot.

2.4.2 Therapeutic modalities

Among all of EAM's various modalities, seven are presented in this book. Using its guidelines, the included techniques of acupressure, bodywork, movement and breathing can all be performed and taught safely to birth team members, as can moxibustion. Acupuncture and electrical stimulation of acupuncture needles require professional training. Auriculotherapy training is easily available online and is important for effective usage, though not strictly required in most countries.

Tuina, sometimes translated as "acupressure," is a medical art used in China for internal medicine as well as orthopedic and muscular complaints. I use it extensively in the hospital for stroke and other neurological and orthopedic conditions. Tuina uses a large repertoire of "hand techniques"; these include various types of finger pressure, each with its own set of operating instructions and therapeutic goals. For this book, "acupressure" designates techniques that stimulate specific acupoints or discrete linear sections of a single channel, while "birth bodywork" indicates larger-scale techniques – those that move or activate the legs, hips or whole lower back. I was lucky enough to do all of my early training with Tom Bisio, one of the leading teachers of Tuina in the West.[3]

Acupressure is unparalleled for its ease of use, with no equipment required and most techniques easy to teach to birth team members. Acupressure does not move the whole body's Qi as strongly as bodywork or movement, nor is it the strongest for nourishing vital substances. However, with hundreds of points to choose from, as well as a variety of stimulation methods, acupressure can be exquisitely precise in its effects – loosening stuck Qi or ligaments in a particular area, or drawing Qi downward to calm the spirit, relieve nausea and/or help the fetal head descend.

Birth bodywork excels at moving large amounts of Qi quickly – when Baby is stuck in the pelvis, for example, or to calm and descend an upward rush of panic. Like acupressure on a larger scale, it also excels for warming the abdomen and softening the pelvic floor, as well as nourishing Blood, and helping the cervix to ripen prelabor or in hospital inductions. Some of the techniques require a little bit of practice – particularly those in Chapter 6 – but the ones presented in this chapter are relatively straightforward and extremely useful both as comfort measures and to encourage progress.

Moxibustion is the longstanding East Asian practice of burning mugwort (*Artemisia annua*) on or near the body to warm and activate specific points or functional areas (such as the lower back, lower abdomen or stomach region). Perhaps its best-known use in the West is for improving the odds of breech babies turning, when burned at the UB-67 point at the back outer corner of the fifth toenail (instructions for this procedure are provided in Appendix B). Moxa is not permitted in most hospitals and many birthing centers, but can be very helpful prelabor, postpartum and during labor in spaces where it is allowed. Its fiery nature makes it most naturally suited to warming Yang and boosting Qi to help a sluggish labor get in gear, but it is also extremely useful for nourishing Blood, prenatally and postpartum. In particular, its use on the point Stomach-36 appears to increase blood flow to the uterus, along with amniotic fluid levels. I suggest it routinely for moms anytime they are told Baby is small or amniotic fluid is low.

Movement and breathing are important EAM therapies that are often overlooked. This book mostly uses movements that are already familiar

---

3   Tom's excellent book *Zheng Gu Tui Na: A Chinese Medical Massage Textbook* (Bisio, T. & Butler, F., 2007) is coauthored with another of my early mentors. As well as teaching the hand techniques, it links Tuina body mechanics to a set of Qigong and standing meditation exercises that are extremely beneficial for health care providers who spend a lot of time on their feet. More information on Tom's Tuina, Qigong and martial arts classes is available at internalartsinternational.com.

to birth professionals – such as Cat/Cow, and rocking the hips – but uses EAM principles to refine their use in two ways. First, each is presented in association with the imbalance and flow problems it is most likely to benefit, and second through more conscious and specific use of the breath. "Qigong" literally means "Qi work," and describes any exercise where the breath and movement are used together to guide Qi flow in specific health-corrective or preventative directions. As many already know, the powerful combination of breath and movement can create dramatic shifts, not only Qi flow through the pelvis, but also in Mom's spirit, the trajectory of the labor and the whole atmosphere of the room.

Diet is an important element of EAM therapy in general, as is "lifestyle medicine" – activity adjustments like morning walks for Yang deficiency, and limiting evening exposure to news or social media for Yin deficiency. These are not relevant to labor, but will be discussed briefly in the "care packages" provided for the different body or *constitutional* types described in Chapter 4.

2.5 The Acupuncture Channels

Some readers may be accustomed to the term "meridians," to describe longitudinal pathways in the body that connect external acupoints, located all along the limbs and torso, with the internal organs and their functions. "Meridians" is a slightly antique translation, conjuring up images of invisible force lines on a map. A more accurate rendering would be "channels," in the sense of agricultural ditches that carry water to fields. Chinese medical and agricultural science both developed extensively in the first millennium BCE, both far in advance of their Western equivalents. Current medical research increasingly associates the acupuncture channels with large planes of fascia, a watery connective tissue that supports and lubricates bones, muscles, internal organs and the nervous system. The fascia is highly responsive to acupuncture-type stimulation, and may explain some of acupuncture's therapeutic effects.[4] As a map of the body,

---

4   For more on this fascinating line of inquiry, see the work of Helene Langevin.

Langevin, H. M., & Yandow, J. A. (2002). Relationship of acupuncture points and meridians to connective tissue planes. The Anatomical Record: An Official Publication of the American Association of Anatomists, 269(6), 257-265.

Langevin, H. M., Churchill, D. L., Fox, J. R., Badger, G. J., Garra, B. S., & Krag, M. H. (2001). Biomechanical response to acupuncture needling in humans. Journal of Applied Physiology, 91(6), 2471-2478.

Langevin, H. M., Churchill, D. L., & Cipolla, M. J. (2001). Mechanical signaling through connective tissue: a mechanism for the therapeutic effect of acupuncture. The FASEB Journal, 15(12), 2275-2282.

the channels help us both to understand where flow is obstructed in the body, and also to target balancing methods to areas where they are needed most. A complete list of acupoints used in this book, along with their abbreviations, is provided in Appendix A.

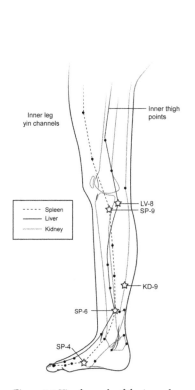

Figure 2.2 Yin channels of the inner leg
– Spleen (SP), Liver (LV), Kidney (KD).

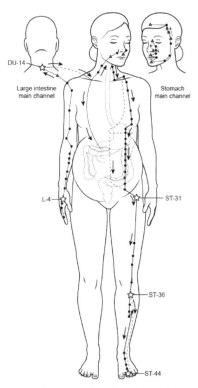

Figure 2.3 Yang Stomach and
Large Intestine channels.

In relation to birth, a few things are most important to know about the channels.

- Each channel has an affiliation with a vital or digestive organ, connecting the region of the torso that contains the organ with the head, arms and/or legs.

  - The Yin channels pertain to the vital organs (Heart, Liver, etc.). The most important ones for birth run up the inner legs towards the torso (see Figure 2.2).

  - The Yang channels pertain to the digestive organs (Large Intestine, Stomach, Gallbladder, etc.). They run downwards, carrying Qi from the head to the feet (see Figure 2.3).

- – In the West, acupoints along each channel are numbered in accordance with its flow (e.g. Stomach-36, or ST-36 for short). A few "extra" points are not located on the main channels, so their Chinese names are used (e.g. Duyin).

- Specific points along each channel can amplify therapeutic effects and carry them elsewhere in the body. For example:

  - – Large Intestine-4 excels at moving stuck Qi downward, particularly in the head, face and lower torso. Self-acupressure can help with headaches, sinus pain, back pain and sciatica.

  - – The Kidney regulates many Yin and Yang functions in the body, and its channel circles the inner ankle (see Figure 2.2); the area is therefore very useful for replenishing weak Yin and/or Yang with acupressure or moxibustion.

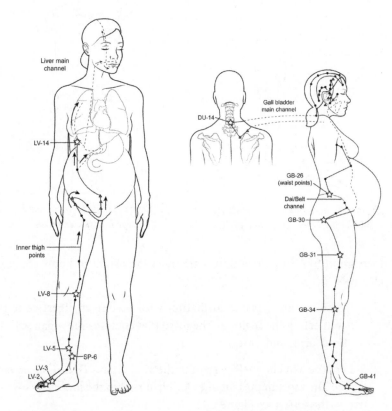

Figure 2.4 Yin Liver channel.

Figure 2.5 Yang Gallbladder channel and Dai (Belt) channel.

Channels commonly used in birth include the following:

- The Liver (LV) channel is the single most influential channel for softening the pelvic floor and cervix. Classically it is said to "wrap the genitals." As can be seen from its pathway in Figure 2.4, it also moves through the groin and inguinal groove. The whole channel region, along the posterior border of the tibia from the ankle to the knee, can be massaged to strongly move Qi and soften the cervix, as well as treat premenstrual syndrome (PMS) and menstrual cramps. Other important points include LV-2 (used for <u>cervical edema</u> and mastitis) and LV-5 (a go-to for acupuncturists treating any vaginitis or pain in the region).

- The Kidney and Spleen channels, seen in Figure 2.2, also run upwards along the inner leg, and can be used to nourish any of the vital substances. The point SP-6, located a hand's breadth above the inner ankle, lies at the crossing point of all three leg channels, and strongly nourishes both Yin and Blood, promoting cervical ripening and dilatation.

- The Stomach (ST) and Large Intestine (LI) channels, seen in Figure 2.3, are powerful both for moving Qi and also for boosting and activating it. Important points include LI-4 on the thumb and ST-36 below the knee.

- The Gallbladder (GB) channel shares a number of points with an "extra" (non-organ-related) channel pathway that encircles the waist, known as the Dai or "Belt vessel," both shown in Figure 2.5. Several Gallbladder points and areas have a strong softening effect on the pelvic floor, including GB-34, GB-41, the iliotibial band above and below GB-31, and GB-30 in the buttocks.

2.6 Locating and Addressing Obstruction in Birth: Bone, Flesh and Spirit

In birth, there is a very specific task at hand: moving the fetal head down through the cervix and pelvis. As seen in this chapter, EAM concepts of insufficiency, accumulation, and stagnation or obstruction excel at sorting out the nature of any obstruction and the therapeutic approaches most likely to help. To do this effectively in birth, it is necessary to be as specific as possible about the location of the obstruction and the type of tissue involved.

The tissues of the EAM body can be understood on a spectrum from most to least substantial, Yin to Yang. At the Yin end, the bones are the densest material in the body, resistant to change and slow to heal. At the Yang end, our spirit, thoughts and the flow of emotions rippling through our bodies have no discernable substance and can change quickly – though as any health care practitioner knows they are quite real. In the middle is the soft tissue, affected by the bones and also the emotions, Qi and Blood. Much of birth work, EAM or otherwise, lies in discerning accurately in the moment what type of obstruction is most likely occurring. The basic framework for understanding and working with obstruction is presented below. Experiential differences among types of obstruction are discussed in Section 4.6. A more detailed guide to differential analysis is provided in Section 6.1.

2.6.1 Bony obstruction

Bony obstruction is familiar territory for birth workers. In some cases the fetal head is actually too big to enter the pelvis, known as cephalopelvic disproportion or CPD. More common is what might be termed functional CPD, when the head approaches the pelvis in a bad position or off angle, so that the force of the contraction presses painfully into the hard bones rather than dilating the cervix. As bony obstruction is the densest, most absolute form of stagnation, gross physical movement is the treatment of choice, shifting the dysfunctional relationship of head, pelvis and gravity in search of one that works. Tuina bodywork is particularly useful in this regard. The forms I learned in particular were developed alongside traditions of martial arts for use with musculoskeletal pain and injuries. They can be particularly useful both in moving the pelvis and sacrum, and also in liberating extra millimeters of extra space by loosening their connecting ligaments. For example, a technique I learned for addressing sacroiliac joint pain – grasping the knee and shaking the femur gently along its long axis[5] – is extremely handy for jiggling the pelvis and encouraging asynclitic (poorly angled) babies to reconsider their approach.

2.6.2 Flesh and flow

When the problem is not with the bones, but with inadequate contractions or cervical dilatation, then there must be imbalance or stagnation of the vital substances, requiring some combination of nourishment and movement. These fleshy obstacles to labor progress are detailed in Chapter 4, but can be summarized as follows:

- Contractions may be inadequate due to insufficiency of Yang or Qi.

---

5   See Section 6.3.1.3

- Accumulated Yin damp may also slow Qi flow, mimicking the symptoms of insufficient Yang or Qi.

- Cervical ripening and dilatation may be slow due to insufficiency of Yin or Blood.

  - When contractions are disproportionately painful for their size, this indicates stagnation of Qi; possible underlying causes include tightening of the tissues by cold, or impaired flow and low resilience due to insufficiency of Yin or Blood.

- EAM does not draw a clear boundary between emotional challenges and physical difficulties; therefore, any challenge of slow dilatation, excessive pain, delayed labor onset or slow progress may also reflect emotional challenges including past trauma (see the section to follow).

- Remember that Qi flow is also the movement of the emotions in the body. Strong emotions such as anger, grief and fear can stagnate the Qi, tightening the inner thighs and pelvic floor and slowing down cervical ripening and dilatation.

2.6.3 Spirit, thoughts and emotions in EAM

The EAM view of the human spirit is remarkably similar to that of the 2017 Pixar movie, *Inside Out*, which itself is creatively inspired by contemporary, evidence-based insights about the nature and development of emotion and cognition.[6] In the movie, emotions such as joy, anger, sadness and fear form a kind of leadership committee for the person, clustering around a control console in the brain as they process information from the senses and send out commands for movement, speech and action. Traditionally, EAM has located its command center in the heart, but the joint leadership structure – with joy at the helm – is identical.

In a healthy state, the five spirits work together to integrate their sensory information and emotional drives into a coherent consciousness and action plan. Under stress, one of the five may filibuster – prioritizing its agenda, and ignoring sensory evidence about the outside world that does not fit its view of how things are and ought to be. This happens in the movie, too – when the characters Joy and Sadness abandon the control room, leaving Anger at the helm. Indeed, habitual anger is the most common of the emotional imbalances, associated with Qi stagnation and the Liver, as well

---

6   https://www.psychologytoday.com/us/blog/if-babies-could-talk/201712/the-science-emotion-the-inside-out

as related emotions such as frustration, self-hatred and depression. Most people have a default emotional orientation, and it is not at all uncommon for anger, fear, grief or anxiety to become "sticky" during a stressful labor, arising more often than circumstances warrant, and sometimes permeating the room. This stickiness usually manifests physically as well as emotionally, in tightness of the chest, abdomen, lower back, pelvic floor and/or inner thighs; and in most cases, using breath, acupressure or needles to work with tightness in the body is a direct and effective way to keep the emotions flowing smoothly.

In some cases, particularly when there is a history of trauma, the emotion will become fully obstructive – with Mom stuck in a distressed state of flashback or reactivity. There are many tight areas, but touching or moving them only worsens the distress. There may be a sense of overload, which operates like Yin deficiency, with any stimulation at all leading to further agitation and lockdown. Or, conversely, Mom may "check out," dissociating from her experience – the emotional version of Yin and Yang not interacting. These challenges are more than just sticky emotions: think of the spirit as the governance structure of the human being, the spark of consciousness and purpose around which balance and flow are organized. When the spirit is dissociated or locked down, it is as though the ruler of a castle has run away or is barricaded in a closet. The immediate priority is creating a safe space and helping Mom back to the seat of power in the center of her body. Acupressure at the point Kidney-1, on the sole of the foot, is so effective for this that one of my colleagues calls it "the Panic Button." Other approaches are discussed in Chapters 4, 5 and 6.

There is considerable overlap between spiritual and emotional challenges – a precise differentiation is both unnecessary and impracticable. What is important to remember is that while strong emotions such as anger and frustration often respond well when treated as Qi stagnation in the flesh, fear and trauma can easily lead to dissociation or lockdown. In those cases establishing a safe healing space is top priority; any physical work will likely be much gentler, as discussed in the chapters to follow.

2.7 Summary Table and Ideas to Remember

With some additions and elaborations, the use of EAM's vital substances and pathological processes to understand and intervene in human health has persisted since at least the 2nd century BCE. EAM thrives worldwide and continues to evolve to meet the needs of cultures as varied as China, Japan, Korea, Vietnam, France, Australia, Turkey, several African nations, the United Kingdom and the United States. It is both the oldest and the most widely practiced system of traditional medicine in the world.

2.7.1 Summary table

Table 2.3 summarizes the healthy function and pathology of the four vital substances, as discussed in this chapter.

Table 2.3 Function and pathology of the four vital substances.

Vital substance	Qi	Yang	Yin	Blood
Functions	Raises & holds Transforms & transports Distributes Yang warmth Protects	Warms Activates	Moistens Settles Cools	Nourishes & moistens Houses the mind Flows with Qi Determines menstruation
Qualities seen in deficiency	Fatigue, reduced function	Qi deficiency plus cold, wet	Hot, dry, restless, sleepless, irritable	Needy, insecure, unsteady
Menstrual cycle in deficiency	Short cycle with prolonged heavy bleeding (e.g. 22/7)	Long cycle with severe cramps	Short or absent cycle with scant, thick, brown colored blood; possible perimenstrual headaches	Fluid is absent, scanty, or pale and watery; cramps late in cycle
Qualities seen in excess accumulation	Pain, anger, frustration, depression, drama	Heat	Cold Excess fluids	Fixed, stabbing pain; Masses (e.g. cancer); Menstrual clots

2.7.2 Ideas to remember

2.1 The four vital substances:

- Yin and Yang represent opposite principles of stillness and activity, while Qi and Blood are substances doing the work of Yin and Yang in the body.

- Yang warms and activates; in birth it initiates hormonal activity including contractions. When it is insufficient the body will be cold, and excess water may build up.

- Qi governs flow, strength and overall vitality; it keeps the other substances moving, and also holds them up and in. Deficient Qi shows in fatigue, brain fog, soft flesh tone and poor digestion.

- Yin governs cooling, rest and moisture; Blood carries nourishment and Yin moisture to the tissues, stabilizing body temperature, Qi and the emotions.

- Deficient Yin and Blood both show in dryness of the tissues, insomnia and anxiety, with deficient Yin tending more to restlessness, heat and impatience, while Blood deficiency tends more to insecurity and poor concentration.

2.2 Balance and flow:

- A healthy body's regulation of body temperature and fluid levels with activity keeps it relatively balanced over time.

2.3 The pathological processes:

- Forms of stuck or disrupted Qi flow include stagnation (partial obstruction of flow), severe obstruction and counterflow (when Qi flows the wrong way, e.g. belching).

- Insufficiency or accumulation of the vital substances may obstruct Qi flow – or vice versa, stagnant Qi may cause local imbalances.

- The menstrual cycle provides an excellent window into balance and flow of the vital substances.

2.4 Overview of EAM therapeutic principles and modalities for birth:

- A variety of EAM therapies can assist the body to rebalance itself, using the core therapeutic principles of nourishing insufficiency, and moving stagnation or accumulation.

- General therapeutic principles are based on the functions of the vital substances that they are restoring.

- Additional, more specific principles are based on the clinical goal to be achieved, e.g. "soften pelvic floor" and "promote cervical ripening."

- Therapeutic modalities for executing those principles include acupressure, Tuina (Chinese medical massage), moxibustion, movement and breathing, as well as acupuncture and auriculotherapy, which require specific training.

2.5 The acupuncture channels:

- The channels serve to amplify and target therapeutic principles to the areas where they are needed, based on their organ affiliations and directions of flow.

- Channels important in birth include the Liver, Kidney, Spleen, Stomach, Large Intestine, Bladder and Gallbladder channels, as well as the extra "Belt" channel, which circles the lower abdomen.

- Acupoints are numbered per channel in its direction of flow, e.g. ST-36.

2.6 Locating and addressing obstruction in birth: bone, flesh and spirit:

- During labor, it is important to understand whether obstruction of progress is occurring at the level of bone, flesh or spirit/emotions, though they can be hard to distinguish.

- Bony obstruction in general is addressed with gross physical movement including EAM bodywork in order to improve the interface of fetal head and pelvis.

- Obstruction at the level of the flesh can be effectively addressed with EAM methods to reestablish balance and flow, as described in Sections 4.6 and 6.1.

- Emotional and spiritual challenges are sometimes responsive to treatment of the vital substances, and sometimes require more specific approaches, as discussed in Chapters 5 and 6.

THE EVENTS OF BIRTH

Chapter 3 Outline

— 3.1 The Baby and the Bones

— 3.2 The Soft Tissues

— 3.3 The Labor Journey

— 3.4 Summary Table and Ideas to Remember

This chapter examines the beginning, middle and end of the birthing process from several different perspectives: what is happening with the bones (mainly Mom's pelvis and Baby's <u>occiput</u>); what is happening with the soft tissue (mainly the uterus and cervix); and what is happening with the hormones, neurotransmitters and local signaling molecules that underlie changes in the soft tissue. Those three perspectives then combine to form an experiential, real-time narrative of how a normal birth unfolds, and where it may go off track.

3.1 The Baby and the Bones

For male mammals, the function of the pelvis is to support and balance the considerable weight of the abdomen, thorax, head and upper extremities as they move around over the legs – a considerable engineering feat. For the female half of the species, that feat is then made all the more impressive by adding a "secondary" function of propagating the species by growing a fetus in the abdomen large enough to survive in the outside world, then moving it out through the pelvis.

There are various strategies among species, for managing the trade-off of development versus ease of birth: bigger, more robust babies have a better chance of becoming adults, while smaller fetuses have a better chance of getting out in good shape (and with a healthy mother). Kangaroos deliver tiny, relatively immature babies, which then live warm and safe in a pouch for some weeks. Horses and giraffes gestate for close to a year, delivering large babies that are ready to walk within the hour – but quadrupeds' pelvises have relatively more space to deliver through, as they don't have to support the full weight of the body.

It is important to understand that upright posture is a relative anomaly in the animal kingdom, and has evolved in relation to a culture of communal living that – like the kangaroo pouch – provides a period of warmth, safety and nourishment for relatively helpless newborns. Even our closest genetic relatives, chimpanzees and mountain gorillas, do not normally walk on two legs for long distances. Humans' exceptionally long childhood compensates to some degree for our upright posture and big brains, by letting babies be born relatively small. However, there is no question that, without medical intervention, some would not survive. On the one hand, birth is an animal event that in most cases flows better with less overthinking and micromanagement. On the other hand, we need to acknowledge that, evolutionarily speaking, it's a tall order to get a viable fetus out of a biped pelvis. For most of recorded human history it has been far and away the primary killer of mothers and babies alike.

This section of the chapter describes in detail the baby's journey through the pelvis – entering, moving down through it and turning to descend out. As we follow that journey, it's important to note the relationship between the shape of the pelvis, and the baby's positioning and movements needed to move smoothly through and out. As will become apparent, babies do sometimes grow too big to get out safely – but often, hang-ups are due to position or problems maneuvering, and could potentially be resolved given an appropriate combination of movement, gravity and time.

3.1.1 Engagement, or entering the pelvis

The obstetrical pelvis is defined as the parts of the pelvis actively involved in childbearing – basically the large oval hole in the bottom of it, and not the hipbones up near the waist. During the 9 months of gestation, the baby floats above the obstetrical pelvis. When the time for delivery approaches – usually a week or two before – the pelvic floor stretches as Baby grows, and his head begins to dip into the bony opening. On examination, once the head can no longer be jiggled or "balloted" from side to side, the head is said to be engaged, meaning that the widest part of the head has entered the obstetrical pelvis.

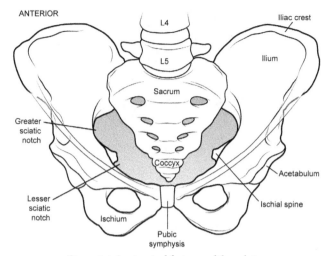

Figure 3.1 Anatomical features of the pelvis.

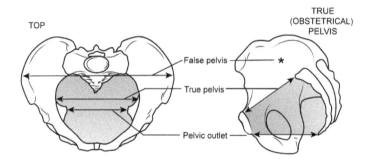

Figure 3.2 The obstetrical pelvis.

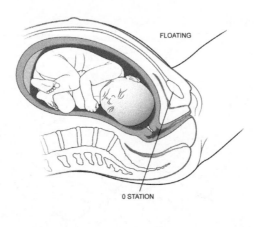

FLOATING

0 STATION

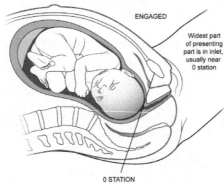

ENGAGED

Widest part
of presenting
part is in inlet,
usually near
0 station

0 STATION

Figure 3.3 The fetal head floating versus engaged.

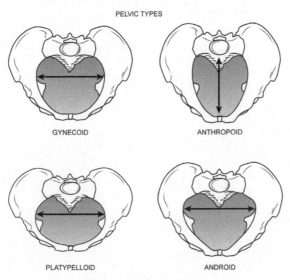

PELVIC TYPES

GYNECOID

ANTHROPOID

PLATYPELLOID

ANDROID

Figure 3.4 Pelvic types.

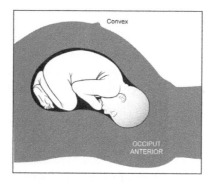

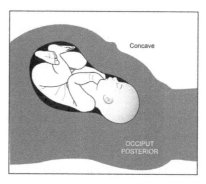

Figure 3.5 Occiput anterior versus occiput posterior – internal view.

The pelvic shape considered most conducive for birth is the vaguely heart-shaped gynecoid pelvis, which provides plenty of space at the front of the pelvis for Baby's <u>occiput</u> to drop into, usually angled toward the front left. There are two main ways that the shape of the pelvis can interfere with engagement:

- A flat (or <u>platypelloid</u>) pelvis is too shallow from front to back, which doesn't leave enough room for baby to drop in.

- A pelvis with a narrow pubic arch may force the baby to enter with its large, protuberant occiput toward the sacrum (the pubic arch is the front portion consisting of the two pubic rami that join at the pubic symphysis). <u>Anthropoid</u> and <u>android</u> pelvises tend to be narrow in front. The resultant *occiput posterior* (<u>OP</u>) position can cause long labors that are quite painful in the back and sacrum, as well as *prelabor rupture of membranes* (PROM).

3.1.2 Moving into the pelvis

Baby's head usually engages with Baby's nose pointed toward one or the other of Mom's buttocks, the occiput obliquely forward. Once the soft tissues are also ready – see Section 3.2 below – the labor can get into gear. This is because, once the head is settled at an appropriate angle in the obstetrical pelvis, its shape naturally funnels the contraction pressure toward the *cervix*, pulling it up against Baby's head so that it is forced to dilate – like a very tight turtleneck. As Baby's head proceeds downward into the pelvis, there is no bony obstacle to progress until halfway down. At that point, the head bumps into the ischial spines, which protrude into the pelvis at its midpoint (see Figure 3.1). In most cases Baby must turn himself to a different angle, with the occiput facing forward, to get between the ischial spines and also the ischial tuberosities (sitz bones).

If Baby enters the pelvis looking forward and out rather than in toward the spine, this is called occiput posterior position – OP or "sunny side up," so called because OP babies are born looking upward, if Mom is on her back. OP contractions cause pain in the sacrum (see Figure 3.1) and lower back, often described as back labor. In the absence of back pain, if there are problems in the labor after engagement, they are likely attributable to soft tissue problems, as there is simply nothing in the pelvis itself to obstruct progress before transition, when Baby turns and descends to exit the pelvis.

Baby's progress through the pelvis is described in terms of the head's location. Using abdominal palpation, the head can be thought of in five segments, each about 2 cm or the width of a large male finger (see Figure 3.6). If most of the head is palpable, the head is still floating; when it is engaged, only about two-fifths are palpable. When midwives or doctors perform a vaginal exam, the head station is assessed directly from within (see Figure 3.7). In this system, the ischial spines are taken as "0" or the center point (a handy mnemonic for acupuncturists is to think of this as the "Point Zero" of the pelvis). If baby is above this point, the head station is a negative number: "−3" indicates that the lowest part of the baby's head is about 3 cm above zero, still floating; by "−2" the head is engaged. It is possible for the lowest part of Baby's head to get past the ischial spines, to "+2" or so, before the narrow space between the spines forces him to turn, a movement called transition (see Figure 3.8). It is transition that allows the baby to exit the pelvis.

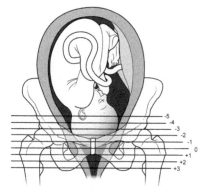

Figure 3.6 Evaluation of fetal <u>descent</u> by external palpatation.

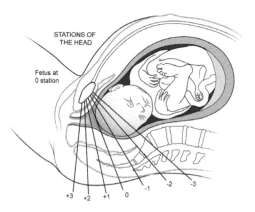

Figure 3.7 Evaluation of fetal descent by internal palpatation.

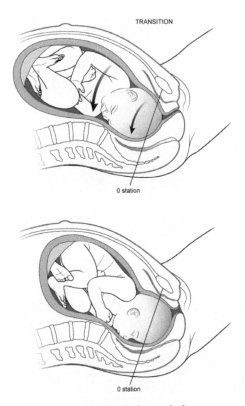

Figure 3.8 Transition, before and after.

3.1.3 Transition: Turning and descending to exit the pelvis

Transition is the point in labor where the shape of the pelvis forces all but the smallest babies to turn from angled to the front left (usually the best way to enter the pelvis) to facing Mom's spine (or OP, if the pubic arch is narrow or Baby is feeling mischievous). Baby's head is relatively long in the front-to-back dimension, and relatively narrow side to side (see Figure 3.9). The opening at the top of the pelvis in most cases starts out wider from side to side, requiring Baby to drop in with the large occiput angled forward. Then the relatively narrow space between the ischial spines and ischial tuberosity forces baby to turn front to back. Transition may occur between 8 cm and 10 cm of dilatation, or after full dilatation is reached, depending on the consistency and construction of the cervix.

Once transition is complete, Baby is in position for delivery with nothing between her and the outside world but the perineum and a tight spot in the vaginal canal where the cervix used to be. If all is going according to plan, Baby dives under the pubic arch and out into the big bright world. However, it is not at all uncommon for babies to get stuck in transition, stalling the labor until something changes – either the right combination of pelvic and fetal movement, or operative intervention. Some of the bony obstructions that can impede transition are discussed below.

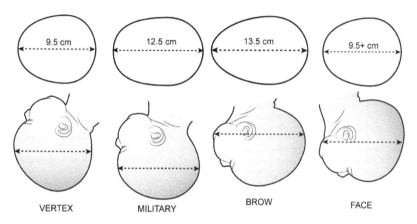

Figure 3.9 Dimensions and presentations of the fetal head.

3.1.3.1 Malposition

"Position" in birth is used solely to describe the *rotation* of the "presenting part" – in most cases the occiput of the head; otherwise the sacrum, if Baby is breech. The position is classified as posterior or anterior based on whether the occiput is in front or in back, and may be further specified as right or left. Left occiput anterior (LOA) is by far the most common position, showing in some two-thirds of births. Right occiput posterior (ROP) is the next most common, occurring in some 25 percent. Persistent occiput posterior (OP) can lead to arrest of labor and Cesarean section. However, vaginal birth is entirely possible in most cases, and in many cases midwives, doctors or doulas are able to suggest movements and positioning for labor and delivery that can help create a little more space for Baby to either turn to a better position or wiggle out the way she is. Due to the angle of Baby's head, pressure is directed in a posterior direction rather than through the cervix and vaginal canal. Severe tearing of the perineum and anal sphincter is therefore more common in OP than OA births.

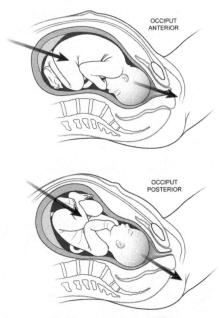

Figure 3.10 Angle of exit in occiput posterior versus occiput anterior births.

3.1.3.2 Malpresentation

Presentation means, literally, the part of the baby that is showing itself to the doctor. Normally speaking, this should be the vertex, meaning the top of the head when it is well flexed, with the chin is tucked down toward the chest. Malpresentation denotes a "bad" presentation, meaning anything that is not the vertex, e.g. the forehead, shoulder or breech (the space between the buttocks). In contemporary practice, breech presentation is generally diagnosed in advance; vaginal birth may or may not be attempted depending on the region and practitioner. Face and brow presentations occur when Baby arches her head back rather than tucking her chin in. Babies presenting their whole face can often deliver vaginally, while brow presentation generally goes to Cesarean section as the chin obstructs progress. Another important type of malpresentation is compound presentation, in which Baby's arm is raised, either up over his head – this usually leads to C-section – or with the palm on his face, which may deliver vaginally.

Box 3.1 Compound presentation.

I have attended two compound presentation births, and in each it was clear that there was some kind of bony obstruction that I didn't entirely understand. In both cases I used predominantly movement techniques to encourage change, such as rocking the hips, as well as acupressure to boost Qi and Yang (these tend to get depleted in a long, slow labor). In the second birth, the pushing stage was particularly rocky, with the fetal heart dropping out on the monitor for long minutes at a time, and the nurse eventually just holding the monitor on Mom's abdomen to catch the heartbeat. That baby came out with not one but two hands on her face, looking like a chubby miniature of Edvard Munch's *The Scream*. The physician supervising the case was the new head of the residency program at the hospital, and I had never worked with her before. She looked at me quizzically and said, "That's a double compound. Double compounds don't deliver vaginally." It was her belief – and mine – that the movement and acupressure had made the difference between vaginal and Cesarean delivery; she went on to refer a number of cases for acupuncture in the years she was there.

3.1.3.3 Asynclitism

In <u>asynclitism</u> the baby's head enters and moves through the pelvis at the wrong angle – essentially the birth equivalent of bad parallel parking (see Figure 3.11). Just as either the curb or the car behind you may prevent you pulling into a space, the baby's head bumps against either the sacrum or the pubic bone as it engages, kinking his neck toward Mom's back or front as he descends into the pelvis. This kinked neck makes transition difficult at best; the head may stay wedged with the occiput transverse and tilted, unable to tuck and turn as it should.

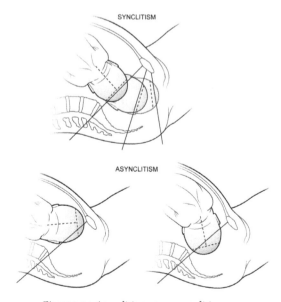

Figure 3.11 Asynclitism versus synclitism.

3.1.3.4 Cephalopelvic disproportion

Cephalopelvic disproportion (CPD) simply means the head is too big for the pelvis. It is frequently cited in hospital paperwork as the reason why a particular delivery occurred by Cesarean section. Moving as I do between home birth and hospital circles, I find it remarkable how differently the term is used and perceived by different birth personnel relative to their life experience. Most doulas and home birth midwives are familiar with the work of Ina May Gaskin, a pathbreaking midwife whose first book, *Spiritual Midwifery*[1] told of her experience in the 1960s and early 1970s delivering over 300 babies vaginally without incident, before the first one needed to be transported to the hospital for Cesarean section. That figure is all the more shocking today, when over 30 percent of US births are by C-section, but it is anomalous even for the 1970s, when the US C-section rate was 5 percent.

Box 3.2 True versus functional CPD.

It is tempting to believe that the body would never grow a baby too large for itself, and that our exploding C-section rate could be reversed entirely by better birth practices. While I have no doubt that the number could be reduced drastically, I have also seen true CPD more times than I can count, in an urban community hospital where many patients are immigrants from countries with different nutritional profiles. Some are young, with their pelvis not fully developed; others endured malnourishment as children (which can reduce pelvic size) or currently suffer from <u>gestational diabetes mellitus</u>, which increases the size of the baby. Even in general populations, babies are growing larger – while an increasing number of moms were themselves born by Cesarean section, meaning that they did not necessarily inherit a favorable pelvic shape from their mother. At the hospital a few years ago, I remember remarking to a nurse that a particular baby looked too large for the mother's body, with her belly stretched so tight that I could see the outline of Baby's shoulder. The nurse, a 30-year veteran, had clearly seen this situation many times over. "You can see the shoulder?" she quipped, "I can see it's a boy. He's way too big." As she predicted, the baby never engaged, and was born by Cesarean section.

Relaxation and movement not only increase soft tissue's ability to stretch around a large baby, but also give Baby time and space to find his way out. In addition to wriggling around to the best angle, babies accommodate to the shape of the pelvis with soft skull bones that slowly change shape with

---

1   Gaskin, I. M. (2010). *Spiritual Midwifery*. Summertown, TN: Book Publishing Company.

pressure (<u>molding</u>), to gain a few extra millimeters of clearance. In that light, it is hard to escape the conclusion that many diagnoses of CPD really reflect lack of movement for a patient stuck in bed, and lack of patience for the doctor. Very early in my career I was at a birth where the medical staff diagnosed CPD and they performed a C-section. The baby weighed 6 lb 1 oz, and had pronounced molding at the side of his head, a clear sign of asynclitism. I had tried everything I knew at the time, and was as surprised as the doctor by the outcome. However, knowing what I know now, I believe I could easily have helped the mom to move and the baby to unwedge herself. Overall, CPD should be regarded as "true" only when the head really is larger than the largest passage through the pelvis. In my vocabulary, the term "functional CPD" describes all the other possibilities – from a small baby with her head wedged asynclitically, to a large one who has a possible route out but isn't finding it yet. The exact purpose of expert labor support is to resolve every possible case of functional CPD – both by introducing movement that can unstick bony problems, and also by helping Mom's soft tissues to stay on track while Baby finds her way out. The more efficiently Mom and Baby can move through <u>latent</u> and <u>active phases</u>, the more energy they will have left for problem-solving in transition and second stage.

The above discussion includes all of the bone-level problems commonly seen during labor. Function and dysfunction of the soft tissues are described below.

3.2 The Soft Tissues

Much more complicated than the structure of the pelvis (and much less well understood by Western science) is what happens in the pelvic floor, cervix and uterus during labor and delivery. This section provides a very brief introduction to a very large topic, focusing on what is most essential to birth work. The first three subsections cover what the uterus, cervix and pelvic floor are made of, and what they do before, during and after birth. A fourth subsection introduces the main hormones and other signaling molecules in the body, whose delicate dance through our tissues is the interface between our human experience of birth and Western medical reality. The final section describes how both of those realities are seen through the lenses of East Asian medical assessment and treatment.

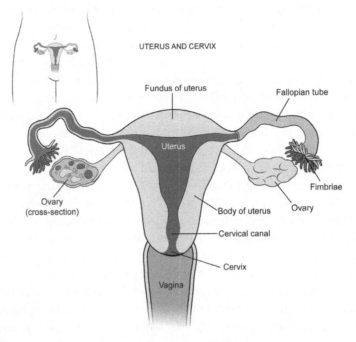

Figure 3.12 The uterus and cervix.

3.2.1 The uterus

Considering its enormous importance, the uterus (Figure 3.12) is a very small piece of tissue. It is pear-shaped, but not pear-sized: before a first pregnancy it is only about 3¼ by 2 in. or 8 cm long and 5 cm wide. Before pregnancy (and depending on the menstrual cycle) it typically weighs 40–50 g, or a little under 2 oz. After pregnancy, it grows larger in all dimensions by a half-inch (1.2 cm), and weighs somewhat over 2 oz (60–80 g). The uterus is sandwiched between the urinary bladder and the rectum, which is why the bladder is sometimes nicked during Cesarean sections and the urge to push resembles the urge to defecate. In EAM, herbs and acupuncture points used to treat constipation are also used to promote labor, and some expert herbalists I know use retaining enemas as the most direct way to treat pain and other symptoms of endometriosis and fibroids. The uterus is made of smooth muscle, similar to that of our hearts and digestive organs; the muscle layer is called the myometrium. The uterine lining, which thickens and sheds with the menstrual cycle, is called the endometrium.

During the first 12 weeks of pregnancy, specialized cells in the placenta burrow into the endometrium and requisition the blood supply, much like a parasite or an invading army. Immune function is lowered in pregnancy (likely to prevent attack of the fetus); response to this invasion may also explain why 80 percent of pregnant patients experience nausea. The blood of Mom and Baby do not normally mix during pregnancy: instead, the capillaries of the placenta run right next to uterine blood vessels so that oxygen, nutrients and waste can be exchanged. Attached to the placenta are membranes that hold amniotic fluid, which supports and protects the baby (the amount of amniotic fluid is commonly quantified using the numerical Amniotic Fluid Index or AFI).

3.2.2 The cervix

The cervix is the firm, knobby opening of the uterus, which protrudes into the vagina (see Figure 3.12). It is 1.5–2.5 in. (3.5–4 cm), about a third of the total length of the uterus, and made of dense connective tissue. For most of the 9 months of pregnancy, it holds its shape firmly in order to keep the baby safe inside. Around week 37 – or sooner, in cases of incompetent cervix or premature labor – the process of cervical ripening begins. Under the influence of multiple hormones and other signaling molecules, the cervical tissue begins to soften and to move forward in the vagina, as the softer tissue is more easily stretched by the baby weight. The cervix also begins to open (cervical dilatation) and shorten (cervical effacement); it may also lose the plug of cervical mucus that has been contained within the dormant cervical opening (cervical os). A complete report of a perinatal vaginal exam (VE) includes cervical dilation (from 0–10 cm), effacement (from 0–100%) and head station, along with cervical quality (soft/mid/firm) and position in the vagina (posterior/mid/anterior).

Table 3.1 Bishop Score.

		Points allocated			
		0	1	2	3
Factor	Dilatation of cervix (cm)	0	1–2	3–4	5–6
	Effacement of cervix (%)	0 to 30	40 to 50	60 to 70	80 or more
	Consistency of cervix	Firm	Medium	Soft	
	Position of cervix in the vagina	Posterior	Mid	Anterior	
	Head station	−3	−2	−1, 0	+1, +2

3.2.3 The pelvic floor

The phrase "pelvic floor" is somewhat of a misnomer. It is generally used to describe a set of muscles around the perineum, vagina and urethra, which stop the flow of urine, close the anal sphincter and pull upward and inward during sex and orgasm (see Figure 3.13). However, these small muscles are contiguous with a larger web of muscles and fascia (connective tissue) that line the lower abdomen and wrap the bladder, rectum, uterus, fallopian tubes and ovaries, holding them upright and free flowing rather than puddled and kinked on the "floor." During pregnancy, weak pelvic floor muscles can cause stress incontinence as well as constipation and an uncomfortable bearing down sensation. Most importantly, lack of support from the pelvic floor muscles can cause excessive pressure on the cervix, which leads to premature shortening and may require bed rest or even stitches to prevent early delivery. Any of these symptoms – particularly the bearing down sensation – should be taken as important warning signs and referred back to the medical provider as well as to an experienced EAM practitioner. When it's really time for labor, the sheer weight of the baby should stretch the pelvic floor, which then puts pressure on the cervix and begins the complex process of cervical ripening, described in the sections to follow.

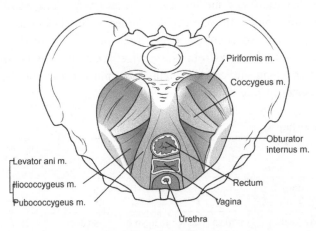

Figure 3.13 The pelvic floor.

3.2.4 The key hormones (and other signaling molecules) of birth

Estrogen and progesterone are hormones critical to initiating and maintaining pregnancy, and their levels must be appropriate for labor to proceed smoothly. Relaxin, oxytocin and small local signaling molecules called prostaglandins are more directly involved in labor initiation and progress. "Signaling molecule" is a generic term for any molecule that originates in one place and acts somewhere else, in effect carrying a chemical message. As will be seen below, the terms "hormone," "neurotransmitter" and "eicosanoid" are subcategories of signaling molecules: hormones originate in glands and act on tissues or organs, neurotransmitters act within the brain and eicosanoids act locally on the cellular level.

3.2.4.1 Estrogen and progesterone

Estrogen and progesterone are two of the central hormones of female reproduction; their levels must be appropriate for labor to proceed normally. Estrogen levels need to be adequate for fertilization to occur; they rise during the pregnancy, and stay high to maintain the pregnancy. No special changes occur around the time of birth, but high estrogen levels are required for the uterus to be sensitive to *oxytocin*, the main hormone that drives uterine contractions.

Progesterone supports and maintains the uterine lining before implantation. In the absence of implantation, the uterine lining sloughs off. However, if a fertilized egg does implant, progesterone levels remain high to support the uterine lining. Progesterone also helps maintain the pregnancy by lowering the immune response, as well as decreasing contractility of smooth muscle, so that labor doesn't start early. In the weeks before delivery, progesterone levels need to drop, allowing the uterus to contract and preparing the body for lactation.

3.2.4.2 Relaxin

As its name suggests, relaxin is a hormone that softens connective tissue in the body. It is present at all times, but fluctuates with the levels of other hormones, peaking at menstruation, in the first trimester and again at delivery. In pregnancy, relaxin softens the cervix so that it can dilate more easily, and softens the pelvic ligaments and pubic symphysis to provide a little extra room for delivery. High levels of relaxin can lead to sciatica, carpal tunnel syndrome and *symphysis diastasis* in pregnancy. Conversely, relaxin may be deficient in patients suffering from diseases that stiffen the connective tissue, such as fibromyalgia and scleroderma.

3.2.4.3 Prostaglandins

Prostaglandins are a class of local signaling molecules, built from fatty chemical building blocks throughout the body. Like B vitamins, there are a number of related prostaglandin types, and they tend to travel and function together. Unlike hormones, which send signals from one system to another, prostaglandins are low down in the body's "chain of command" and regulate actions between neighboring cells or within a single cell. Prostaglandins are very important in inflammatory and immune responses: their signaling serves to initiate and perpetuate the classic redness, swelling, heat and pain signs that show the body's reaction to a perceived injury or threat of infection. Prostaglandin E2, the main prostaglandin involved in cervical ripening and uterine contractions, also induces fever. Its action is inhibited by aspirin and other non-steroidal anti-inflammatory drugs (NSAIDS).

To understand the actions of prostaglandins during labor, it is important to remember how all signaling molecules work. They do not just carry information, like computer communications on a wireless network. They are physical objects that function mechanically within the cell, like three-dimensional keys that fit into keyholes in the cell membranes, called binding sites. What's more, once a signaling molecule fits into its binding sites, it changes the shape of the membranes around it, which then affects potential binding sites in the area. For example, when levels of progesterone in the body are high, the progesterone molecules bound into uterine and cervical tissues prevent prostaglandins from binding in large numbers, as they will during labor. It's not that prostaglandin binding sites are closed by progesterone – it's that when progesterone is bound, the cell membranes are entirely the wrong shape for prostaglandins to bind into. Like train platform 9¾ in the Harry Potter books, the binding site is just not there until the conditions are right.

With all that in mind, let's look at how prostaglandins act in the cervical connective tissue and pelvic floor muscles. As progesterone levels drop toward the end of pregnancy, the baby is also getting large enough to stretch the tissue. Prostaglandins are automatically released from the muscle, and local connective tissues are stretched. And then, because progesterone is low, there are binding sites available for those same prostaglandins to bind back into. What happens when prostaglandins are bound into those binding sites? The tissue softens, meaning that the same baby weight stretches them more, which then leads to more prostaglandin release, which leads to more tissue softening, and so on.

It is worth noting that East Asian medical reasoning relies heavily on this kind of self-perpetuating cycle. Patients who tend to be angry often make themselves angrier by dwelling on infuriating subjects. Those who have fatigue and low energy often make matters worse by avoiding exercise. With the understanding that stretching the connective tissue stimulates prostaglandin release while prostaglandin uptake makes tissue stretchier, we promote cervical ripening with bodywork that jiggles and stretches the hips and bottom.

In the cervix, this virtuous cycle of tissue stretching, prostaglandin release, tissue softening and more stretching is one and the same as cervical ripening. In the uterine muscle layer, stretching and softening also take place as progesterone drops and the baby gets larger. However, there is one important addition to the picture: once prostaglandins are bound in their binding sites, this opens up binding sites for oxytocin.

3.2.4.4 Oxytocin (as a hormone)

Heart muscle cells are unique in the body, in that they both propagate and respond to electrical signals that tell them to contract rhythmically. Other muscle cells in the body don't contract until nerves tell them to, but the heart's pacemaker cells keep a rhythm going without external stimulation. Uterine tissue is also quite special: like the heart it has the ability to contract rhythmically, but, unlike the heart, it only does so when the hormonal and local tissue conditions are right.

What are the right conditions?

- Systemic estrogen has to be high (as it is in pregnancy).

- Systemic progesterone has to be low (it drops toward the end of pregnancy).

- Prostaglandins have to be bound in their binding sites, so that...

- Oxytocin is bound in the cell membranes of the muscle cells. This can only happen when prostaglandins are bound in the tissue *and* oxytocin is systemically high.

Under all of those conditions, the uterine muscle then begins to contract rhythmically – just as though it were a second, slower, heart. The binding of oxytocin and onset of contractions is contiguous with the process of cervical ripening described above, and usually happens gradually. Especially in first-time moms, the tissue has never done this before, and takes a while to figure it out. The phenomenon can be compared to a stadium full of novice sports fans, mostly inexperienced in doing "the wave." It would take a while for the old hands in the group to explain the principle – just stand up and raise your hands as soon as the person next to you does it. Throughout the arena there would be pockets of people doing it right, mostly clustered around the experienced folks. Those clusters would be isolated at first, and it would take quite some time for word to travel from neighbor to neighbor, so that the wave could propagate successfully around the stadium.

In just the same way, contractions start out small and irregular – just a handful of muscle cells activating when enough oxytocin is bound that that they contract. Those cells tug on neighboring cells, which in turn stretch, bind prostaglandins and oxytocin, and begin rhythmically contracting and propagating the electrical signal. Two heart cells in a Petri dish will beat at different rhythms if they are not in contact, but once they are pushed together they will synchronize, taking the faster of their two rhythms.

Similarly, in early labor the uterus will have multiple initiation sites at different, quite slow rhythms – 151 minutes here, 98 minutes there, so that the result is weak, irregular contractions that stretch the tissue but do not cause much sensation or movement. The force of an individual muscle fiber's pull in the uterus never does change – one fiber can tug only as hard as one fiber tugs. What changes is the *coordination* of the pulling action, and the number of cells participating. As the cells of the uterus progressively soften and stretch under the influence of prostaglandins, then activate under the influence of oxytocin, a higher and higher proportion of uterine muscle cells contract and then rest in time with each other. It is this coordinated activity – ideally initiated right at the top of the uterus – that pushes the baby down while pulling the cervix up.

Oxytocin is secreted from the pituitary gland, located just below the hypothalamus at the base of the brain. In addition to acting on the uterus, it also acts on other tissues in the body, including the mammary glands (which contract rhythmically to secrete milk). It is secreted at the time of orgasm in both sexes and in males appears to facilitate erection and accelerate ejaculation (oxytocin antagonists can prevent premature ejaculation). Its precise role in orgasm and ejaculation is not well understood[2] scientifically, but there is no lack of clarity on the part of birth professionals that smoochy kisses, sexual activity and orgasm are excellent ways to promote and prepare for labor.

3.2.4.5 Oxytocin (as a neurotransmitter)

Our nomenclature for signaling molecules is based on where they are secreted and where they act. When molecules are secreted from a gland and take action in tissue elsewhere in the body – such as the uterus – they are called hormones. When signaling molecules are secreted and act within the brain, they are called neurotransmitters. Because oxytocin is secreted in the pituitary gland, which is in the brain, it is called a hormone when it acts on the uterus

---

2   Jong, T. R., & Neumann, I. D. (2015). Moderate role of oxytocin in the pro-ejaculatory effect of the 5-HT1A receptor agonist 8-OH-DPAT. *The Journal of Sexual Medicine*, *12*(1), 17–28.

and a neurotransmitter when it acts on the brain. The fact that it is present at high levels during birth, orgasm and breastfeeding cannot be entirely coincidental; experientially these are not unrelated processes, but moments of ultimate intimacy. Oxytocin, as a neurotransmitter, does indeed appear on the scene at times when people are usually thought to be feeling warm, loving feelings: in happy relationships, breastfeeding, falling in love, etc. Oxytocin levels are usually higher in monogamous animals than non-monogamous ones, and when mother sheep are given oxytocin antagonists, they refuse to mother their own young. Oxytocin levels are generally higher in women than men, and oxytocin is thought to be a major modulator of stereotypically female behaviors – just as testosterone factors into stereotypically male behaviors. On closer research, our idea of the "fight-or-flight" response to adrenaline appears to be better understood as the typical response to adrenaline plus testosterone, whereas the typical response to adrenaline plus oxytocin appears to be the more feminine "tend and befriend."

Oxytocin's role as a neurotransmitter is important to birth in several ways. First, oxytocin levels rise as Mom goes into labor, and they peak at delivery. This makes sense: it is oxytocin that is making the contractions happen. So by keeping the hormone/neurotransmitter connection in mind, we can often notice that when a mom is getting ready to go into labor, she feels quite emotional and loving, and often displays chatty, extroverted "tend-and-befriend" behavior (whether or not this is her normal state). Second, it is not at all uncommon for moms to get into a great contraction pattern at home, then head in to the hospital only for contractions to stop upon entering the scary, antiseptic-smelling building. Stress inhibits oxytocin, which makes perfect sense, as any mammal in the wild might start going into labor only to be stalked by a predator. The ability to stop labor and then restart again would have been an important survival mechanism.

One final way in which it is important for birth support personnel to remember the relationship between oxytocin's hormonal and neurotransmitter functions is what happens after the administration of synthetic oxytocin.[3] Oxytocin was the first human hormone to be synthesized – Vincent du Vigneaud won a Nobel Prize for it in 1955 – and in the decades since, these synthetic versions have been used for the *induction* and *augmentation* of labor. Oxytocin is given intravenously, at concentrations that are low relative to most drugs, but quite a bit higher than what occurs naturally. The IV oxytocin usually does its job of making the uterus contract more strongly. However, there are several side effects – most

---

3   Pitocin and Syntocinon are commercial names for synthetic oxytocin.

notably that as oxytocin levels spike higher than normal, the pituitary gland stops releasing it. Which, because oxytocin is a large molecule that does not cross the blood/brain barrier, means that for the first time in her life Mom finds herself experiencing the world with little or no oxytocin in her brain. If one were going to try out a new drug that radically affected one's perception of the world, labor is not the time one would typically choose to try it. We have some idea what high levels of oxytocin do to our experience: they make us feel happy, open, trusting and resilient. In other words, exactly what is needed during the exciting, but intense and potentially quite frightening experience of birth.[4]

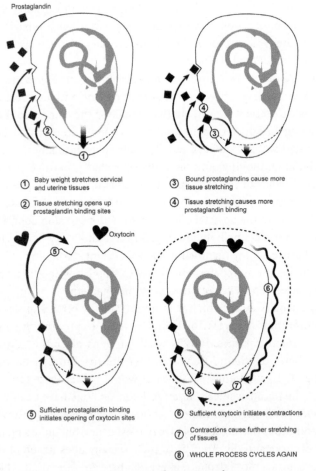

Figure 3.14 The cervical ripening cycle.

4   In Yin/Yang terms, synthetic oxytocin performs oxytocin's Yang function, making the uterus contract, but not its Yin emotional function of supporting love and bonding.

3.2.5 The cervical ripening cycle

The "cervical ripening cycle" is a (greatly oversimplified) graphic depiction of some of what happens in the soft tissues during early labor (Figure 3.14). Within the graphic, the base represents the pelvic floor, the left-hand side reflects the cervix and the right-hand side represents the uterus. In Step 1, the pelvic floor is stretched by increasing fetal weight, which (Step 2) stretches the cervix and other tissues, opening binding sites for prostaglandins and other inflammatory cytokines that help to soften the cervical tissue once bound (Step 3). In Step 4, the softer tissues stretch more, opening yet more binding sites. This self-perpetuating cycle is the "first gear" that gets labor going. In Step 5, sufficient binding of prostaglandins in the uterine tissue opens binding sites for oxytocin, which, once bound in sufficient amounts, initiates contractions (Step 6). These contractions in turn begin to dilate the cervix (Step 7), which is the "overdrive" of labor really kicking in (Step 8).

3.3 The Labor Journey

The preceding sections have introduced the bones and soft tissues of the pelvic area as they relate to birth. In this section, that information is used to describe the sequence of events of birth in detail, as they unfold in healthy labors. Also described is where the process can break down leading to "dystocia," or dysfunctional labor.

The entire labor and delivery process is conventionally divided into three stages. As a matter of usage, I have always heard these described as first, second and third stage, never as stage 1 or stage 3. The first stage of labor and delivery comprises everything from the first progressive contractions through full cervical dilatation, with the baby fully turned and ready to be pushed out – in other words, nearly all of "labor." Clinically, first stage is further divided into latent phase, active phase and transition. The second stage then specifies simply delivery of the baby; colloquially it's often referred to as "pushing." Optimally, this should be relatively fast, although in practice many factors can prolong it. The third stage specifies delivery of the placenta, and control of postpartum bleeding.

3.3.1 The first stage – labor

As described above, the first stage is conventionally subdivided into three phases: latent phase, active phase and transition. At least in the US, these terms are always used, never "phase 1" or even "first stage, third phase."

One would simply say, "latent phase" or "transition." Average duration of the stages and phases of labor is shown in Figure 3.15. This "labor curve" (sometimes referred to as the "Friedman curve") shows the relative rates of change in cervical dilatation and head station as the labor progresses. It is worth noting that these values, which have been conventionally accepted in most countries for decades, are currently undergoing a renegotiation based on newer observational data.

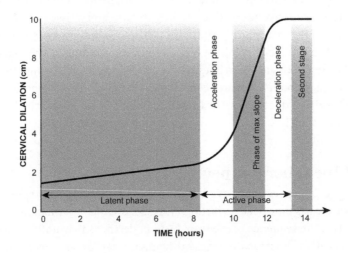

Figure 3.15 The labor curve.

3.3.1.1 Latent phase

Latent phase, also called early labor, begins when contractions become strong enough to dilate the cervix – a notoriously slippery metric. Mild cramping sensations are not always recognized as contractions, and may begin gradually in the week or two before labor. Progressive contractions – that is, contractions long and strong enough to dilate the cervix – last 30 to 45 seconds and can be felt from outside as a hardening of the abdomen. The end of latent phase is the beginning of active phase, when the rate of dilatation begins to accelerate (a landmark that has been reevaluated in recent years, as will be discussed in the section to follow).

A key maxim for understanding functional latent phase is, "latent phase should stay latent." For almost 9 months, the cervix has had one single job: holding the baby in. Over the course of latent and active phases, the cervix will not only soften and stretch, but literally disappear into the walls of the birth canal, becoming merely a tight place that the baby passes through on his way out. The transition from latent to active phase is thus a sea change energetically and experientially as well as hormonally. Contractile activity is a part of this change: as seen in the cervical ripening cycle, Section 3.3, contractions help gravity to stretch the cervix. Under natural circumstances, contractions only begin when cervical ripening is underway such that oxytocin can bind in the binding sites of uterine tissue, and they strengthen holistically in tandem with further cervical ripening. When contractions are too strong, too soon – as can happen with use of synthetic oxytocin – the result is pain, as the uterus pulls on a hard, unyielding cervix. Pain typically leads people to tighten rather than relax, further impeding cervical ripening. The softer the cervix is, the less force is required to dilate it – and therefore the less pain with contractions, and the more easily Mom can relax into them.

Remembering that oxytocin is a neurotransmitter as well as a hormone, an ideal latent phase takes place at home, under safe and loving conditions that allow Mom to relax fully into the experience. One's oxytocin levels are highest when kissing, falling in love, experiencing orgasm and eating chocolate; therefore, during latent phase, a dreamy, loving mood is clinically optimal. Massage, nipple stimulation and even sex – as long as the membranes are not ruptured – can further enhance the natural onset of contractions together with cervical ripening. By contrast, acupuncture techniques such as electrical stimulation in the sacral foramina, which are thought to stimulate contractile activities, may not be appropriate before the cervix is ripe (more on this discussion, along with acupuncture/acupressure to promote cervical ripening, can be found in Chapters 6 and 7).

Dysfunctions of latent phase include premature labor, prelabor rupture of membranes and postdates or prolonged pregnancy (where labor does not begin until after the estimated due date EDD). Functional but suboptimal latent phase presentations include cervical ripening without onset of contractions, and contractions that are painful before the cervix is ripe.

PREMATURE ONSET OF LABOR

Prior to 37 weeks of gestation, the baby is considered premature. When progressive contractions start before 37 weeks, the mom is generally admitted to the hospital, where the baby can be closely monitored and emergency Cesarean section, specialized pediatric care and a neonatal intensive care unit (NICU) are available if necessary. Depending on the gestational age and other clinical signs, medications may be used to stop contractions and/or accelerate maturation of the fetal lungs. In many cases, contractions subside and the pregnancy can continue. Premature contractions are particularly common during summer, when dehydration can increase the "irritability" of the uterus. Rest and rehydration can often stop the contractions. Premature contractions may also indicate inflammation, infection or other irritation of the uterus; Mom and Baby are therefore monitored for fever or other signs of infection before release.

Box 3.3 How premature is premature?

I had a colleague whose baby was born at 8 pm on the night of the sixth day of her 36th week – in other words, 4 hours premature. However, the designation of "premature" is a binary, so all precautions were taken – meaning that although she had planned to deliver in a birthing center, she was transferred to the hospital instead. Applied to any particular case, this determination may seem excessively strict. However, the line has to be drawn somewhere – if 4 hours premature is not treated as such, then what about 6 or 8 hours, or 1 or 2 days? In addition to being small, premature babies are fragile: their lungs may not be ready to breathe air yet, and they are at elevated risk for infections and brain hemorrhages.

PRELABOR RUPTURE OF MEMBRANES (PROM)

By the 38th or 39th week, if the baby's head is reasonably well positioned to put pressure on the cervix, and hormone levels are appropriate, then cervical ripening will likely already have begun. The amniotic fluid is rich in prostaglandins, so if the membranes rupture at this point, the steady drip of fluid onto the cervical tissue will accelerate cervical ripening and contractions will start. If contractions start within 4 hours of membrane rupture, then this is considered to be a normal initiation of labor via spontaneous rupture of membranes (SROM). If contractions do not begin within 4 hours of membrane rupture, then the event will be termed prelabor rupture of membranes (PROM). Management of this situation varies regionally and by practitioner. Aggressive management in some United States hospitals may include labor induction at 4 hours post-rupture and Cesarean section at 24 hours if vaginal birth is not expected within a few hours. A more conservative approach would consist of hydration and bed rest – to replace lost fluids and minimize further loss – along with close monitoring of Mom's temperature. Infection sometimes causes membrane rupture in the first place, and can also occur post-rupture. To minimize risk of infection, vaginal exams are kept to a minimum in moms with ruptured membranes, and sex and immersion in birthing pools are contraindicated. Antibiotics may be administered prophylactically, and labor may be induced if it does not start after 24–48 hours. The decision about whether and when to induce depends mainly on gestational age.

Membrane rupture before 37 weeks is termed PPROM (premature prelabor rupture of membranes). Before 34 weeks, it is considered that the benefits of continued intrauterine pregnancy outweigh the risks of infection (assuming antibiotic prophylaxis). In some cases, the membranes may even heal – they are, after all, living tissue. After 34 weeks, large-scale analysis finds better outcomes with <u>induction of labor</u> than with expectant management. When the membranes rupture after 37 weeks but contractions don't start, a common reason is OP position: as discussed in Section 3.1.3.1 and seen in Figure 3.10, when Baby is faced backward in the pelvis, the pressure of her head is directed more posteriorly than normal. In addition to being painful, this posterior pressure is not as effective at ripening the cervix, and may actually cause a tear by compressing the membranes against the bony sacrum.

Box 3.4 Ruptured membranes and infection.

The placenta and/or membranes can become infected when membranes are ruptured, which is called amnionitis or chorioamnionitis . The severity of this risk is increased when Mom is colonized with Group B streptococcal bacteria – as some 20–40 percent of women are. Once membranes are ruptured, vaginal exams should be kept to a minimum, and any other activity that can introduce bacteria into the vaginal canal should be avoided – including baths or birthing pools, as well as vaginal intercourse. However, erotic intimacy is still one of the most effective ways of encouraging labor onset, and it should be noted that seminal fluid is rich in prostaglandins, which can increase contractile activity whether added to the system orally or topically.

POSTDATES

Delayed initiation of labor is a common dysfunction of latent phase, often leading to labor induction. Although "latent phase should stay latent," contractions *should* kick in once the cervix is ripe, if Baby's head is putting appropriate pressure on the cervix. Other than occiput posterior or other problems with the bony interface of baby and pelvis, Western medicine does not have a clear explanation for why some women do not go into labor even though the cervix is ripe and Baby is engaged, and others are slow to engage, soften and/or dilate. As will be seen in Chapter 4, principles of Yin and Yang have clear analyses for these two situations, and can be of considerable help in moving the labor forward.

3.3.1.2 Active phase

The concept of an active, or "acceleration," phase is based on the work of Dr. Emmanuel Friedman at Columbia University in the 1950s. Friedman observed that the rate of dilatation increased markedly once the cervix was dilated 3–4 cm, and slowed again at transition, creating a distinctive S-shaped curve when dilatation was graphed against time. Patients would be said to "fall off the curve" if they were too far behind the expected pace of a centimeter per hour, and might be sent to Cesarean section for "failure to progress." Over the past decade, however, a number of studies have demonstrated that labors progressing slowly before 5 or 6 cm do not differ statistically in outcomes from those that accelerate. The result is that previous norms are being questioned internationally, and patients are more likely to be allowed to deliver vaginally with a slow labor. Evidence is particularly clear that the Friedman curve does not accurately characterize the labor course of women of African descent. With that understanding, my clinical experience among a patient population of widely varying race and ethnicity has been that in uncomplicated, unmedicated births, a perceptible acceleration of progress often (though by no means always) takes place at around 3–4 cm, once the head is engaged and contractions are adequate. The phrase "active phase should be active" thus characterizes an optimally robust active phase, while accepting that slower dilatation may not be inherently pathological.

When a labor arrests in active phase and the patient is sent for a Cesarean section, the indication for the surgery is reported as "failure to progress." However, there are two key subtypes to this disordered labor, with different associated scenarios. In some cases, contractions are strong and regular, but the cervix does not dilate. If the vaginal exam remains unchanged for 4 hours, in the presence of "adequate" contractions, failure to progress is diagnosed unless it is thought that a change of plans (e.g. addition of epidural analgesia) will shift the situation.

In other cases, contractions are weak and/or irregular, but can be augmented with oxytocin. A first step to diagnosis of labor dysfunction is thus often placement of an internal contraction monitor, which records the contraction strength reliably (versus external monitors, which are reliable only for frequency and duration of contractions). If contractions are found to be less than adequate, then oxytocin is administered either until progress is seen or until the baby shows signs of distress. Other than OP (which manifests in back pain as the baby's large occiput presses into the sacrum) there are no bony obstacles to progress in active phase. Active phase dysfunction can thus in general be attributed to either failure of the cervix to relax or failure of the uterus to produce adequate contractions. Within Western medicine, stress and fatigue are seen as possible contributing factors, to arrested dilatation and inadequate contractions, respectively; however, they are not disease entities that can be diagnosed and treated. By contrast, East Asian medical concepts do offer a range of possible reasons why the soft tissue might struggle to function appropriately at this challenging time, and in my experience a correct EAM diagnosis and acupressure or acupuncture can result in extraordinary shifts.

3.3.1.3 Transition

"Embrace intensity" is a key phrase for transition – particularly important for first-time moms who have not experienced this extraordinary sensation before. As Baby turns to exit the pelvis and descends, her head presses into the rectum and the feeling of pressure inside becomes a massive, irresistible urge to push. In hospitals with continuous fetal monitoring, sudden spikes in the contraction pattern may appear to indicate that Mom has instinctively begun pushing.

The intensity of transition is emotional as well as physical. A seasoned birth worker can usually recognize transition by a shift in the patient's manner. In active phase, adequate contractions are generally recognizable in that Mom is "non-distractible" during the surge, since she's naturally focusing on the intense sensations within her and is not particularly responsive to events in the room. During transition, this focused quality no longer comes and goes between contractions but remains, as the pressure of Baby's head against the rectum and pelvic floor demand full attention. If the fetal head is large in relation to the pelvis, or angled badly, the pressure may make the woman feel like she is about to burst. Birthing people facing exhaustion and/or pain may find themselves also facing their worst combinations of fear, self-doubt and helplessness. "I can't" is a refrain not uncommonly heard, and many midwives describe this as signaling a necessary process of letting go, allowing one's body to do the work it was designed for, rather than attempting to mastermind the process from one's own willpower or cerebral cortex. "Emotional dystocia" is sometimes used to describe a stall in labor progress, typically at 7–10 cm, where the patient has difficulty overcoming fear or other emotions, as might occur as after stillbirth or sexual trauma.

In addition to emotional intensity, most of the bony problems described above announce themselves at transition, including OP, asynclitism and other causes of true or functional cephalopelvic disproportion. Much of the birth bodywork described in Chapters 5 and 6 addresses bony issues, while acupressure and acupuncture are extremely helpful for emotional challenges.

3.3.2 The second stage – delivery

The second stage is colloquially described as "pushing." An optimal second stage does not last long: if transition has fully occurred (a big "if"), then – in my experience – pushing takes an hour or less in nulliparas (first-time moms), and half that in multiparas. However, in hospitals, second stage is frequently quite a bit longer for several reasons. First, pushing is sometimes started before the baby has fully turned and descended, possibly with bony problems that actually prevent transition. Second, epidural analgesia appears in some cases to slow down the second stage by impairing Mom's ability to feel herself pushing – although current evidence appears to show that epidural does not lengthen second stage. Interestingly, it has been our anecdotal experience at the hospital that patients who receive acupuncture and/or bodywork alongside the epidural often have extremely rapid second stages – sometimes literally just a few pushes.

In a second stage where everything is going according to plan, the contractions have become quite strong and frequent, and the pressure of the baby's head on Mom's rectum triggers reflexive "Valsalva maneuvers," the technical term for what happens with the breath and abdominal muscles during defecation.[5] The cervix should be entirely dilated by now, its connective tissue absorbed into the wall of the birth canal until it is merely a tight place. With transition, the baby should have rotated from occiput facing sideways, to occiput forward. In addition to rotating forward, it's quite important that the baby tuck his chin down. Try this yourself: put your hand on your occiput and appreciate for yourself what a mountainous protuberance it makes, then tuck your chin and feel it disappear into a smooth little foothill. If the occiput is forward and appropriately tucked, then with a few pushes it should cruise through the tight area where the cervix used to be.

At this point, the head is in the vaginal canal; it pushes the labia open so that it is visible both during and between pushes. The feeling of internal stretch is usually intense, so that Mom has a strong urge to push, but as she pushes, the perineum is stretched painfully. The phrase "ring of fire" is sometimes used to describe this unique sensation; I am told it originates with a tradition in some Native American cultures that the burning feeling is the heat of the baby's soul entering his body.[6] Once the head is out – often looking alarmingly purplish – there is a quick, urgent moment where the midwife or doc checks whether the cord is wrapped around the neck, and slips it over the head if possible, otherwise clamps and cuts it. Also in progress is the complicated dance where the shoulders need to do everything the head did to get out, but in reverse – since they are wide side to side, whereas the head is long front to back. So the head starts to comes out, then rotates a quarter turn to allow the baby's front-facing shoulder to pull under the pubic bones, followed by the back shoulder, which slides along the sacrum.

---

5   I am told that "Valsalva maneuver" is also the name of a punk rock band.

6   Prenatal perineal massage is outside the scope of this book, but a number of my patients have found it extremely helpful in preparing for this intense experience, as well as reducing tears.

Ideally, the baby cries at this point, or (even better) looks around alertly at the bright new world she has entered. Depending on the birth setting, there may now be a flurry of nose- and throat-suctioning, cord clamping and cutting, or baby may be sweetly placed on Mom's bare chest. If the baby looks blue, sleepy or "floppy" (a disconcerting, boneless slackness suggesting unconsciousness), then the baby is suctioned, chafed and patted sharply in an attempt to arouse him; usually he awakes, cries, and "pinks up" within a few minutes. The Apgar Score evaluates five markers of the infant's well-being including activity, pulse, reactivity, skin color and breathing. It is assessed at 1 and 5 minutes after delivery; fairly often the 1-minute score is alarmingly low but the 5-minute score is a perfectly healthy 9. (The scale actually goes to 10 points, but it is quite normal for babies' hands to remain bluish for more than 5 minutes.)

A number of issues can complicate the second stage. They are described below.

3.3.2.1 Cervical edema

It sometimes happens that moms feel an urge to push before the cervix is fully dilated (FD). If the tissue is soft, and relatively close to full dilatation (8 or 9 cm), the body's natural pushing impulse may accelerate dilatation without causing problems. However, if the cervix is hard and/or pushing is forceful, the cervix can easily become irritated and swell, actually impeding progress. (Cervical edema is another area where Western medicine has no recourse, but acupuncture or acupressure can be extremely helpful.)

3.3.2.2 Incomplete transition

If Baby's head is not appropriately faced and tucked (i.e. transition hasn't finished, or can't, due to bony problems), then pushing can go on for hours with little progress. These cases are particularly heartbreaking for moms and birth teams, as they have been focusing on 10 cm as the finish line – it's like turning the corner on a long line at an airport or amusement park, and seeing hundreds more people in front of you. The baby's head will usually be visible during pushes, and then disappear behind the labia between contractions, only heightening the sense of "so close and yet so far."

If pushing goes on for some time with little visible progress, one of two things is happening. Progress may be happening, but slowly: in this case, there is usually some visible movement of the head during pushes, either downwards or rotationally until transition is complete and the baby can emerge. Or, the baby may be genuinely stuck, unable to tuck or rotate in such a way as to dive under the pubic arch. If this is the case, then the scalp usually begins to swell from trapped blood and fluids (called caput succedaneum).

Caput is distinct from molding of the head, the gradual flexing of baby's soft skull bones that in some cases provides enough wiggle room for Baby to scoot under the pubic arch and make her escape. Another sign that Baby may be well and truly stuck is that Mom's external genitalia swell even more than usually (which is considerable already). In general, the more progressive the birth professional, the earlier they are likely to consider positions that change pelvic geometry (e.g. squatting, rotating the hips) as well as positions that raise Mom's hips above her shoulders and may provide a "reset" for truly stuck babies.

3.3.2.3 Shoulder dystocia

The moment between delivery of the head and delivery of the front-facing shoulder is a critical one. Baby is not particularly stable right now: she's in transition between the old and new ways of getting oxygen, and compression on the neck, chest and/or umbilical cord may make both difficult. If Baby is large, then either the front shoulder may wedge against the pubic arch or, less commonly, the rear shoulder may catch on the sacrum. The best-case scenario here is that a careful and attentive birth professional cautions Mom not to push, and gently tractions the head until the shoulder slides out. However, if the shoulders are really too big to slide out without further assistance, then the result is shoulder dystocia, a dire obstetric emergency. With an inadequate oxygen supply to Baby's brain, an 8-minute count is started until <u>hypoxic brain injury</u> must be assumed. As those excruciating minutes tick by, the birth team tries to resolve the impasse.

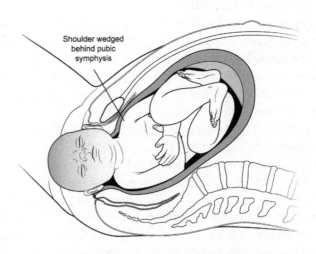

Shoulder wedged behind pubic symphysis

Figure 3.16 Shoulder dystocia.

The usual first-line approach is the "McRoberts maneuver," which looks strikingly similar to the yoga pose "happy baby." Mom is placed in an exaggerated <u>lithotomy position</u>, on her back with two helpers holding her knees bent and pushing them back toward Mom's chest to rotate the pelvis up as far as possible, while another presses down on Baby's shoulder hoping to pop it out. The majority of incidents are resolved this way in less than a minute. At home, or in a situation where there are few personnel for McRoberts, another possible approach is the Gaskin maneuver,[7] where Mom is helped into a hands-and-knees position and encouraged to arch and flex her back as far in each direction as possible (i.e. the yoga "Cat/Cow" pose). This movement, plus the gentle traction of gravity through the baby's head, can create the space for Baby to descend. After the Gaskin maneuver, approaches vary and may include snapping the baby's collarbone to ensure timely delivery. Although this sounds extreme, the collarbone heals quickly in babies, and the fracture is considered preferable to risks of permanent brain damage, or permanent damage to the brachial nerve (<u>Erb's palsy</u>) if the shoulder is forced out intact. In the United States, shoulder dystocia is epidemically on the rise, currently affecting 1 in 100 births. One apparent reason for this is that gestational diabetes (also rising fast) leads not only to high birth weight, but also to an altered fat distribution with more bulk on the shoulders, making shoulder dystocia even more likely.

3.3.3 The third stage – delivery of the placenta

It seems odd, at first, to think that delivery of the placenta or afterbirth constitutes its own stage. However, a brief look at the underlying anatomy and physiology makes it clear why the third stage is actually one of the most critical points of the birth process.

The placenta is like a silent sibling, taking up some 30 percent of the uterine wall and not all that much smaller than the fetus (it usually weighs about 1 lb at birth). It forms along with the fetus, and works hard to deliver oxygen and nutrients, as well as to hold a safe space in which the pregnancy can grow. The placenta also synthesizes a number of the hormones – such as estrogen, progesterone and relaxin – that drive physiological processes in pregnancy. At 40 weeks, the placenta is usually oval in shape, 4–6 in. (10–15 cm) in diameter and 1 in. thick (2.5 cm), with the umbilical cord protruding from the center on the fetal side.

---

7   Bruner, J. P., Drummond, S. B., Meenan, A. L., & Gaskin, I. M. (1998). All-fours maneuver for reducing shoulder dystocia during labor. *The Journal of Reproductive Medicine*, 43(5), 439–443.

Once the baby is delivered, the uterus begins to reduce in size – indeed, "contractions" are nothing other than uterine muscle fibers pulling against each other to make the muscle layer thicker and reduce space inside. During first stage, contractions pulled the cervix up against the baby's head so that it dilated; during second stage they pushed the baby down and out. Many women are surprised that the contractions don't stop after the baby is born – indeed these "afterpains" can be quite uncomfortable, and may intermittently recur for a week or more. Once there is no baby stretching it out, the uterus should shrink with each contraction. As the uterus reduces in size, the placenta is naturally pushed off the uterine wall as the space it was attached to becomes smaller and smaller. Delivery of the placenta usually occurs within 15 minutes. If it is not out by 30 minutes, incidence of postpartum hemorrhage increases greatly, as the uterine arteries cannot close properly with placental tissue still in place.

Third-stage contractions are important to clamp down on any uterine arteries that may have been torn as the placenta separates (remember that the uterine vessels have been greatly expanded by the placenta's initial invasion). When the uterine muscles are fatigued from a long labor (or from excessive use of oxytocin) and cannot contract properly, there is significant danger of maternal hemorrhage. A full bladder may also stop the uterus properly clamping down on the blood vessels. Maternal hemorrhage is a leading cause of fatality in home birth – I have a colleague who had a near-death experience this way – and is also a serious concern in hospitals. For this reason, home birth midwives carry injectable oxytocin, and most hospitals have standard protocols for immediate postpartum administration of oxytocin or other uterotonics (contraction-inducing drugs).

3.4 Summary Table and Ideas to Remember

This chapter has briefly introduced the Western perspective on the main events of labor, for the purpose of informing birth with EAM approaches. It should not be mistaken for a complete or authoritative biomedical monograph.

Table 3.2 summarizes the labor journey in detail, specifying events or "landmarks" in the process, along with the diagnostics typically used to evaluate them, underlying physiological or pathological causes, and medical interventions ordinarily taken.

Table 3.2 The Western labor map: Key landmarks and possible problems.

	Landmark (*Possible Problem*)	Diagnostics	Causes/conditions	Medical interventions
Preterm	*Early shortening of cervix*	Vaginal exam	"Incompetent cervix"	Bed rest, cerclage
	Prelabor rupture of membranes (PROM)	Fern test, fetal fibronectin	Trauma, infection, OP	• Antibiotics if fever • Steroids for lung development
	Preterm contractions	Tocometer	Infection, inflammation	• Antibiotics if fever • Tocolytics and/or steriods
First Stage, Latent Phase	Hormones shift to potentiate labor	n/a	• Progesterone drops, relaxin increases • Local prostaglandins with tissue stretch • Rise in fetal oxytocin	May suggest relaxation, lovemaking, prenatal yoga, etc.
	Braxton–Hicks contractions	Patient report	Hormonal shift	
	Cervix softens	Vaginal exam	Hormonal shift	• Cervical ripening agents: misoprostol, dinoprostone • May suggest movement, breathing, dancing, etc.
	Engagement • Baby often moves to face occiput transverse or left occiupt anterior	Vaginal exam External palpation	• Combined fetal weight, pelvic floor relaxation and tissue stretch • Head must be proportional to pelvis and appropriately positioned	
	Cervix moves anteriorly	Vaginal exam	• Bag and head dropping into pelvis • Posterior pelvic floor release	
	Cervix begins shortening, opening		Hormones & tissue stretch	
	True contractions initiate	• Patient report • Tocometer	• Prostaglandins allows oxytocin to bind • Rise in fetal and maternal oxytocin	Oxytocin
	Contractions increase in strength, regularity	• Patient report • Tocometer/ palpation	Accelerating cycle of prostaglandins, oxytocin, tissue stretch	

	Mom copes well with contraction intensity	Patient report	• Rule out OP • Emotional resilience • Appropriate prenatal education	• Comfort measures • Obstetric analgesia
First Stage, Active Phase	Contractions are regular, 2–5 minutes apart	• Patient report • Tocometer • Provider palpation	• Head is well applied to cervix due to malposition, malpresentation or non-engagement • Patient is not fatigued	Oxytocin
	Contractions have duration/ strength (~1 minute)			
	Progress is palpable, ~1 cm/ hour or greater (especially multips)	• Vaginal exam • Progressive intensity	• Head is well applied to cervix • Cervix is sufficiently softened • Pain does not exceed "copeability"	• Expectant management • Labor augmentation (oxytocin) • C-section for "failure to progress"
	As cervix dilates toward 10 cm, head descends to mid-pelvis (zero station)	• Vaginal exam • Provider palpation	• Head and pelvis are proportional • Appropriate position, presentation, attitude	• Expectant management • Labor augmentation • C-section for "failure to progress"
	Cervical lip/rim	• Vaginal exam	• Anterior lip – laboring supine • Pelvic or musculoskeletal asymmetry • Past surgical trauma to cervix	• Expectant management • Manual reduction by provider
	Transition phase of first stage – fetus may turn between 7 and 10 cm, head drops from 0 to +2	• Rectal pressure • Intensity remains between contractions • Vaginal exam	Fetus may not turn due to: • Cephalopelvic disproportion, asynclitism, malposition, malpresentation • Short or wrapped cord	• Expectant management • Labor augmentation • C-section for "failure to descend" ("failure to progress" if <10 cm)
Second Stage	From full dilation to crowning	• Visibility of head between pushes	Head pushes through pelvis and dilated cervix into vaginal canal	• May pause to allow uterus to contract around fetal body
	Birth of head	Grossly observable	• Labia & perineum stretch to accommodate emergence of head	• May apply lubricant, perineal pressure
	Shoulder dystocia	Shoulder stuck on pubic arch after head delivers	• Fetal macrosomia (large size) • More common with gestational diabetes	• Positional manipulation, pressure at fundus and above pubic symphysis

Third Stage	Birth of placenta	Provider assesses for intactness	• Contractions reduce size of uterus, pushing off villi and closing blood vessels	• May guide (not pull) cord • Fundal massage
	Bleeding	Provider assesses location/severity	• Some vaginal bleeding from lacerations is common • Uterine bleeding may result from retained placental tissue, inadequate contractions (tone) or bleeding disorder	• Fundal massage, etc. to increase contractions • Oxy, rectal misoprostol, etc. • Possible transfusion, artery ligation, etc.

Important ideas to remember from this chapter are:

3.1 The baby and the bones:

- The interface of pelvis and fetal head creates a three-part labor journey – engagement, descent, and transition.

- Depending on pelvic shape, transition or (occasionally) engagement may be a challenge.

- True CPD occurs when the head is too large to move through the pelvis. Other forms of bony obstruction, where the head is functionally too big due to angle or other factors include:

  - OP position, where the fetal occiput faces the sacrum causing back pain and difficult delivery

  - asynclitism, where the fetal head engages at an angle incompatible with the curve of the pelvis, getting stuck and causing severe, bursting pain and/or arrest of labor.

3.2 The soft tissues:

- The uterus and cervix are more complicated than the pelvis. During pregnancy, the uterus stretches passively while the cervix holds tight; during labor, the roles switch, mediated by a number of signaling molecules. These include:

  - prostaglandins, local inflammatory molecules that ripen the cervix and open uterine binding sites for oxytocin

  - oxytocin, which causes uterine contractions and contributes to maternal trust and bonding instincts.

- When oxytocin is given intravenously, contractions are increased while trust and bonding are reduced.

3.3 The labor journey:

- The process of labor and delivery is discussed in three stages.

  - The first stage is by far the longest, and comprises the entire journey from unripe cervix, with no contractions, to the cervix fully dilated and Baby turned in position to deliver.

  - The second stage consists of delivery of the baby, and may be lengthened by epidural analgesia.

  - The third stage denotes the placenta's delivery, which needs to happen in a timely manner and presents the risk for maternal hemorrhage.

- The three phases of the first stage of labor are:

  - latent (cervical ripening and onset of contractions)

  - active (regular, strong contractions with rapid dilatation)

  - transition (slower progress as Baby turns and descends within the pelvis to prepare for delivery).

Chapter 4

YIN BIRTH, YANG BIRTH

The Five Main Birth Types and Their Challenges

Chapter Outline

- 4.1 Qi-Deficient Births

- 4.2 Yang-Deficient Births

- 4.3 Yin-Deficient Births

- 4.4 Blood-Deficient Births

- 4.5 Qi Stagnation Births – Constitutional Type

- 4.6 Additional Qi Stagnation Presentations: Bony Obstruction, Accumulation, Stuck Spirit, Indeterminate Obstruction

- 4.7 Key Points to Remember

- 4.8 Summary Table

This chapter examines the specific roles played in birth by Yin and Yang, Qi, and Blood. For each of these four vital substances, we look at how the overall experience of birth tends to be affected by insufficiency, along with specific dysfunctions at prenatal, intrapartum and postpartum stages. Stagnation or obstruction at the levels of bone, flesh and spirit is also discussed as a fifth type of birth. For each birth type, key therapeutic methods and a "care package" of useful home care techniques are introduced. These are drawn from Chapter 5, and marked with section numbers for easy reference. All point locations used in this chapter are briefly described; for a fuller description and illustration, see Appendix A.

The most important thing to remember about these basic birth types is that if you are clinically active – whether in birth or as an East Asian medicine (EAM) practitioner – you already know them experientially. Far from being abstract medical concepts, these types represent the essential qualities of the substances in deficiency and obstruction, as they play out in daily life as well as birth. For example, Yang-deficient people generally look slower and softer than Yin-deficient people, who tend to be restless, thin and dry. Yang-deficient people should probably exercise more, but they never get around to it; Yin-deficient people keep their commitments to work out, but may forget to eat. In birth, Yang-deficient moms benefit from warmth, praise and stimulating touch – all of which would be annoying to Yin-deficient moms, who tend to prefer low lighting and quiet voices.

These are all stereotypes of course, and have their limitations when applied to real human beings. But it can be useful to develop a sharp eye for personality types and their challenges – for example, when managing colleagues, or selecting committee members or roommates. Similarly, recognizing the faces of Yin, Yang, Qi, and Blood in birth can help all practitioners to be more effective in helping moms prepare for birth, and more on target with their comfort measures and therapeutic methods during labor.

4.1 Qi-Deficient Births

The defining qualities of a Qi-deficient birth are weakness and fatigue. Qi's nature is to flow, and to get work done – like a bountiful river carrying fish, redistributing silt and stones, and pushing a water wheel. In Qi deficiency, it is as though the volume of water is inadequate, so that the water wheel moves slowly if at all, and the fish are trapped in stagnant puddles. The Qi of the labor flows in the waves of the contraction. If the contractions are ineffective – whether because of Yin, Yang, or Blood deficiency – then their Qi is also insufficient.

A pregnant person may head into birth Qi deficient, with underlying congenital weakness, chronic illness, lack of sleep, lack of exercise or inadequate nutrition due to poor appetite, nausea/vomiting or improper diet. Qi deficiency will likely also arise during any long labor, simply because labor is hard work with limited opportunity for rest and replenishment. Perinatal challenges for Qi-deficient moms include:

- musculoskeletal complaints in pregnancy (sciatica, lower back pain, rectus or symphysis diastasis, etc.)

- sagging tissues – varicose veins, swollen ankles, hemorrhoids

- premature cervical shortening or membrane rupture

- weak contractions

- postpartum hemorrhage.

4.1.1 How to recognize insufficiency of Qi

Qi's functions are to transform ingested food and drink into abundant Blood and strong flesh, and to move Blood and fluids around the body and hold them in place. When food is incompletely transformed due to weak Qi, several things happen:

- Not enough blood gets to the head: energy sags, the face may be pale and thinking may be unclear.

- Stools are loose and/or frequent, often with gas and/or bloating.

- Tongue changes may include pale color, scalloped edges (due to teeth marks) and/or a thick coating (which indicates suboptimal digestive functions).

- Flesh tone may become poor, with more sagging than is age-appropriate and/or a soft, weak look overall.

- Posture may be slouchy, and tendons and ligaments may be slack, with patients prone to dislocation injuries, sprains and strains.

- Clinical or subclinical depression is common, with a vicious cycle of fatigue, inactivity and cardiovascular deconditioning.

- Allergic rhinitis (with pronounced fatigue) and/or catching cold easily.

In reproductive health and pregnancy, the main challenges for Qi-deficient moms tend to be:

- History of menses that are excessively heavy, long and/or frequent due to Qi not adequately holding the Blood (or else scanty and pale in color, due to not enough blood being made).

- Premature shortening of the cervix (almost always a Qi deficiency problem).

- Threatened or recurrent miscarriage, as deficient Qi fails to "hold up" or maintain the pregnancy (though there are many other possible causes).

- Fatigue and nausea/vomiting in pregnancy. The fatigue can be debilitating, or nausea/vomiting can escalate to hyperemesis when Qi deficiency is severe (as may occur in twins, or close-together pregnancies without sufficient uninterrupted sleep to recover).

4.1.2 Key experiential qualities

Experientially, whether a labor is going well or badly, its Qi tends to fill the room, a little buzz in the air immediately palpable on walking in – like walking into a great party, or a boring one, or one where a couple has just had a screaming, drunken argument. What is experientially most notable about Qi deficiency in birth is that it doesn't show up to be assessed. When there's not much of a feeling at all in the room, likely either the patient is Qi deficient, or else the labor isn't going anywhere yet – in other words, the labor itself lacks Qi. Our team works with a large number of patients who are being induced with an unripe cervix, meaning that they have far to go before hitting active phase. They are not all Qi deficient, but there is a notable absence of anything palpable when one enters the room. Conversely, a Qi-deficient patient may be at 8 cm with intravenous oxytocin and an epidural, and still it doesn't feel like she's in labor. At home, Qi-deficient moms are vulnerable to a vicious cycle of fatigue and stalling out: their legs tire easily from squatting, and there is a sense of passivity, with less effort, or less focus, than other births. This passivity may be present throughout the labor, or may crop up at the end with fatigue in moms who do not have Qi deficiency signs at baseline.

4.1.3 Prenatal challenges for Qi-deficient patients

During the first trimester, Qi-deficient patients may be prone to severe fatigue and/or morning sickness. Fatigue becomes a central challenge for Qi-deficient patients again in the third trimester, as the weight of the pregnancy challenges their muscles, and the upright integrity of their bony structure. Vigorous deep-tissue massage and strong acupuncture treatments are effective for musculoskeletal pain in robust patients, but Qi-deficient moms do better with gentle bodywork and Qi-boosting treatments. Qi-deficient moms are prone to early cervical shortening and/or membrane rupture, as tissues sag. I therefore consider musculoskeletal pain as a potential warning sign for these problems – though it is a common and relatively benign in the absence of marked Qi deficiency signs. In 15 years I have yet to see a case of cervical shortening *not* associated with Qi deficiency signs and symptoms – in many cases also with concurrent deficiency of Yang, Blood or, occasionally, Yin.

4.1.4 Working with Qi deficiency in labor

The great gift of Qi deficiency is that, although energy pushing the labor forward is relatively low, the energy holding the cervix closed is also relatively low (in contrast to other presentations such as Yin deficiency or Qi stagnation). Energy is not wasted on clenching, and tissues are generally softer and more pliable, meaning that less force is needed to dilate the cervix and descend the baby (hence the association with prematurity described above). In Qi-deficient labors, gravity is our best friend – with loving, proactive labor support a close second.

The optimal position for combining both these elements is the Helper Hang (Section 5.5.4), where Mom has her arms around the birth partner's neck and feels supported to let go and just hang. The birth partner supports her torso, massages the sacrum if possible, and shifts side to side in a relaxing rhythm that is comfortable and sustainable (and perhaps even a little sexy) for them both.

Once active labor has started, I find that short periods of deep relaxation work better for Qi-deficient moms than long naps, although this is not an absolute rule. Breathing and inward focusing work can also be extremely helpful. The Miles Circuit[1] is also a terrific resource here, using deep relaxation to open optimal flow through the pelvis.

As an alternative to relaxing the baby out, another possible approach is to pump more Qi into the labor. This is where loving, proactive labor support comes in. Chafing downwards along the outer shin from Stomach-36 (Section 5.1.1.4) and hip rocking (Section 5.1.1.2) are both great ways to literally put more Qi into the labor, adding birth team members' energy to Mom's. However the addition needs to be made sensitively, like an appropriate piano accompaniment – not galumphing in with a tuba or electric guitar. This listening, harmonizing quality is the same one that distinguishes a good from a bad backrub, and many health care professionals are great at it – but not all partners are.

When there is a contraction monitor running, it is amazing to see the immediate strengthening of contractions when the outer shin is chafed, and this is a good technique to teach partners. Hip rocking is a little more challenging: the right-sized pushes for Qi-deficient patients can be amazingly small, but being small they are quite rapid, faster than her heartbeat and therefore have an activating effect. Hip rocking that is well "tuned in" to Mom's needs can boost contractions extraordinarily, while out-of-key rocking can visibly reduce them. It is therefore critical both to check in with Mom and also to self-evaluate: after a period of 5–10 minutes of rocking, do contractions feel stronger? If not, the method may not be helping.

---

1   The Miles Circuit is a sequence of simple exercises and relaxing postures to encourage optimal fetal positioning; see also Section 5.6. www.milescircuit.com

---

Box 4.1 Qi deficiency care package.

For basic home care:

- Chafing downwards along the outer shin (Section 5.1.1.4).

- Round rubbing at the mid-back (Section 5.3.1.2).

- Moderate, regular cardiovascular exercise, e.g. at least two walks per day of at least 15 minutes' duration.

- Also consider structured physical activities, e.g. yoga, belly dancing, etc. or Cat/Cow (section 5.5.1).

- Avoid cold or raw foods, particularly if there is nausea, poor appetite or loose stools; meals are ideally hot, flavorful (ginger, curry, etc.) and moderately sized. If hot food is not available, eat with ginger or other tea.

For common Qi deficiency symptoms, add:

- For fatigue, add moxibustion on Stomach-36 (Section 5.4) and/or Cat/Cow (section 5.5.1).

- For morning sickness, try cinnamon gum or ginger tea, candy, etc.

For labor preparation starting daily at 39 weeks, or every 4 hours if induction is imminent, add:

- Acupressure, 5 minutes each on bilateral Large Intestine-4 (at the base of the thumb), Spleen-6 (behind above the inner ankle bone).

- Thumb circles (Section 5.2.2.2) and chafing (Section 5.1.1.4) around the sacrum.

- Both repeated daily, or every 4 hours if induction is imminent.

4.1.4.1 Weak contractions, fatigue and Qi deficiency

Fatigue and weak contractions are the characteristic signs of Qi deficiency during labor. That said, some fatigue is entirely normal toward the end of a long labor regardless of Mom's constitution. In practice, three distinct cases should be considered:

- Toward the end of a long labor, Mom feels tired and contractions reduce in size or apparent effect (without changes in frequency and regularity). This is straightforward Qi deficiency due to hard work, regardless of patient constitution. The treatment goals are to boost Qi and push it into the contractions. The most useful approach in this case is to chafe the outer shin between contractions, and stimulate Large Intestine-4 on the webbing of the thumb or Duyin at the distal crease on the underside of the second toe (Section 5.2.1.2) about 30 seconds before contractions are due.

- Around when transition is due (usually 7–10 cm dilated), contractions both weaken and slow down, without obvious signs of maternal fatigue. This is most likely to bony obstruction, rather than Qi deficiency.

- The labor has been sluggish and difficult to initiate throughout. This may indeed be constitutional Qi deficiency. However, as discussed below, Yang deficiency and/or damp should also be considered as possible culprits or co-conspirators.

4.1.4.2 Ineffective pushing
Ineffective pushing due to Qi deficiency is extremely common – whether due to constitutional deficiency or fatigue. The problem is most effectively addressed through judicious alignment with gravity, with squatting or other upright positions. It may also be useful to chafe down the outer shin between contractions and stimulate LI-4 or Duyin during contractions.

A related situation is ineffective pushing due to epidural analgesia. Depending on the density and location of numbness, moms with epidural often lack sensory feedback with which to guide their effort. This lack of feedback may itself be the problem or may complicate Qi deficiency. I find that gentle pressure or a needle pointing forward at Du-20 on the top of the head (Section 5.2.2.1) can be helpful to give Mom a sense of focus (and to focus Qi at the perineum, which is directly opposite Du-20). I also find that pressure directly downward at Gallbladder-21 in the belly of the trapezius muscle with each push (Section 5.2.2.1) may be very useful in helping Mom to direct Qi downward.

4.1.4.3 Postpartum hemorrhage
Postpartum hemorrhage is a potentially lethal result of Qi deficiency in general, and fatigue due to protracted labor in particular. Qi deficiency leads to weak contractions, most particularly at the end of long labors when the muscle fibers themselves are exhausted. If uterine blood vessels should be damaged as the placenta pulls off, the main way that that the uterus normally stops that bleeding is through contraction of the muscles to compress the blood vessels. When contractions are weak, blood flow is not effectively stopped. Contraction-stimulating points such as LI-4 and Duyin may be combined with chafing down the outer shin to boost Qi and promote contractions. Experience has also shown that strong pressure with a fingernail on Spleen-1 at the inner corner of the great toenail can slow down blood flow.

4.2 Yang-Deficient Births

During birth, we can think of Qi as the gas in the tank, and Yang as the actual spark and fire that initiate the car's movement. The two are often combined in the term "Yang Qi," and a person with Yang deficiency by definition is also prone to symptoms of Qi deficiency. In birth, Yang deficiency's experiential quality is sluggish and hesitant; Mom is often fearful as well. Yang's specific birth responsibilities are:

- initiating contractions and keeping them regular

- keeping the cervix warm enough to stretch

- ripening the cervix (this is a joint project with Yin; Yang provides the chemical energy to synthesize the complex hormones needed and the body heat to stimulate the chemical reactions).

Yang-deficient births are therefore characterized by slow or irregular contractions, and cervical ripening may be behind schedule. Indeed, Yang-deficient people are often behind schedule in daily life; asking this question can be a useful diagnostic – and also helps to lessen anxiety over late labor onset or slow progress, by normalizing it in the context of other life activities.

It is also important to remember that the flow of Yang Qi can be blocked by the accumulation of damp or cold – so that it is insufficient in its function. These moms may present with some signs of stagnation (see Section 4.6), but as a rule of thumb, anybody who is cold or edematous can be helped by warmth and movement.

4.2.1 How to recognize Yang deficiency

As discussed in Chapter 2, Yang's functions include warming the body, initiating action and metabolizing excess fluid. Yang also drives development and reproduction, together with Yin. In general, hypo-function, or slow initiation of metabolic processes, suggests that Yang is unable to do its job, due to deficiency or blockage. Common signs and symptoms of Yang insufficiency include:

- pale face, tendency to be overweight

- large, pale, wet tongue

- feeling cold, particularly in the feet, hands, lower back and buttocks

- undigested food in the stool (more than occasionally)

- ankle edema

- clear, copious urination (often without excessive water intake)

- pulse slower than 64 while pregnant (or slower than 74 in labor)

- long menstrual cycles (over 30 days)

- menstrual cramps that improve with heat (or are worse on cold days)

- hypothyroid or other low endocrine function.

4.2.2 Key experiential qualities of Yang-deficient births

It is normal for the body to become hot during labor, since labor itself is an inflammatory process. When Mom's own Yang is insufficient, the labor is slow to heat up as well as to get properly moving. A telling sign of deficient Yang is when Mom prefers to stay fully covered during active labor, rather than throwing clothes off. There is often also a timid, hesitant quality to the labor's progress, which may show in Mom's affect.

Yang-deficient moms are prone to accumulation of Yin cold and/or damp. When there is cold in the uterus, contractions are excessively painful – only exacerbating the tendency for yang-deficient labors to be fearful and hesitant. When the movement of Yang is blocked by damp, the experience of hesitancy is similar, but the emotional valence is quite different. Damp has a palpable sluggishness to it, as though the labor is wading through deep water. It also resists treatment: everything we try seems to help for 10 minutes and then the sluggishness returns. It is easy to become frustrated in these labors, and important to keep one's own Yang and Qi moving with breaks, walks and coffee as needed.

Yang-deficient moms are also prone to lack of progress because the fetal head is not well applied to the cervix, typically because of occiput posterior (OP) position, or a swayback posture due to weak or tight back muscles. This is like a toy not working because the battery is not properly seated: the circuit is broken and therefore Yang Qi can't flow through the labor.

4.2.3 Prenatal challenges of Yang deficiency

Painful dysmenorrhea and infertility are frequent manifestations of Yang insufficiency or cold excess. Once pregnant, Yang-deficient moms may have difficulty maintaining high hormone levels to hold the pregnancy. During the second trimester, severely Yang-deficient patients may lack the Qi to hold the baby in, and be sent to bed with a diagnosis of incompetent cervix. Babies small for their dates are also prevalent with Yang deficiency.

By the third trimester, most challenges are structural. Yang-deficient moms tend to back pain and excessive lordosis or swayback posture, which may lead to *diastasis recti* and can delay labor initiation. Their ankle swelling is earlier and more severe than other types. Yang-deficient moms frequently go past their due dates, although early cervical shortening and labor may occur if Qi deficiency is severe. Polyhydramnios (too much amniotic fluid) is most prevalent in moms who are Yang deficient and/or damp. It responds extremely well to EAM dietary therapy, using a traditional recipe for carp and white radish soup,[2] along with the recommendations in the "care package" (see Box 4.2).

4.2.4 Working with Yang deficiency in labor

The main therapeutic principles for working with insufficient Yang in labor are warmth, activation and movement. Yang's chief responsibility in birth is to maintain the rate and regularity of contractions (strength belongs to Qi). Hip rocking (Section 5.1.1.2) along with chafing at the ankles and sacrum (Section 5.1.1.4) can be helpful in activating Yang. The "Handwich" (Section 5.3.1.1) is also key for addressing Mom's fear and painful contractions.

Box 4.2 Yang deficiency care package.

For basic home care, use Qi deficiency methods diet plus:

— Morning sunshine: at least one 15-minute walk within an hour or two of rising, particularly in damp weather.

— Chafing on inner ankles, lower back and sacrum (Section 5.1.1.4).

— Soak feet in hot water deep enough to cover 4–6 in. (10–15 cm) above the ankles. Ideally, start with warm water and add hot water to keep as hot as comfortably tolerated for 10–25 minutes. For ankle edema, Epsom salts can be added.

— Avoid cold or raw foods, particularly if there is nausea, poor appetite or loose stools; meals are ideally hot, flavorful (ginger, curry, etc.) and moderately sized. If hot food is not available, eat with ginger or other tea.

— Also consider structured physical activities, e.g. yoga, belly dancing or Cat/Cow (Section 5.5.1).

— Stay comfortably warm, turning the heat up if necessary.

— For morning sickness, try cinnamon gum or ginger tea, candy, etc.

---

2   This recipe for carp and daikon soup can be made with any whole white-fleshed fish and/ or ordinary red radishes, if the original ingredients are not available. Fluid usually begins reducing within a day or two of the first dose. https://www.whitepinehealingarts.org/ polyhydramnios-and-koi

> For labor preparation starting daily at 38 weeks, or every 4 hours if induction is imminent, add:
>
> — Heating pad at sacrum (5-minute sessions only) or Handwich (Section 5.3.1.1).
>
> — Daily hot foot soaks or extra chafing at inner ankle.
>
> — Acupressure, 5 minutes each on bilateral Large Intestine-4 (at the base of the thumb), Spleen-6 (about 1" behind and 3" above the inner ankle bone).
>
> — Thumb circles (Section 5.2.2.2) and chafing (Section 5.1.1.4) around the sacrum.

During transition and pushing, the two main concerns for Yang-deficient moms are poor fetal positioning and keeping contractions adequate. The two problems mimic each other, as contractions tend to slow down when the labor is blocked by OP, asynclitism or malpresentation. One rule of thumb is that the contractions tend to be more painful if there a bony obstruction, and less so if they are simply petering out. Bony obstruction in general is addressed with gross bodily movement – lunging and climbing stairs if Mom is mobile, positional change and bodywork if not. Sluggish contractions due to Yang deficiency can be addressed with chafing at the ankles and/or shins as well as acupressure at LI-4 or Duyin (Section 5.2.1.2).

4.3 Yin-Deficient Births

Yin governs receiving, opening and relaxing. Stretching and flexibility (physical and emotional) *allow* the birth to happen. However strongly Yang contractions may push, the birth will not move forward without Yin physically and emotionally permitting the cervix to dilate.

Insufficient Yin may well be the most problematic presentation in pregnancy and birth, simply because so many tasks of pregnancy are Yin in nature, and require abundant Yin in order to proceed well. These tasks include receiving, holding and nurturing the embryo as it grows; the accumulation of fluid; the stretching and quiescence of the uterus (until labor); and the extraordinary effacement and retreat of the cervix during labor. Yin emotional qualities are also required: the patience to accept a gradual, less than optimally comfortable experience over which one has little conscious control; and the resilience to accept and live contentedly in whatever reality presents itself, rather than insisting on what should, could or would be the case. For Western providers of women's health care, this type of patient is among the most important for early referral to EAM care.

4.3.1 How to recognize insufficiency of Yin

As discussed in Chapter 2, Yin's functions include resting and relaxing, cooling, taking in nourishment and nurturing others, and appropriately inhibiting or stopping Yang actions or processes such as inflammation. A person's ability to "power down" from a big work day and get to sleep at night is a direct expression of their Yin function. If too wound up to settle down, something of a Yin nature may help – meditation, chamomile tea or perhaps warm milk – nature's original Yin tonic. If moms still can't sleep (or if something disrupts the sleep cycle, like the artificial light and agitating content of Facebook), then the Yin functions of patience, acceptance and resiliency may well be impaired the next day. Thus, although pregnancy is an inherently Yin condition, once it reaches the last month when hardly anybody sleeps well, Yin flexibility and resilience can get stretched rather thin, and Yin qualities of patience and acceptance can break down even in a person whose Yin has historically been fine.

Signs and symptoms of insufficient Yin include:

- Restlessness, irritability or inability to settle down: these are the main signs that warn of Yin deficiency in birth. A history of extreme or excessive exercise may reflect lack of interest in rest.

- Anxiety is also common, though a little more difficult to use diagnostically. Blood-deficient and Qi-deficient patients also have anxiety, though the flavor of it in these cases is more helpless and less impatient. Yang-deficient patients may also be fearful, but, again, the quality differs.

- Dryness anywhere – dry skin, eyes, lips, throat, mucus membranes or (most commonly in menopause) vaginal secretions, dry/difficult stools or constipation.

- History of inflammatory or autoimmune disorders, including chronic soft tissue inflammation such as carpal tunnel syndrome or plantar fasciitis.

- Night sweats and/or tendency to feel hot, particularly in the late afternoon. Menopausal hot flashes are often ascribed to the decline of Yin and its cooling function (though it can be more complex than that).

It is of course normal for women to feel warm during pregnancy, so we should ask about their previous history as well.

- The tongue may be extra red in color, it may be smaller than most and its fur may have peeled patches.

- The pulse will be somewhat rapid. Most importantly, on palpation the artery itself will be narrow and not particularly forceful –a healthy pregnant pulse should be both large and exuberant.

4.3.2 Key experiential qualities

The overall quality of a Yin-deficient birth is restless or impatient, and moms often have an anxious edge (though anxiety is not unique to Yin deficiency). Key experiential qualities of empty Yin are:

- Restlessness, crankiness and impatience with the birth process (or people). As birth team members we may find our own selves cranky and impatient in these labors, and partners commonly find that whatever they do to try to help, it isn't right.

    - Anxiety is often a part of this picture – and is also very contagious, easily transferred to the birth team.

    - It is useful to contrast this impatience and lack of acceptance with the vulnerability we see with Blood deficiency, or the frank fear that characterizes Yang deficiency.

- Lack of acceptance can mean:

    - Refusing to accept what's happening, e.g. refusing transport to the hospital when midwife suggests it.

    - Not accepting nourishment – this can be food/drink, or care and love from birth partners and professionals.

- Slow, difficult cervical dilatation:

    - This is the lack of relaxation inside, exacerbated in severe cases by dryness and tightness of the tissue itself.

    - A slender build and sinewy flesh tone can be an external flag for this presentation.

4.3.3 Prenatal challenges of Yin deficiency

Prenatal challenges for Yin-deficient moms are considerable. They may be caused by constitutional tendencies, excessive work with insufficient sleep or other life stressors. There may also be a cascade effect where inability to hold down food in the first trimester depletes Yin for the rest of the pregnancy. Maternal/fetal health challenges seen commonly (though not exclusively) in Yin deficiency include:

- hyperemesis gravidarum (severe nausea/vomiting that threatens the pregnancy)

- insufficient weight gain during pregnancy

- intrauterine growth restriction (IUGR, where a baby is in the smallest 10 percent for its gestational age)

- *preeclampsia*

- insufficient amniotic fluid (oligohydramnios)

- preterm contractions.

Yin deficiency is a common and important cause of hyperemesis gravidarum; Qi/Yang deficiency or stagnant fluids may also be involved. Regardless of cause, however, the loss of fluids, emotional distress and lack of rest can devastate even previously healthy Yin. Vomiting easily injures the Stomach Yin, as does extreme dieting, diarrhea or laxative use – so patients with a history of eating disorders are at particular risk for developing hyperemesis gravidarum. It is common for nauseated patients to be told to drink ginger tea; indeed, one study showed that a group of hyperemesis sufferers had been told it an average of 20 times! Ginger may indeed be of help for patients who have nausea due to Stomach Qi or Yang deficiency. However, ginger's warm spicy nature will make the condition worse for patients with Yin deficiency: peppermint gum, mints or mint tea (sweetened to taste) are all better choices.

4.3.4 Working with Yin-deficient births

The two problems most commonly seen in Yin-deficient births are difficult dilatation and hyper-response to pharmaceutical therapies used in labor such as misoprostol, dinoprostone, oxytocin and epidural analgesia. Anxiety and impatience can exacerbate either of these problems, as can lack of sleep. In most situations the primary therapeutic goal with Yin-deficient patients is to calm and settle the nervous system, in order to promote rest and dilatation. Dimming the lights and keeping voices low, as well as acupuncture, footrubs, auriculotherapy and acupressure at SP-6, a hand's breadth above the inner ankle bone (Section 5.2.1.1), should be considered as first-line therapies. Birth team members can be coached that they may need to manifest extraordinary flexibility, so as to head off potentially scratchy interchanges. Annoying or extraneous personnel may be sent on long errands.

If reducing stimuli and nourishing Yin do not result in easier dilatation, then possibilities for further assistance include deep breathing, the Handwich (Section 5.3.1.1) and gentle Liver Gummies (Section 5.1.1.3).

Another obstacle to dilatation may be a dysfunctional Yin-deficient contraction pattern, often exacerbated by oxytocin or cervical ripening agents (as will be seen in the next section). Like the weak, rapid pulse characteristic of Yin-deficient patients, this contraction pattern is rapid in frequency and small in amplitude. The uterus is unable to fully relax between the rapid waves, and therefore cannot generate useful force when contracting.

Box 4.3 Yin deficiency care package.

For basic home care:

- Yin footrubs (Section 5.3.1.3).

- Warm (not hot) foot soaks before bed. Can add essential oils. If there are leg cramps, can add small amount (one or two tablespoons) of Epsom salts.

- Moderate exercise: at least one 15-minute walk outdoors per day; also consider restorative yoga, deep breathing, meditation.

- Sleep hygiene: avoid screens, news and weighty conversation after dinner.

For commonly occurring challenges:

- For morning sickness or heartburn, *avoid* ginger: try mint or lemon instead – fresh in water, or in gum, candy, essential oil, etc.

- For constipation, chafe downward along outer shin; also try pear juice, avocados, nuts, dried fruits, especially goji berries, and okra (if tolerated).

- For anxiety: Belly Breathing (Section 5.5.7).

- If fluids or fetal weight are low, use moxibustion at Stomach-36 or chafing down outer shin (Section 5.4); if tolerated drink pear juice, coconut water or miso soup.

For labor preparation starting at 37 weeks, add:

- Gentle acupressure on Kidney-1, at the sole of the foot, and Spleen-6, behind and above the inner ankle, 5 minutes once or twice daily.

— Hula Hips (Section 5.5.2) and Belly Breathing (Section 5.5.7).

— At 39 weeks, add:

  * Mom's choice of Hip Openers (Section 5.5.6).

  * Acupressure, moderate pressure 5 minutes each on bilateral Large Intestine-4 (at the base of the thumb), Spleen-6 (behind and above the inner ankle bone).

  * Thumb circles and strong pressure for 5 minutes each at sacral points (Section 5.2.2.2).

  * Gentle Liver Gummies as tolerated (Section 5.1.1.3).

  * All repeated daily, or every 4 hours if induction is imminent.

4.3.4.1 Adverse responses to misoprostol, oxytocin, epidural analgesia

In my experience, patients with insufficient Yin have an elevated likelihood of hyper- or adverse response to certain medications. This relates to Yin's job of appropriately inhibiting processes in the body.

As of the time of writing of this book, misoprostol (brand name Cytotec) is approved to promote cervical ripening in the EU, but not in the US. It is a synthetic analogue of prostaglandin E1, and can therefore play a similar role in cervical ripening to prostaglandin E2, whose actions are described in Chapter 3.[3] It is well understood that cervical ripening agents can cause uterine hyperstimulation and/or tachysystole. Tachysystole is Greek for "overly fast contractions" and is defined in the US as more than six per 10 minutes; hyperstimulation is only diagnosed if the fetal heart tracing becomes abnormal. A systematic review of the literature in 2006[4] concluded that, in comparison to dinoprostone, misoprostol caused more instances of both tachysystole and hyperstimulation. My personal experience is that Yin-deficient patients have a much higher incidence of both, and particularly with misoprostol. It makes sense that Yin-deficient moms would be prone to rapid contraction problems, as the Yin-deficient contraction pattern is already rapid, and their body lacks Yin to balance the action of the newly introduced hormones. It is also my experience that, the stronger and faster

---

3 Cervidil/dinoprostone is a Prostaglandin E2 analogue, and it seems to cause somewhat fewer hyper-responses.

4 Crane, J. M. G., Butler, B., Young, D. C., & Hannah, M. E. (2006). Systematic review: Misoprostol compared with prostaglandin E2 for labour induction in women at term with intact membranes and unfavourable cervix: A systematic review. *BJOG: An International Journal of Obstetrics & Gynaecology, 113*(12), 1366–1376.

these contractions are, the more the Yin-deficient patient simply tightens up against them rather than dilating. The approach that seems most useful in tachysystole with misoprostol is to needle or gently press Yin-nourishing points on the inner leg – usually SP-6, a hand's breadth above the inner ankle bone, and KD-1 on the sole of the foot – as well as auriculotherapy if possible (see Chapter 6). For hyperstimulation, Spleen-4 should be used instead – though it is more difficult to locate, on the medial surface of the foot in the hollow just anterior and inferior to the base of the first metatarsal bone (see Appendix A).

Yin-deficient patients often respond quite strongly to oxytocin, sometimes resulting in fetal heart rate changes and withdrawal of the oxytocin without useful clinical effect. From a Yin/Yang perspective, oxytocin is potently Yang in its contraction-inducing function. It is therefore seldom the treatment of choice for a Yin-deficient patient whose lack of progress is due to poor dilatation more than lack of contractions, and it is no wonder that the effect is both strong and clinically unhelpful. An EAM-informed set of guidelines for administration of oxytocin would likely advise lower initial dosage (and trial of acupressure first!) for all patients with history of disorders suggestive of Yin deficiency, such as hyperemesis, low weight gain, oligohydramnios, preterm contractions or IUGR.

A number of moms receiving epidural analgesia will have a blood pressure drop of greater than 20 percent. Such a drop sometimes leads to fetal heart rate changes and an emergency C-section. The main mechanism of the drop is thought to be vasodilation, and a recent study suggested that compression of the lower legs could reduce the effect.[5] Administration of intravenous fluids beforehand can also reduce incidence of the problem,[6] though there is some evidence that the optimal amount to prevent adverse events differs considerably between individuals.[7]

In my experience, it is most commonly Yin-deficient patients who suffer large blood pressure drops with adverse events such as loss of consciousness

5   Steinmetz, M. M., Shelton, J. A., Watt, S. A., & Johnson, J. R. (2017). Lower limb compression prevents hypotension after epidural in labor patients: A randomized controlled trial. *Obstetrics & Gynecology, 129*, 3S.

6   Loubert, C., Gagnon, P. O., & Fernando, R. (2017). Minimum effective fluid volume of colloid to prevent hypotension during caesarean section under spinal anesthesia using a prophylactic phenylephrine infusion: An up-down sequential allocation study. Journal of *Clinical Anesthesia, 36*, 194–200.

7   Xiao, W., Duan, Q. F., Fu, W. Y., Chi, X. Z., Wang, F. Y., Ma, D. Q., ... & Zhao, L. (2015). Goal-directed fluid therapy may improve hemodynamic stability of parturient with hypertensive disorders of pregnancy under combined spinal epidural anesthesia for Cesarean delivery and the well-being of newborns. *Chinese Medical Journal, 128*(14), 1922.

or abnormal fetal heart tracing leading to C-section. A Western clinician who also recognized signs of Yin deficiency might do well to make sure that those patients received extra fluids as well as leg compression. Birth team members could elevate the legs immediately post-procedure and vigorously chafe the ankles, to raise Qi and fluids.

4.3.4.2 Postpartum challenges

Yin-deficient patients' greatest vulnerabilities postpartum are fluid loss leading to constipation and difficult lactation, as well as difficulty sleeping and postpartum depression. Coconut water, miso soup and pear juice are all exceptionally good at replenishing fluids, but any liquid intake will do and should be encouraged.

Difficulty sleeping and the attendant challenges to overall coping are more concerning, and should be addressed aggressively to prevent more severe problems. The needs of newborns make sleep difficult, so if at all possible, family and friends should step in to make room for naps and self-care (including acupuncture office or home visits).

4.4 Blood-Deficient Births

In EAM theory, Blood carries Yin moisture to the body tissues, so Blood-deficient moms may present with dry skin and a tough cervix. Blood also "roots the spirit" – providing emotional grounding and stability. The main challenges of Blood-deficient patients during the perinatal period include:

- insomnia and anxiety

- muscle cramps, numbness/tingling of extremities

- contractions experienced as disproportionately painful, fatigue, and/or low "copability" during transition and pushing (due to some combination of lactic acid buildup in tissues, tight cervix and lack of emotional grounding)

- slow or arrested dilatation (due to tight cervix, clenching due to anxiety)

- a fetal heart rate tracing that is overly variable or reactive

- insufficient lactation

- postpartum depression

- postpartum constipation.

It is important to note that a Western diagnosis of anemia overlaps with EAM Blood deficiency, but is not equivalent. Many patients suffer signs and symptoms of Blood deficiency with normal or low normal blood counts, while a number of patients diagnosed with anemia present with Qi or Yang deficiency signs and symptoms rather than Blood deficiency (Blood deficiency and Qi or Yang deficiency also co-occur frequently). It is normal for pregnant people's hematocrit to drop in the last trimester of pregnancy, to levels that approach the cutoff for anemia in a non-pregnant person. It is thus the norm that some otherwise healthy moms develop both Western anemia and EAM-defined blood deficiency in their final month of pregnancy. Western medicine addresses this with iron supplementation – a suboptimal solution, as constipation is common in both Blood deficiency and pregnancy in general. It is also the case that Blood deficiency is difficult to address during labor (relative to, say, Yang deficiency, where warmth can be added). Therefore, anticipating and addressing Blood deficiency early on, with home moxa and/or referral to a qualified Chinese herbalist, can make an enormous difference in a given birth.

4.4.1 How to recognize insufficiency of Blood

In clinical practice, signs of Blood deficiency include:

- Pale face, lips, and inner eyelids, with or without a Western diagnosis of anemia. Most anemic patients show signs of Blood deficiency, but not all; some are Qi deficient.

- Moms may have a history of scanty or pale-colored menstrual blood, bleeding only 1–3 days or not at all, reflecting the insufficiency of available blood. Conversely, excessive bleeding (due to fibroids or other causes including Qi deficiency) also causes Blood deficiency due to constant depletion.

- It is not so easy to distinguish deficiency of Blood and Yin, because Yin deficiency includes Blood deficiency and can be thought of as a further pathological development. Symptoms in common include insomnia, anxiety and dry skin. However:

  - Blood deficiency is temperature neutral (patients often feel cold but are also intolerant of heat), while Yin-deficient patients tend to feel hot and suffer night sweats. Also, Blood deficiency makes the face and tongue pale, while:

  - Yin deficiency leads to redness on the cheekbones and tongue, which may also be small in size, or show cracks on the surface, or peeling of the coat.

4.4.2 Key experiential qualities

The key emotional quality of the Blood deficiency birth is anxiety, with a flavor of neediness, helplessness or insecurity. This is distinct from the anxiety that moms sometimes experience in Yin-deficient births, which has more of an impatient edge to it. Blood-deficient moms may also present as "checked out," particularly if there is an epidural on board.

In birth, there may also be a sense that Blood-deficient patients feel emotionally victimized by the contractions, seeking somehow to run away from them, either by clenching and resisting or by dissociating emotionally. Acupuncturists may share my sense that Blood-deficient patients are also more than usually needle sensitive. As it happens, the shape of a Blood-deficient contraction is remarkably similar to that of the "choppy" pulse in EAM, which is common in Blood deficiency. In Blood-deficient births in particular, pain and clenching tend to escalate and exacerbate each other, a snowball effect that if unchecked may tumble into epidural and/or Cesarean section.

4.4.3 Prenatal challenges for Blood-deficient patients

Prenatal challenges for Blood-deficient patients include:

- muscle cramps, numbness/tingling of extremities

- prenatal anxiety, depression and insomnia.

4.4.4 Working with Blood-deficient births

Like Yin-deficient patients, Blood-deficient moms are slow to dilate. They also tend to experience more pain with contractions than other birth types.

My favorite hand technique for Blood deficiency is round rubbing on the mid-back (Section 5.3.2). The slow circles are extremely calming, and seem to literally relax the liver (which stores blood for release during exercise) as well as the diaphragm (which allows for deeper breathing). Moxibustion on UB-17 (right behind the diaphragm) and SP-3 behind the base of the big toe, are also extremely effective for building blood prenatally (see Section 5.4.2). During labor, SP-6 acupressure and/or Liver Gummies generally produce immediate results with dilatation. Gentle squeeze and release on the Liver channel of the inner leg and thigh can also be quite beneficial. However, attention must be paid to the overall pain management situation if contractions are already at the limit of copability, as increased dilation will intensify the sensation. Also, Blood-deficient moms generally crave contact and thrive with bodywork, in direct contrast to Yin-deficient patients who by and large don't love to be touched. New practitioners need to be somewhat careful with Blood-deficient moms, not to become emotionally over-attached or energetically drained.

Box 4.4 Blood deficiency care package.

For basic home care:

— Moxibustion at Stomach-36 (Section 5.4).

— Chafing downwards along the outer shin (Section 5.1.1.4) then upwards along the inner shin (this is the Liver Gummy area, Section 5.1.1.3).

— Round rubbing at the mid-back (Section 5.3.1.2).

— Moderate, regular cardiovascular exercise, e.g. at least two walks per day of at least 15 minutes' duration; also consider social activities, e.g. yoga, belly dancing.

For other commonly occurring challenges:

— For constipation, chafe downwards along outer shin; also try pear juice, avocados, nuts, dried fruits, especially goji berries, and okra (if tolerated).

— If fluids or fetal weight are low, use moxibustion at Stomach-36 or chafing down outer shin (Section 5.4).

— For first-time moms with concerns about contraction intensity, consider training tolerance with perineal massage or ice cube training (see Appendix A).

For labor preparation:

— Starting at 37 weeks, add:

　* Hula Hips (Section 5.5.2) and Belly Breathing (Section 5.5.7).

　* Massage or chafe gently upwards along the inner shin (Liver Gummy area, Section 5.1.1.3).

— Starting at 38 weeks, add:

　* Mom's choice of Hip Openers (Section 5.5.6).

　* 5 minutes each of moderate pressure on Large Intestine-4 at the base of the thumb (Section 5.1.1.1) and Spleen-6.

— At 40 weeks or if induction is imminent, add Liver Gummies (Section 5.1.1.3), thumb circles and pressure at sacral points (Section 5.2.2.2), 5 minutes each, daily to every 4 hours depending on time pressure.

4.4.4.1 Contractions experienced as disproportionately painful

At the hospital, where our team often meets patients for the first time while they are already laboring, Blood-deficient patients may already be struggling at 3 or even 2 cm dilated. In some cases, we can help our patient to interrupt the cycle of physical and emotional distress and get back onto the track of productive laboring. Bodywork, ear seeds (see Section 6.4) and/or needles can successfully interrupt the escalating cycles of distress and pain. In these cases, head station, cervical dilation and rate of progress become important considerations. If the head is dropping and Mom progresses to 5 or 6 cm within a few hours, then she is having a relatively healthy labor despite extra discomfort from Blood deficiency. Conversely, if progress is slow and/or the head is still unengaged, then a high level of distress may not be realistically sustainable for the amount of time it will take to get to full dilation, transition, descent and normal vaginal birth. While I am no great proponent of epidural analgesia personally, I do encourage some first-time moms to reevaluate their pain management plans in light of how their physical experience is currently unfolding. If they are already distressed at 2–3 cm, I advise them that sensations may get more intense before they get easier, and that requesting an epidural in a busy hospital is like ordering pizza on a rainy night – best not to wait until one is desperate, as immediate availability can't be counted on.

4.4.4.2 Overly reactive or otherwise non-reassuring fetal heart rate tracing

Broadly speaking, the fetal heart rate monitor is looking for evidence of interruptions in blood flow to Baby, or low blood flow over time. These are shown by "decelerations" (dips in the heart rate) and low variability (variability being the little ups and downs that a normal heart makes in response to fluctuating metabolic demands as well as to ambient sounds, maternal movements and whatever thoughts are coming and going in the fetal head). High variability (lots of little upticks, or "accelerations") and reactivity (accelerations in response to stimuli) are considered as signs of fetal well-being – in moderation, of course. Excessive variability or reactivity can also raise concern that something's not right.

In Blood-deficient births, my experience is that the fetal heart tends to be more reactive overall. Conversely, fetal heart rates in Blood-deficient births also seem quicker to show low variability toward the end of labor, a sign of fetal fatigue or lethargy due to insufficient oxygen. Remember that Baby's blood flow comes through the uterine arteries to the placenta, and that the uterine arteries sit inside the uterine muscle. Toward the end of labor, when contractions should be coming every 2–3 minutes and lasting a full minute, blood flow to the fetus becomes intermittent. Healthy babies can tolerate this mild "insult," but it makes sense that with a background of Blood deficiency, Baby was less well-perfused to begin with, so symptoms of low blood flow might show up sooner.

This collection of tendencies exemplifies the potential utility of EAM prognostic thinking, even in a highly medicalized setting. If we know a patient to be Blood deficient, then even if the tracing appears normal at the outset, we can be aware that they are at elevated risk for Cesarean section due to "non-reassuring fetal heart rate." Warming the point Stomach-36 with the palm of the hand, and chafing from there down the Stomach channel are simple hand techniques easily taught to birth team members that will improve blood flow to Baby throughout. Somewhat more aggressive treatments to promote labor progress are also warranted. With Blood-deficient patients – because of the reactive fetal heart rate, and the susceptibility to exhaustion late in labor – time is not on our side. In general I try to intervene as little as possible, empowering the partner or birth family through exercises and simple acupressure. However with Blood-deficient births, I do tend to keep a close eye on progress, ready to jump in and keep the labor flowing.

4.4.4.3 Postpartum challenges
Insufficient lactation, postpartum depression and constipation are all common problems for Blood-deficient patients. Warming the point UB-17 with moxibustion (Section 5.4.2) can be extremely helpful.

4.5 Qi Stagnation Births – Constitutional Type
This section describes the specific Qi stagnation type – a strong personality that expresses itself boldly in daily life and in birth, as distinct as any of the deficiency types above, and extremely common. Indeed, most of us become "Qi stagnation types" when stressed or angry. Qi stagnation becomes an ongoing problem with physical symptoms mostly in young, robust people when stress, anger or other strong emotions permeate life, or when they cannot be expressed, so that the body begins to act them out over time.

Used more generally, the term "Qi stagnation" simply describes any situation where Qi cannot flow freely. There are a number of situations in birth where Qi flow is obstructed by deficiency or accumulation of one or more vital substances, by physical and/or emotional trauma, or by poor interface of the fetal head and pelvis. These are discussed in the section to follow.

4.5.1 How to recognize Qi stagnation

Qi stagnation may be the most commonly diagnosed pattern of disharmony by acupuncturists across the globe; its manifestations are both emotional and physical, reflecting the fact that those two constructs are not strongly distinguished in EAM. When an acupuncturist feels the pulse, she is first and foremost evaluating this flow – is it slow or fast, strong or weak, rough or smooth? The pulse quality associated with Qi stagnation is "wiry" – meaning that it feels like a piano string under the fingers, taut and rigid rather than flowing in a smooth wave. An acupuncturist looking for signs of Qi stagnation in the abdomen would similarly check for rigidity, particularly around the diaphragm, as holding or stopping the breath is a common and important manifestation of Qi stagnation ("Qi" also means "air" and "breath"). Any tight muscles anywhere indicate localized friction or stoppage of Qi flow. Finally, any symptom that appears or is worsened with stress can safely be diagnosed as at least in part attributable to Qi stagnation. Patient complaints typically associated with Qi stagnation include:

- tension headaches and neck tension, jaw pain, migraine headaches

- constipation

- irritable bowel syndrome or any gastrointestinal symptoms worse with stress, including heartburn

- moodiness including anger outbursts, anger turned inward (e.g. depression, excessive tendency to drama and/or low self-esteem)

- hypertension.

In reproductive health, commonly encountered manifestations of Qi stagnation include:

- premenstrual syndromes including moodiness, breast tenderness and headaches

- irregular menstruation, i.e., variable cycle length

- menstrual cramps (any pain indicates that Qi is stagnant; however, cramps may also be caused or complicated by cold or other factors)

- dyspareunia (pain during sex)

- subfertility (though Qi stagnation is not the most common cause)

- depression during pregnancy and postpartum depression (Qi stagnation is almost always a factor, but usually in combination with deficiency, particularly postpartum).

4.5.2 Key experiential qualities of Qi stagnation

Our human reaction to unwelcome events or sensations is typically to clench our muscles – as we hunch our shoulders when confronted with a non-consensual shoulder rub. When we tighten up to signal that we don't want to play along with whatever game is being proposed, we are rejecting some part of reality. This rejection is the essence of Qi stagnation: by rejecting the situation that is unfolding, we are obstructing its Qi. In the case of the prospective shoulder rubber, the rejection plays out socially: we are letting him know that we do not share his vision of the immediate future, and it is his Qi that gets obstructed as his backrub plan is thwarted. However, when I clench my shoulders on reading the morning newspaper, this is a rejection of things that have already happened, so the only Qi that gets obstructed is mine. Those who use their life energy to work for positive change, rather than rejecting the world as it is, are to be greatly admired.

In social situations, the feeling of Qi stopped in its tracks is palpable. Sometimes there is a strong flavor of anger or frustration, and sometimes there's just a dead zone, where something probably ought to be said but everything you can think of seems wrong. The same is true of labor: sometimes frustration, anger or disappointment hangs heavy in the air, and sometimes there's just a stuck feeling. Beware – the feeling is contagious! In one case I remember vividly, my brilliant and consistently cheerful colleague Melani came storming out of Room 2, complaining angrily that the patient *insisted* on pushing when she'd been told *multiple times* that her cervix was still thick and *only 6 cm* dilated and would *swell* if she kept pushing. This physical presentation is absolutely typical of Qi stagnation, and the patient did indeed have a wiry pulse, but I had suspected the diagnosis before I entered the room, simply from Melani's uncharacteristically cranky demeanor.

With constitutional Qi stagnation, there are several quite distinct "flavors" of experience, depending on Mom's constitution, culture and socialization, as well as any other imbalances she may be carrying. Typically one or more of the following occurs:

- a high level of interpersonal drama, which may involve family or members of the birth team, and may have an angry, fearful or frustrated quality to it

- quiet internal tension, with fear, anxiety, frustration or grief locking up Qi flow. (Strong, active people stuck in bed may also experience this.)

- a vicious cycle of pain and clenching with each contraction. As in the example of the backrub that is being rejected, this Mom is physically fighting the contraction even as it happens, which both tightens the cervix and makes the pain worse.

4.5.3 Working with Qi stagnation in birth

Whether stagnation expresses itself emotionally, physically or both, the main therapeutic principle is moving Qi through the body in general and through the Liver, Gallbladder and Dai or Belt channels in particular (see Figures 2.4 and 2.5). It is just a question of choosing between the gross bodily movement of exercises and breathing, the inner Qi movement of acupressure and acupuncture, or bodywork, which combines elements of both.

As a general rule, if Mom can get up and move, then exercises and breathing (Section 5.5) are the most direct way to circulate a large amount of Qi through the body. Sumo Walking and Cat/Cow (with deep inhales and exhale) are particularly strong to break up any unpleasant internal or external dynamics, and also to help the labor move forward. Gentle bouncing followed by a supported Cat/Cow or squat helps Qi to flow directly through the pelvis, often breaking the cycle of clenching and pain, allowing Mom to consciously breathe into the belly and soften the pelvic floor. The Duplex Lion Pose, followed by Horsey Lips, also excels for this purpose.

If Mom is stuck in bed, then Cat/Cow can be modified to a seated or reclining position (or possibly performed on hands and knees). The hospital workout consists of walking forward and backward on the sitz bones, which moves and stretches the cervix and pelvic floor; Duplex Lion and Horsey Lips are also useful. Hip rocking is also a useful way to move Qi in lateral recumbent position, particularly if it's possible to alternate sides.

There are a few reasons why one might choose acupressure or bodywork over exercises. Sometimes, it is not the whole person that is tight, but mainly the cervix and/or pelvic floor. Liver Gummies between contractions (Section 5.1.1.3) and strong pressure at Large Intestine-4 during contractions (Section 5.1.1.1) both move Qi to strongly dilate the cervix and reduce pain. The pelvic floor usually softens with movements such as Hula Hips, Cat/Cow and the Sumo Squat, but sometimes gentle hip rocking with acupuncture or acupressure along the Gallbladder channel is useful instead or in addition. It may also be that Mom's emotional journey requires her to "go inside" and feel the stuck place for herself so that she can release it; strong steady pressure on points such as Kidney-1 on the sole of the foot and Spleen-6 above and behind the inner ankle can help to keep the Qi moving as she breathes into the experience. Acupuncturists will find needles useful in this situation, more so than when Mom is moving (though a number of the needles can be taped down for pain and/or Qi moving effects); auriculotherapy can also be helpful for any kind of Qi stagnation.

Overall, without overlooking the seriousness and sacredness of birth, it can be possible to engage the Qi flow of the labor as similar to walking a tired, cranky child home through a shopping mall. Opportunities for distraction, obstruction and heartbreak abound, but the goal is to stay happy and keep moving – so it's necessary to have a repertoire of little games on hand, and the ability to switch from one to another without going too deeply into the details of what was wrong with the previous one. In general big physical movements are extremely useful for "changing the channel" on a conversation, letting conflicts drop if they are extraneous, while subtler techniques of acupressure and bodywork can help to focus the conversation on what's important.

Box 4.5 Qi stagnation care package.

For basic home care:

— Ensure regular exercise including at least two brisk walks per day, the first within 1–2 hours of rising; consider belly dancing or other rhythmic movement.

— Find and massage tight tender points on inner thigh and knee, calf, neck, shoulders and back, particularly along the course of the Liver and Gallbladder channels (see Figures 2.4 and 2.5).

— For emotional discomfort (frustration, anxiety, resentment, etc.): consider Hula Hips (Section 5.5.2), dancing (5.5.3) and/or gentle bouncing (5.5.5). Seek out acupuncture or professional prenatal massage if possible. Also encourage conversation with friends and family; if not resolved consult primary care provider.

For labor preparation, add:

— Starting at 37 weeks:

* Mom's choice of Hip Openers (Section 5.5.6), particularly Sumo Walking and Stair-Crabbing.

— Starting at 38 weeks, add:

* Liver Gummies (Section 5.1.1.3).

* 5 minutes of moderate pressure on Large Intestine-4 at the base of the thumb (Section 5.1.1.1); 5 minutes each of thumb circles and strong pressure at sacral points (Section 5.2.2.2).

> * Belly Breathing (Section 5.5.7).
>
> — At 40 weeks or if induction is imminent, increase frequency to every 4 hours and add one or two more hip opening exercises.

4.6 Additional Stagnation Presentations: Bony Obstruction, Accumulation and Qi Stagnation, Stuck Spirit, Indeterminate Obstruction

As discussed in Chapter 2, the main dysfunction of the labor process is simply that it isn't moving forward – "baby stagnation." Developing a sense for exactly what is stuck and why is the main learning curve of labor support. Having looked at the experiential qualities of constitutional Qi stagnation above, this section introduces other types of Qi stagnation that arise during labor. These are more varied, but there are a few recognizable cues that can be of help in sorting out what exactly is obstructing labor progress. These are summarized in Table 4.1, and their experiential characteristics are described below. A guide to differential analysis and assistance of obstruction in birth is provided in Section 6.1.

4.6.1 Bony obstruction

As discussed in Chapter 3, sometimes the fetal head is actually too big to pass through the pelvis (known as true cephalopelvic disproportion or CPD) and other times the head is not absolutely too big, but is interacting with the pelvis in a manner that will not let it through (we're calling this functional CPD). These two are difficult to distinguish clinically, so as a policy we treat as though the problem is functional, making every attempt to resolve the situation non-surgically.

Bony obstruction has two basic presentations. The most distinct and characteristic presentation of bony obstruction is severe pain during active phase, either in the back due to OP position, or with a bursting feeling as an asynclitic head presses into the pelvis at an angle, pushing the sacrum away from the pelvis. Less commonly, bony obstruction pain wanders around the pelvis at transition, as Baby tries different angles of exit; or there may be pain at the diaphragm or ribside area, as the top of the uterus presses down on a baby that has nowhere to go. Bone pain will usually break through epidural analgesia, so bony obstruction should always be suspected if a previously adequate placement stops working – and moms should be aware of this important limitation of the method's capabilities. The silver lining of bony pain is that it gives immediate feedback as to where the obstruction lies and whether our intervention is helping. Strong stagnation wants big movement. All of the exercises discussed above to promote Qi flow through the pelvis – squatting, Cat/Cow, etc. – can often nudge Baby in the right direction. For OP, hip rocking with Mom lying on her right side often resolves it; details are in Section 7.1.2, along with additional bodywork to jiggle the pelvis and facilitate fetal reorientation.

The other presentation of bony obstruction is that the uterus will sense the futility of the situation and decline to contract. This typically happens at engagement – in which case contractions just don't start – or at transition. As discussed in Chapter 2, the fetal head pressing straight into the cervix with each contraction is like a battery making contact with both terminals: if the angle is off and the circuit is broken, electricity may not flow. It is perfectly normal for contractions to ease off slightly around transition, allowing Baby a little space to reorient for exit. However if contractions cease completely, usually either Mom is exhausted and needs a nap, or there is a bone, flesh or spirit challenge to address. As a rule of thumb, once a contraction pattern is established, moms' bodies are quicker to let it drop when they are deficient, particularly with Qi or Yang deficiency, or damp accumulation. Stronger, younger moms will tend to endure painful, unproductive bony obstruction contractions for longer. Oxytocin augmentation may also produce bony obstruction-type contractions.

With no contractions at engagement, two types of bony obstruction are easily spotted. The first is OP, where the bump is generally too high and in the center, with a hollow at the navel (see Figure 3.5). The second is "swayback" presentation or excessive lordosis, where Mom's back tightens and weakens as the pregnancy pulls it forward, so that it is arched more than it should be and the baby bump points more forward than usual. In this situation, Baby lies at a flatter angle, with too much weight pushing outward against the abdominal muscles, and not enough pushing downward into the pelvis. In this situation, Cat/Cow and any type of massage along the muscles of the back can be helpful; see Appendix A for specific techniques.

4.6.2 Obstruction in the flesh

Throughout all our discussions of the four deficiency types, Qi stagnation has hovered like an evil elf waiting for an opportunity to hex the labor. Deficiency or accumulation of one or more of the vital substances may obstruct Qi flow – causing some combination of delayed labor initiation, pain and slow progress. Accumulation of Yang, in the form of heat or fever, can also impact the labor.

Other types of obstruction at the level of flesh include cervical tightening or discoordinated contractions with underlying physical causes, cervical edema and "strong woman syndrome," when a body in the habit of holding its Qi up has trouble letting it go for labor.

4.6.2.1 Qi Stagnation, deficiency and accumulation

Cold accumulation can arise with Yang deficiency, or due to repeated chilling of the legs or lower back – such as with sports in the cold wind. It tightens the uterus cervix, causing excessive pain with contractions. Occasionally, someone goes into labor while suffering a cold or flu with muscle aches; this may cause painful contractions, or occasionally the whole back and neck may spasm. In any of these cases, the clear solution is warmth. Heating pads at the lower back and/or abdomen should be used with care, at moderate settings in 5-minute intervals so as not to overheat Baby.

Some accumulation of Yin fluids during pregnancy is normal, with swollen ankles and general puffiness in the last few weeks. Severe fluid accumulation can arise with any combination of Qi or Yang deficiency, obesity, humid summer weather or diet skewed toward cold, raw or other hard-to-digest foods. In addition to being uncomfortable, the excess fluids impede the flow of Yang Qi, meaning that pregnancies frequently go postdates (i.e. past the due date) as the cervix ripens and Baby drops but contractions cannot initiate. The extra fluid can be moved by alternating frequent short walks, elevation and hot foot soaks above the ankle with bath salts.

Blood flow easily becomes stagnant when either Qi or Blood is deficient; or there may be preexisting Blood accumulation including fibroids, endometriosis and other painful gynecological conditions. The excessively painful contractions and low emotional resilience of Blood deficiency also appear when Blood flow is obstructed, and can be addressed in labor with the same movements and acupressure used for Qi stagnation, but executed more gently in light of the lower pain threshold.

Yin deficiency dries out the muscles and connective tissue, predisposing them to Qi stagnation, with excessive sensitivity to the small contractions of latent phase, and a stronger tendency to delayed labor onset. Moving the Qi with exercises, breath and acupuncture is the treatment of choice, but will need to be negotiated carefully as most Yin-deficient patients have a low threshold for external stimulation.

When Yang Qi accumulates in the body – due to Qi stagnation, deficient Yin, infection or other causes – it manifests as fever. EAM does not strongly distinguish between feeling hot and the measurable elevation in temperature we call fever. Indeed, during labor it is often possible to feel heat rising off Mom as her blood vessels dilate to shed excess heat, hours before the thermometer shows anything. In general, heat speeds up flow in the body; it therefore does not slow down the labor. A temperature elevation in labor may be a benign reflection of labor's Yang, inflammatory nature – particularly for moms who tend to be hot, who are heavy or who have an epidural in place.[8] However, intrapartum fever is a common first sign of chorioamnionitis, where the membranes become infected. Infection may cause new onset symptoms of headache, nausea or general unwellness, but these are often hard to pinpoint during the chaos of labor. Acupressure and/or needles at the "foot heat points" between the first, second and third toes (Section 5.2.3.2) can sometimes reduce fever considerably, even when the cause is infection. Other methods for reducing fever are discussed in Section 6.2.6.

4.6.2.2 Physically based cervical hardness or discoordination of contractions

In some cases, the cervix dilates slowly either due to discoordinated contractile activity or else due to tightness in the cervical tissue. Discoordinated uterine contractions may be caused by emotional Qi stagnation itself, or there may be a more straightforward physical cause. A C-section scar or fibroids may cause the uterus to contract unevenly, the equivalent of squeezing a toothpaste tube asymmetrically. In EAM terms, patients who suffer painful dysmenorrhea alleviated by heat (i.e. Yang deficiency or excess cold) may also show discoordinated contractions, as the cold inhibits the smooth flow of Qi through the uterine muscle.

In some cases, contractions are fine but the cervix is slow either to dilate or to contract, for reasons that are physical rather than emotional. Procedures such as cryosurgery or LEEP (loop electrosurgical excision) that freeze or burn off abnormal cells may leave the cervix understandably cranky. Termination of pregnancy procedures that involve mechanical dilatation of the cervix, and cervical cerclage procedures may also result in a tight, stagnant cervix. In these cases, I first try rubbing out Liver Gummies (which are usually plentiful and quite tender). If this doesn't work, I usually needle the points Liver-2 and Liver-5, and use electrical stimulation between them.

Although most manifestations of Qi stagnation appear early in labor, the appearance of a cervical lip may also be a physical Qi stagnation sign. Cervical lip is when most of the cervix is fully dilated, but one part of it is still thick and

---

8   From an EAM perspective, epidural seems to reduce the body's ability to shed heat through sweating; if there is lack of sweating or fever, acupuncturists may choose to "release the exterior" with such points as LI-4, TH-5 and SI-3.

hard enough to block progress. Among patients in the hospital lying on their backs with epidural analgesia, this lip is typically anterior due to the uneven application of gravity. If it is on one side or the other, a cervical lip is typically due to some anomaly or injury to the cervix, as described above.

4.6.2.3 Cervical edema due to early pushing

In general, Mom's body is wise, and if she feels the urge to push before full dilatation, as long as she is gentle, the pressure simply helps nudge the labor forward. However, it sometimes happens that Mom's urge to push gets ahead of the cervix's readiness to dilate. If Mom pushes too fast, or if the cervix still has a thick or hard lip, it will become irritated and swell, further obstructing the labor. In this situation, famous Canadian obstetrical acupuncturist Jean Levesque needles the point Liver-2, above the webbing between the first and second toes. In most cases I have tried, this quickly resolves the edema; however, in a few cases where it has not, I have run electrical stimulation at 2 Hz between the Liver-2 points, and it has then resolved. If needling is not an option, strong acupressure with a probe, pen, toothpick or other semi-sharp object would likely also help.

4.6.2.4 "Strong woman syndrome"

In some cases, there are no signs of Qi stagnation drama, nor evidence of physical clenching per se, and yet the labor refuses to start, or with what seem to be perfectly fine contractions, it refuses to progress. Practicing in New York City, the Acuteam commonly sees this presentation as "strong woman syndrome." Dancers, serious yoga practitioners and other people accustomed to holding their Qi tightly in control may often have difficulty letting it drop. As discussed in the section on Qi deficiency, the normal mechanism of labor initiation involves Mom's Qi losing its grip on things in the face of Baby's increasing weight. Moms deeply accustomed to holding their Qi up may actually have quite a hard time letting go.[9] Strong pressure or needling seems to help with this, as well as the Handwich and Belly Breathing (Section 5.5.7), and hip rocking (Section 5.1.1.2). The other therapy I have seen to be effective in helping these moms to relax their abdomen is the "nuclear option" of epidural analgesia.

4.6.3 Stuck spirit

The Chinese word "Shen" is usually translated as "spirit" and sometimes as "mind"; "consciousness" might be more accurate, though it's awkward to use clinically. In EAM diagnostic terms, Shen is the conscious presence of

---

9   Difficulty letting go may also be a symptom of past trauma; see the section to follow.

the person in the room with you, the spark in their eyes that makes and enjoys interpersonal connection. Shen is considered weak or absent when the patient withdraws and avoids eye contact, and it is present when their gaze and facial expression are communicative and responsive to others. I have had stroke patients who have plenty of Shen even though they cannot find a single word; with their right brains intact, they are vividly present, responsive and expressive with their eyes, faces and hands. Conversely, the empty slack-jawed look of a healthy person gazing at her smartphone is an example of absent or deficient spirit – the body is present but the consciousness is far away. Consciousness is the part of our being that we strengthen when we practice meditation or other disciplines that train focus and presence.

Helping Mom to be as conscious and present as she wishes to be, throughout the birth process, is a prime directive of labor support. When the intensity of birth challenges Mom's ability to cope, there are three main ways in which the spirit may be less than present, or may even obstruct labor progress. These spirit challenges arise most commonly in moms with a history of trauma, those with deficient Blood or Yin, and in births that are unusually fast, painful or disorienting due to unexpected or poorly delivered medical care.[10] Emotions may become stuck in a particular dynamic or story, Mom may dissociate, or she may go into a state of overload and lockdown – where every contraction, and every attempt to help, feels like an assault. In each case, skillful EAM assistance involves some combination of working with the Qi flow in the body, and helping to shift the narrative frame that is shaping Mom's thoughts.

4.6.3.1 Sticky or obstructive emotions

As discussed in Chapter 2, human consciousness is a steering committee of five members, each with her own emotional priorities – namely, joy, anger, fear, grief and worry. In healthy life, joy is in the driver's seat, while the others shout advice from the back seat. The Western idea of "operating from a place of love rather than a place of fear" similarly seeks to locate leadership in the heart.

During the intensity of birth, either traumatic memories or habitual emotional patterns may jump into the driver's seat, with fear, anger, grief or worry not only steering the car but also determining what is seen through the windshield. When we are frightened, everyone around us is threatening; when we are angry, everyone is infuriatingly incompetent. What is most

---

10 An excellent resource for working with trauma and other issues of disempowerment during birth is Penny Simkin's book *When Survivors Give Birth*. Simkin, P. and Klaus, P. Seattle, WA: Classic Day.

distinctive about this pattern is that the person in the grip of it is not able to be fully present in the current moment, because she is stuck responding to emotional challenges of the past, or projecting challenges into the future.

These habitual distortions of thought and emotion are common in daily life, and acupuncturists are accustomed to working with them in office visits with specific types of points on each emotion's associated channel to drain energy from the tyrant and nourish appropriate leadership.

During birth, I tend to focus on moving Qi in the body, redirecting Mom's attention and energy in the positive direction of meeting her baby sooner. Along with direct questions about Baby's name, sex, and sibling and cousin status, this shift is most directly accomplished through movement and breathing – the more vigorous the better – e.g. Sumo Walking or Stair-Crabbing (Section 5.5.6.2).

4.6.3.2 Deficiency and dissociation

During birth, intense sensations or strong emotions, such as fear and anxiety, may agitate the spirit such that it wants to run away from the experience – to dissociate, in Western terms. Blood is primarily responsible for rooting the Qi and spirit in the body, hence the low resilience that often accompanies Blood deficiency. For this reason, many of the therapeutic methods used to address pain and fear also function to calm and root the spirit – including pressure on Kidney-1 (Section 5.2.2.1), the Handwich (Section 5.3.1.1) and Belly Breathing (Section 5.7).

When Mom is dissociating, there is a feeling that she is not entirely in the room with you – whether stuck in the past, worrying about the future or just elsewhere. When I first started practicing, there were televisions in each room and they were a primary route of dissociation; now, it's smartphones. It is a general rule of thumb that, under stress, all deficiency types except Yin deficiency will gravitate toward dissociation, simply because they have less total energy with which to fight reality. Stronger, more robust moms tend to sticky emotions, which if severe turn into the presentation of overwhelm and obstruction (below). Yin-deficient moms are also more prone to overwhelm and lockdown than to dissociation, as Yin governs acceptance and flexibility.

4.6.3.3 Overwhelm and obstruction

Most of us are familiar with the angry, inconsolable sobbing of an overstimulated infant or toddler. Everything is awful, the cries seem to say – everything hurts, nothing helps, every stimulus is noxious. This is the feeling state of overwhelm, and recognizing it is a critical skill in labor support. Pain is stuck Qi, and the therapeutic method that unsticks Qi is movement, but when Mom's spirit is stuck in a state of overwhelm, movement is hateful and threatening, so it will be counterproductive unless very skillfully introduced.

Obstruction in EAM is directly related to Western concepts of trauma. When Mom's spirit is in an obstructed state, the body is tight, attempting to control the flow of Qi and emotions by locking it down. The issue of control is key here: when in this state, Mom is experiencing a terrifying sense of uncertainty and lack of control, often based on negative childhood experiences, which may or may not be consciously remembered. When Mom is in this acute, locked-up physical state, it is safe to say that either past trauma is being triggered, or a new trauma is unfolding – often both.

Box 4.6 Three steps for working with stuck spirit during birth.

First, make a safe space. The direct antidote to uncertainty and lack of control is to identify a space and time that is genuinely safe. During labor, this is often the time between contractions: you can ask, gently, "Does anything hurt right now?" If not there is an opportunity for you to help her recognize that in this moment she is okay. (Showing her that you can be counted on to help with the next contraction is the next step.) In hospitals, the trigger for a traumatic response may be an unskillful vaginal exam or other painful interaction with medical and nursing staff. In this situation it's important not to overpromise: it's tempting to say "I won't let her do that again," but not always realistic.

Second, find a working connection. Once there is a small space that is not threatening, it is possible to connect there, physically and verbally, showing Mom that you can be counted on to help. During transition or back labor, when there may not be full respite between contractions, these two steps may combine and the safe space may simply be your therapeutic presence: let her know that you are there for no other purpose than to help, and you won't do anything she doesn't prefer; she has nothing to fear from you. Simply working with her to locate the pain and placing a gentle hand on it is an active demonstration of a completely benign therapeutic relationship, and is extremely calming in and of itself. When I meet a laboring patient already in pain, often my "safe space" is to let her know who I am and that I'm here to help, and my second step is to ask if I can press her bilateral Large Intestine-4 points during her next contraction. This almost always helps enormously (assuming she's not OP), and the whole thing takes less than 4 minutes.

Third, use the "Three Rs" of Relaxation, Rhythm and Ritual. The Three Rs come from Penny Simkin, pathbreaking doula and author of several excellent books on labor support; she also has videos on her website. "Relaxation" is simply making use of the respite between contractions, helping Mom to relax deeply in that quiet time, rather than using up energy worrying about the next one. "Rhythm" refers to Simkin's observation that moms who are coping well with intensity tend to use some kind of rhythm to get through the contractions. This may be by repeating a phrase silently, belting out a catchy tune with the birth team or rocking her own body. Hip rocking (Section 5.1.1.2) and other EAM bodywork can be very helpful in assisting Mom to find her own rhythm; quite often, once we start a rhythmic movement, she will adjust it and make it her own.

4.6.3.4 Shadow emotions and obstruction

It is important to emphasize the three steps described above are not only useful for moms with a documented traumatic history. Indeed, with years of habit they have become my way of approaching nearly every patient on any unit. The truth is there is no knowing who has survived what traumatic experiences; much better to assume that everybody is vulnerable, and can benefit from extra care around safety and the forging of a therapeutic bond.

The stuck spirit presentations described above are in their acute form, but with time you may come to recognize their shadows all around. For example, strong woman syndrome, described in Section 4.6.2.4, describes a situation where moms accustomed to feeling in control of their lives are unwilling or unable to let go and allow labor to progress. In many cases, hip rocking and strong stimulation of Qi moving points helps to soften the pelvic floor; in other cases it doesn't, in which case a gentler approach taking the spirit into account may be more helpful. Any time stuck Qi doesn't resolve as expected with moving strategies, consider the possibility that the spirit is involved. The most common times for obstruction at the level of spirit include:

- engagement: the cervix may soften, but the pelvic floor does not allow Baby to drop and contractile activity remains negligible, as Mom's spirit declines to enter into the uncertainty of labor

- early active phase, as contractions begin in earnest

- transition, which requires a new level of internal relaxation and acceptance

- pushing, where sensations are suddenly quite strong.

4.6.4 Indeterminate obstruction including short cord and not ready

One last type of labor obstruction is really a composite of multiple different problems where it's clear that something is obstructing the labor, but it's not at all clear whether it is one of the factors above, or something different.

At engagement, when labor just refuses to start, if there are no signs of OP or swayback and no symptoms of constitutional imbalance or Qi stagnation, then nothing can be known. This could be true CPD, or something strange with Baby's disposition in the uterus, such as her neck arched back or an arm thrown over her head. It could be stuck spirit or strong woman syndrome. In some of these cases Mom goes into labor and a problem either does or doesn't appear. Other times, after a failed induction, a Cesarean section is performed and the umbilical cord is found to be the problem. If it is exceptionally short, then it holds Baby back from entering the pelvis. More commonly, the cord is only functionally short – ordinary length, but wrapped one or more times around the neck or torso, preventing downward movement.

A short cord (true or functional) is somewhat easier to spot during active labor, though there are no certainties until after delivery. When Baby has enough slack to get into the pelvis, but cannot descend all the way through, then distinctive decelerations will usually appear on the heart rate monitor. True or functional CPD may also cause decelerations, though there is usually more pain in those cases. Stuck spirit is also a possibility for a labor arresting, but in that case decelerations are less likely.

Another cause for labor not initiating, is simply that Mom isn't ready. This may be due to inaccurate estimation of her gestational age, or Yang deficiency slowing down her internal clock, or emotional factors such as not having fully processed a previous loss. There is also considerable overlap between categories of "not ready" and dissociation. As will be seen in Chapters 6 and 7, it is not usually possible to identify one single factor as the cause of all the problems. Most effective is usually to systematically consider and rule out bony, flesh, spirit and these miscellaneous types of obstruction, checking and rechecking the textbook presentations against the live situation as it unfolds until a pattern emerges.

4.7 Key Points to Remember

4.1–4.4 Qi-, Yang-, Yin- and Blood-deficient births:

- The five main birth types include one each for Qi, Yang, Yin and Blood insufficiency, plus one for Qi stagnation without underlying deficiency.

    - Each birth type has commonly seen physical characteristics and perinatal challenges.

- Qi-deficient births are characterized by fatigue and weak contractions, with a risk of premature cervical shortening. Movement and touch are helpful.

- Yang-deficient births include Qi deficiency symptoms. Moms may also have excessively swollen ankles, feel cold or have a history of severe menstrual cramps alleviated by warmth. Labor is often slow to initiate and contractions may be slow, irregular and/or painful. Warmth is essential; movement, touch and encouragement are helpful.

- Yin-deficient births may present with low fluids, low maternal and/or fetal weight, slow cervical ripening and dilatation, with small contractions closely spaced and a risk of premature contractions; they are prone to side effects such as tachysystole with oxytocin or cervical ripening medications, and blood pressure drop with epidural. Low lighting and soft voices are usually best; movement or acupuncture may be helpful, touch is usually not.

- Blood-deficient moms are often anemic; in birth they may dilate slowly with high pain sensitivity and/or low emotional resilience. Touch and encouragement are usually essential.

- Challenges of one birth type may easily cross over to another, or crop up in robust moms during a long labor; they can be addressed with the same care package. In particular:

  - Yang deficiency presentation includes Qi deficiency.

  - Fatigue, weak contractions and other symptoms of Qi deficiency are common late in labor.

  - Yin deficiency signs such as irritability and slow dilatation are often seen with lack of sleep.

  - Qi and Blood deficiency frequently present together.

- To generalize, Qi- and Yang-deficient labors are challenged by insufficient contractions, while slow cervical ripening and dilatation is characteristic of Yin-deficient, Blood-deficient labors and Qi stagnation labors.

  - If contractions are inadequate but there are no other signs of imbalance, consider bony or other obstruction.

4.5 and 4.6 Qi stagnation type and additional Qi stagnation presentations:

- Qi stagnation births are typically seen in young, robust moms who are stressed out or prone to drama; they present as slow dilatation despite strong contractions. Movement, acupuncture and strong acupressure are helpful.

- Other factors may stagnate Qi flow during labor, including bony obstruction, excess fluids or traumatic history.

- EAM has two basic therapeutic strategies:

  - Stagnation is addressed with movement, to restore flow.

  - Insufficiency is addressed by nourishing whatever substance is deficient, to restore balance.

4.8 Summary Table

Table 4.2 summarizes the birth challenges described in this chapter. For each of the main events or "landmarks" of birth, as described in Chapter 3, dark shading indicates a relatively high prevalence of difficulties while paler shading indicates challenges that sometimes arise.

Table 4.2 EAM pathology in birth: Comparative labors of birth types.

	Birth landmark	Yang deficient	Qi deficient	Yin deficient	Blood deficient	Qi stagnation, other
Preterm	Short cervix	High risk				
	Prelabor rupture			High risk		Acupuncturists: "wood invading earth" type may rupture early
	Preterm contractions					
First stage, latent phase	Pelvic floor softens Engagement	Sometimes late		Often late	Sometimes late	Often late
	Cervix softens	Sometimes late		Often late	Often late	Often late
	Cervix moves anteriorly	Cervix not moving anteriorly as cervix ripens is the less common interior manifestation of swayback due to Yin, Yang or Qi deficiency (see Section 5.6.1)				Possible local stagnation after coccyx injury
	Cervix begins shortening, opening	Sometimes late		Often late	Sometimes late	Often late
	True contractions initiate	Often late				
	Contractions increase in strength, regularity	Contractions slow, irregular	Contractions weak, short	Contractions rapid, weak	Contractions not well tolerated, unproductive	

	Birth landmark	Yang deficient	Qi deficient	Yin deficient	Blood deficient	Qi stagnation, other
	Mom copes well with contraction intensity	Often fearful	• "I can't do this" • Sense of powerless-ness, giving up	• Often impatient, irritable, easily frustrated • Lack of sleep depletes Yin in any constitution	• May present as anxious, needy or checked out • Craves touch, reassurance	Qi and Blood deficiency often present together
	Engagement	Sometimes late		Often late	Sometimes late	
First stage, active phase	Contractions have adequate frequency, regularity, duration, strength	Contractions slow, irregular	Contractions weak, short			
First stage, active phase	Progress is palpable, ~1 cm/hour or greater (especially multips)			Any cervix misbehavior is stagnation in the Liver channel, often with underlying Yin or Blood deficiency		
First stage, active phase	As cervix dilates to 10 cm, head descends to mid-pelvis (zero station)					
First stage, active phase	*Cervical lip/rim*					
First stage, active phase	**Transition** fetus may turn anywhere between 7 and 10 cm					Pelvic floor release and successful transition depend on Belt channel softening
Second stage	From full dilation to crowning	• Strength of contractions and pushing rely on Qi • Qi may be deficient in any constitution due to fatigue			Often co-presents with Qi deficiency	
Second stage	Birth of head					
Third stage	Birth of placenta					Elevated risk of retention for Qi stagnation moms
Third stage	Bleeding	Deficient Yang/Qi may lead to uterine fatigue/atony and increased risk of hemorrhage				Heat may also cause postpartum bleeding

Chapter 5

BIRTH BASICS

Core Methods for Integrative Labor Support

Chapter Outline

- 5.1 EAM Labor Support: Comfort, Flow and Balance

- 5.2 Acupressure

- 5.3 Birth Bodywork

- 5.4 Moxibustion

- 5.5 Movements and Breathing

- 5.6 Chapter Summary

For those not already familiar with it, labor support is the art and science of being helpful during labor, providing physical, emotional and/or educational resources before, during and after the birth to help Mom progress with as much awareness and comfort as possible. Comprehensive instruction in the skills and sensitivities of this important work is outside the scope of this book; however, basic competence in labor support should be considered as a prerequisite for advanced problem-solving in labor. I therefore recommend that anyone not already working in labor and delivery, who is serious about doing so, should consider attending a doula training as a useful experiential introduction to the world of birth. For those still exploring the possibility of birth work, or just helping friends and family, the brief introduction in this chapter may suffice, although additional research is recommended (see the Resources section). The excellent app, "Acupressure for Natural Pain Relief in Labour," may also be of help, with videos for finding and stimulating points by situation.

The first section of this chapter lays out the basic principles of labor support, along with a set of four indispensable acupressure and bodywork techniques that are flexible enough to be of use in nearly any labor situation.

Sections 5.2 through 5.5 introduce the therapeutic modalities in detail, providing instructions for a core set of therapeutic methods for use in birth. All points introduced in this chapter are listed in Appendix A.

5.1 EAM Labor Support: Comfort, Flow and Balance

As discussed in Chapters 2 and 4, East Asian medicine (EAM) therapies in general seek to maintain Qi flow and Yin–Yang balance within the body – or to restore it, when disrupted by the pathological processes of imbalance and stagnation. Getting oriented to what's happening in the birth and using human touch, warmth and movement to help Mom avoid or get through rough patches is different from the diagnosis and treatment of disease. Labor is not an illness. When we use EAM principles in birth to characterize a laboring Mom as a Yin-deficient type, we open a treasure chest of historically and experientially based insights as to what her labor challenges may be and what therapeutic methods may bring her comfort and help the labor to progress.

5.1.1 Getting started: Come find birth love

In the acute situation of birth, start with comfort: if there is pain, or if the labor is not progressing well, then Qi is stuck and some kind of movement is needed, to free up flow as much as possible at the levels of bone, flesh and spirit. This includes the vital substances: are there signs of imbalance or stagnation? If so, then acupressure and other comfort measures, which nourish or move whatever's insufficient or stuck, will also help the labor to progress. Finally, it's important to keep reevaluating – always looking at Mom's progress and responses to what we've done so far, always seeking to learn more about her constitution and the labor's own Qi as it unfolds. This process of assessment, orientation, action and reevaluation continues until the baby is out, and is the functional core of EAM labor support. The key words for the process are: comfort, flow, balance and learning more. An easy mnemonic for them is "come find birth love."

Box 5.1 The "Core Four."

My aunt Pam is one of the most intelligent people I ever met – and most definitely not the domestic type. She once remarked to me that she would love to have a cookbook that *really* started with the basics; for example, "First, face the stove." I cribbed this joke for years, when describing how our acupuncture program in the hospital's neurological and orthopedic rehabilitation unit taught students the nuts and bolts of inpatient care from the ground up – "First, face the patient." One day when a school administrator nodded sagely and

---

remarked how he wished that developing compassion had a higher priority in all the clinical programs, I realized that the phrase's double meaning was one that had been present all along, though too large for me to consciously articulate. The first, most important task of helping out in acute situations is to be fully present, doing one's best and paying careful attention to positive and negative changes. The simpler the therapeutic framework, the less opportunity there is to intellectualize or distract oneself by focusing on diagnostic minutiae.

To teach acupuncture students to engage actively with the intensity of labor in the moment, I coach them in four basic methods: LI-4 pressure, hip rocking, Liver Gummies and ankle chafing. Each of these methods is so flexible that it can be adapted to nearly any combination of bone-, flesh- or spirit-level challenges. The methods are also easy enough to teach to other birth team members. Together, I think of them as a four-legged stool – a solid platform on which to sit and be fully available to help, confident that even if the technique isn't helpful in the first minute I choose it, I can easily adapt or choose another, informed by what didn't work with the first. With modifications, the Core Four probably account for 80 percent of what the Acuteam does. They are nearly always what we start with, proceeding to more specific techniques as need determines.

The four treatment methods below – the Core Four – are a quick way to implement EAM labor support (see Boxes 5.1 and 5.2). Like a chain necklace or charm bracelet, they are ready to wear as is, but also create a space for holding future additions.

5.1.1.1 Pain and contractions: Acupressure at Large Intestine-4

As acupuncturists know, LI-4 is a highly influential point on the Large Intestine channel. Its tendency to strengthen and unblock the downward flow of Qi during labor is a natural extension of its more usual work treating constipation. Strong, steady pressure on LI-4 is a comfort measure well known to doulas, and to anyone who has used Debra Betts' seminal handout on acupressure during birth. With different stimulation, I also use the point to strengthen contractions.

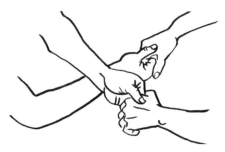

Figure 5.1 Strong pressure on Large Intestine-4.

As a comfort measure, LI-4 works best when used on both hands simultaneously, and when squeezed between thumb and forefinger – pinched, really, not just pressed from above. Pressure should begin just as the contraction is starting, and continue until it has mostly subsided. Between contractions, the point can be gently massaged or left alone. Best ergonomics (and Qi flow) are achieved when the practitioner faces Mom, and crosses their own arms so that right hand squeezes Mom's right hand and left squeezes left – a technique I learned in a doula training in 2007 from the (now) internationally known birth activist Debra Pascali-Bonaro. At that time Debra was giving postpartum surveys in her doula practice, regarding what had been most helpful to moms, and she had yet to receive a response that did not rank LI-4 as favorite or a close second.

Stimulating LI-4 with small, lively pulses, two or three per second, can be very useful in boosting weak Qi and strengthening contractions. This works best using the same good body mechanics described above – think of actively pumping warmth and good cheer into Mom's energy banks, straight from the heart, rather than just pressing someone's thumbs with your fingers. The pulses can be used between contractions, and can switch to steady pressure for comfort as needed. When Mom is Qi deficient and/or exhausted after a long labor, it can also be helpful to start this pulsing during or after delivery – if it's not too much of a distraction – to encourage the uterus to contract and prevent postpartum hemorrhage.

5.1.1.2 Movement and comfort: Hip rocking

Hip rocking can function to move Qi or to boost it, depending on the rate and size of the rocking motion. With practice, the methods can also be extremely relaxing, and very sensitive to intention regarding location of effects. As a comfort measure, hip rocking moves Qi to reduce pain and will be quite familiar to most birth workers. With Mom in a side-lying position, legs bent, the practitioner gently and repeatedly nudges the hips forward – like pushing a child on a tiny swing – until a comfortable rocking rhythm establishes itself all along the body. It's difficult to overstate the power of this simple treatment method to completely shift a rough labor. It is as though, by finding and encouraging a waveform that Mom's body likes, we are helping the body to be more receptive to contraction waves (and to respond to them by dilating). Along with pressure on LI-4, hip rocking is almost always the first method the acupuncture team uses when meeting a new patient in the hospital. In the vast majority of cases, within 5–10 minutes the contraction monitor shows smoother waves that are stronger, while Mom experiences them as easier.

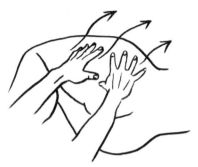

Figure 5.2 Hip rocking.

For readers not familiar with some version of hip rocking, it's hard to explain without a video. Several examples can be seen on my teaching website at Citkovitz.com. It's extremely intuitive, once you get the hang of it – I strongly recommend lots of practice on friends and family (they won't mind one bit). It's important to practice on lots of diverse hips including genetically male ones, because while some hips are quite easy to rock, some (including many male and/or Yin-deficient ones) are tight and require considerable finesse to get going. Others are so loose that it's hard to find an appropriate rhythm without getting lost. As well, perhaps one person in nine just plain doesn't care for this kind of work, and lets you know by tightening up. In these cases there is often some Yin deficiency involved, plus or minus any history of traumatic injury (which tends to locks down the lower back or pelvis). It's therefore extremely important to work on one's skills for getting the movement going, in an exploratory way that leaves space for a nice rhythm to develop if that works for the recipient, without committing to the technique prematurely.

The key point of understanding about rocking is that it is truly a waveform – meaning that amplitude (size) and frequency (speed) are interdependent, and that finding the right size and speed of rocking for a particular patient is exactly like tuning in a radio station.[1] Yin-deficient patients and those with tight hips tend to respond to very small, rapid waves. Qi- and Yang-deficient patients have slacker tissue, which responds to a bigger, slower wave and may have trouble carrying a coherent signal at all. In each case, our therapeutic goal is to meet the person where they are and then gradually nudge them toward health. For Yin deficiency and stagnation, the direction of health is relaxing into larger, freer waves. For slack tissue, the direction of health is finding greater energy and structural integrity by vibrating at a higher frequency.

---

1   This comparison may be less useful for younger readers, who have never had to "tune in" a radio station by turning a dial up and down to control the frequency of waves received, while listening for the sweet spot with the least static.

It is my experience that working with constitution in this way tends to improve the characteristic constitutional problems in the contraction pattern itself – slow for Yang deficiency, rapid for Yin deficiency, etc.

Getting started:

1. Invite the recipient to lie on their side facing away from you. This will likely require some arrangement of pillows between the knees for comfort. The top hip can be straight above the bottom hip, or relaxed forward with support. The head should be supported with a pillow or two and everything tends to work better if the buttocks are not naked and vulnerable, unless that's what Mom prefers in the moment.

2. Establish contact using "good hands." By this I mean, the same caring touch that you use for loved ones and/or patients. This might take 30 seconds and it can include anything you might normally do to relax a tight back; I use round rubbing, described below.

3. Start a rocking rhythm, letting it grow out of whatever movement you have been doing. Start with a very small rocking rhythm, and rather rapid (i.e. appropriate for Yin deficiency and stagnation) and then slow down and increase the size of the wave as the tissue allows it. If you don't immediately find the "sweet spot," then do a little bit of regular massage on the lower back, perhaps some thumb circles on the sacrum, and then try again with very tiny, very rapid rocks, watching for the moment when the ribcage starts to move in sync with the hips, meaning that the body is now engaging the waveform. If the body just doesn't want to engage, then don't push it, just do a little more massage of some other type and move on.

Hip rocking is the tool of choice when there are possible signs of occiput posterior (OP) or other bony obstruction.[2]

- For OP, rocking with the right side down should lead to improvement in back pain within one or two contractions. If it gets worse, turn immediately to the left side down. If there is no change on either side, alternate hip rocking with Cat/Cow and other standing exercises that open space in the hips (see the sections to follow), or check Chapter 7 for more specific guidance.

- For severe pain or other signs of possible non-OP bony obstruction, alternate rocking on either side with standing Hip Openers, changing

---

2   Several variations of hip rocking for specific types of bony obstruction are seen in Chapter 6.

every 8–12 minutes or as Mom prefers. Pay attention to whether one side feels better than the other.

Hip rocking is also indispensable in births where Mom chooses to lie down, or is not free to get up. In particular, I find that it greatly accelerates hospital inductions using topically applied prostaglandins and/or internal balloons for cervical ripening: small, gentle rocking movements seem to jump-start the cycle of tissue stretch and prostaglandin binding described in Chapter 3. With practice, in addition to being a phenomenal comfort measure, hip rocking is useful to locate and break up bony and soft tissue obstruction. Because it takes some practice, hip rocking is not always the best technique to teach to others on the spot. However if a birth team member is a bodyworker or seems to have good hands, it's worth a try with a little initial oversight.

5.1.1.3 Dilatation: Spleen-6 and/or Liver Gummies

Spleen-6's point name, Three Yin Crossing, refers to its location at the confluence of all three of the Yin channels on the leg. Gentle pressure on the point can draw Qi down from the Yang areas of the head to nourish Yin and Blood, and promote Yin functions – particularly cervical dilatation. Indeed, several clinical trials suggest that steady pressure on SP-6 during contractions can reduce the experience of pain and shorten duration of labor.[3]

As discussed in Chapter 4, Yin and Blood deficiency both predispose to painful contractions with slow cervical ripening. In my experience, these moms thrive with gentle pressure on SP-6 during contractions, alternated with footrubs in-between. For moms who present with more stagnation than deficiency – or in situations where time is of the essence – Liver Gummies are a less comfortable technique that "dredges" the Qi of the Liver channel to encourage cervical softening and dilatation.

The "Gummies" themselves are actually nodules, easily felt by running a thumb along the inner back edge of one's shinbone, from right above the ankle bone to right below the knee, just where the flesh meets the bone (see Figure A6). In general, the more gynecological Qi and Blood stagnation is present (or the tighter the cervix), the larger and more tender the nodules will be. I began to notice the tender nodules early on, when palpating for the point Liver-5 in order to needle and apply electrical stimulation – my go-to treatment for softening a tough cervix, at the time. Over the years I found that in most cases the needling wasn't necessary: the cervix would dilate if I

---

3   Smith, C. A., Collins, C. T., Crowther, C. A., & Levett, K. M. (2011). Acupuncture or acupressure for pain management in labour. *Cochrane Database of Systematic Reviews, 7*. DOI:10.1002/14651858.CD009232

just massaged the nodules away, in an upward direction using the side of the thumb against the shinbone to press them out.

An important note for using Liver Gummies is that care needs to be taken to adjust the speed and level of pressure to Mom's constitution and tolerance. Deficient patients can benefit from the technique when done quite lightly, while robust moms with Qi stagnation – particularly those stuck in bed – may do well with strong pressure, just as some people enjoy vigorous deep-tissue massage. "It helps a lot with dilating the cervix, and it feels great when I stop" is something I often say.

Box 5.2 Liver Gummies for home care.

Prenatally, Liver Gummies are an excellent way to promote cervical ripening. I teach them at 37 or 38 weeks, with instructions to go gently at first, starting with 3 minutes each leg and increasing a minute or two each week. As most moms are not flexible enough to reach their own shins by this time, the session becomes an opportunity to practice communication with the partner or birth team member about finding the right pressure. Alternatively, starting at about 39 weeks the strong sensation can be used as practice in working with contractions: 1 minute on, 4 minutes off, provides a visceral way of teaching the body that a minute isn't forever.

Perinatal care aside, the technique is also terrific for moving stuck Qi in menstruation. In teaching it over the years, I have frequently had students report that menstrual cramps resolved or a delayed period came on, after they received the treatment in class. I have since started giving Liver Gummies out as a self-care method, starting after ovulation for any patient with premenstrual syndrome (PMS) or dysmenorrhea. The results have been strikingly good.

5.1.1.4 Boosting vital substances: Chafing

Western medicine has no way to add energy to the system. Chafing can do this – and what's more, when taught to family members it grants their deepest wish, providing an entry point through which their love and support can actively nourish the birthing person. Chafing is done by pushing away from oneself with the "palm root," meaning the base of the palm nearest the wrist. Body alignment and relaxation are important: the upper arm should be moving straight out and back as though swinging one's arms while walking, not angling toward or away from one's own center line. Following the specified direction of the push stroke is important, so it may take a little extra moving around to find an appropriate position. The forearm and hand should be completely relaxed, with the fingertips settling into comfortable contact with the patient and going along for the ride as the palm root drives the warming action.

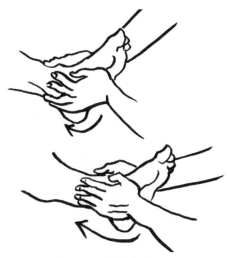

Figure 5.3 Ankle chafing.

Chafing is useful anytime, and on any surface that wants to be warmed or nourished. When applied to the Stomach channel at the outer shin it can nourish Qi and Blood. Applied to the Kidney channel at the inner ankle, it can nourish Yin or Yang selectively based on speed and pressure.

- Qi and Blood: Down the outer shin (for acupuncturists, ST-36 to ST-37). The Stomach channel travels down along the tibialis anterior muscle, just outside the shinbone; the muscle fits neatly in the cleft of the palm, and chafing here feels pleasantly warm as it boosts Qi and supports Blood flow to uterus. Chafing from the knee about halfway down the shin is an excellent way to nourish Mom and support baby, particularly if there is Qi and/or Blood deficiency, fatigue or a fetal heart tracing that doesn't look great.

- Yin or Yang: Up the inner ankle (for acupuncturists, KD-1 to KD-8). The Kidney channel runs from the sole of the foot up behind the inner ankle and shinbone, the perfect place for a relaxed hand to tuck in and chafe upward. The palm root travels from the sole of the foot up to where the palm comfortably cups the ankle bone, while the rest of the hand stays in relaxed, comfortable contact with the channel up to about the level of SP-6. Fast strokes with strong pressure generate friction that quickly warms the channel and activates Yang. Slow, gentle strokes are relaxing, encouraging rest and nourishing Yin.

Box 5.3 Using the Core Four in birth.

These four therapeutic methods are presented in the order in which they are normally deployed, from a simple comfort measure, to supplementing weak qi, to learning more about what might help a problem labour.

— If a patient is already in pain when we meet her, we start with LI-4 pressure and hip rocking immediately, often with immediate results.[4]

— If contractions are weak, LI-4 pulsing and vigorous ankle chafing help to boost Qi and Yang. If contractions are adequate but dilatation is slow, SP-6 and/or Liver Gummies are likely to help.

— In the absence of excessive pain or impeded progress, all four methods can be used as comfort measures, to move stuck Qi, or to selectively nourish Qi and Blood, Yin or Yang.

The chapter sections to follow introduce approximately 20 more techniques, grouped by modality as well as function. This is still a relatively small set, but enough to be confusing if added all at once. My suggestion for those genuinely new to birth is to work with the first four techniques for several births, bringing in new techniques at a leisurely and comfortable pace.

5.2 Acupressure

Acupoints do not work like elevator buttons, with a single function that arrives when summoned, independent of the quality of touch used. In practice acupressure works more like speech, where words have a range of possible meanings, but are given life by the speaker's tone of voice and relationship with the listener. For example, strong pressure on the point LI-4 is commonly used to reduce pain with contractions, but when activated more gently with light pulses of pressure, it can increase contraction strength.

Two main factors determine how touch will function. First is the amount of pressure: this is the difference between a whisper and a shout. Second and equally important is the *responsiveness* of the touch to the texture of tissue underneath it, and how it changes when manipulated. This is the difference between empathetic listening and unsolicited advice. In general, a lighter, more inquisitive touch tends to nourish the system by drawing Qi toward it, as though the body is leaning in for an intimate conversation. Movements such as chafing or pulsing can increase warming or activating effects.

---

4   Indeed, I remember once starting my two students with LI-4 plus vigorous hip rocking for a mom with severe pain stalled at 7 cm for 6 hours; she felt better by the second contraction. I ran out of the room to file the consent paperwork and log us into the case on the computer, and returned to find Mom ready to push.

Moderate pressure is used to direct Qi up, down or away from a tight area, while heavy pressure is used to clear heat or reduce pain. Specific techniques are described below.

5.2.1 Nourishing and warming techniques

The human touch brings warmth and nourishment, both physical and experiential. Simple placement of a fingerpad or palm onto a point, with calm and attention but no special effort is already extremely warming and nourishing. It is very much like holding hands, but with a therapeutic goal. As a rule, the more relaxed the operator's arm and shoulder (as well as heart), the more Qi flows through the hands and the more nourishing and relaxing the touch will be. Pulsing and tapping can selectively amplify the nourishing, warming and/or activating capacities of simple touch.

5.2.1.1 Gentle pressure

Gentle pressure is appropriate for any presentation with a component of insufficiency. Its effectiveness can be increased by choosing constitutionally appropriate acupoints. Its most common uses are:

- SP-6, with thumbs – to nourish Yin and Blood support cervical ripening/dilatation in deficient patients (use stronger pressure for stronger moms).

- Lower back and abdomen, with palms – (also known as the Handwich – see below under birth bodywork), to calm the spirit, warm and nourish all vital substances and relax the pelvic floor.

- ST-36, with thumbs or palms – to supplement Qi and increase blood flow to the uterus. This method has the same goal as chafing the area (as previously introduced) or warming the point with moxibustion. It is not as strong, but is useful when Mom is asleep or the mechanics are not right for chafing.

5.2.1.2 Pulsing

Pulsing works best with the thumbs, just adding little squeezes to gentle pressure to boost Qi and Yang. When used on certain points, it seems to initiate or strengthen contractions. The technique is used often on:

- LI-4, to boost Qi and strengthen contractions

- Duyin, to strengthen contractions.

One situation where pulsing does not work well is during contractions. Ironically, pulsing pressure seems to be a natural impulse for friends and family helping in labor, when rhythm is very helpful in coping. However repeated experience has shown that the point's reducing pain function requires strong, steady pressure; pulses during contractions are generally perceived as ineffective and annoying. Team members can be coached that pulsing on LI-4 between contractions is a fine way to boost Qi and prepare the contractions to be more effective, but that pressure during contractions, needs to be steady and strong.

5.2.2 Moving techniques

Moving stuck Qi and nourishing insufficient Qi are oppositional principles of treatment even though deficiency often leads to stagnation and vice versa. When there is an excess of stuck Qi, acupuncture excels at moving it along and rebalancing the system, as one might find and break up a beaver dam to restore flow in a previously thriving river. However, when deficiency is the primary problem, it is acupressure that excels. Acupuncture's basic nature is to move Qi around, while acupressure's is to nourish. It is therefore possible to perform a hand technique that directs Qi out of a stuck place, while still overall adding energy to the system rather than subtracting from it. Moreover, the proportion of moving to nourishing can be titrated as appropriate to the constitution and situation. The techniques below are presented in order from most nourishing to most moving.

5.2.2.1 Redirecting pressure

Points such as GB-21 and PC-6 have a natural propensity to move the Qi in a specific direction, so that moderate pressure from any birth team member will usually have the desired response. "Redirecting pressure" is a two-part technique of acupressure stimulation that becomes habitual when practiced regularly, and seems to greatly enhance effectiveness of acupressure stimulation. For fans of Debra Betts' acupressure guide and app (including me), the technique is applicable to all the points in it, particularly those listed below.

The first step is simply gentle pressure, making contact between the thumbs and the point, and listening carefully to the tissue underneath. The tissue may soften, inviting the touch deeper – or it may resist the touch, possibly even tightening more. If the tissue does relax, then the thumbs should take up any slack as soon as it is provided, but no faster. This is a very slow and deliberate way to enter someone's personal and therapeutic space, and the body seems to find it quite trustworthy – much as animals are reassured by slow, predictable movements that allow them to make the first move. In this way the thumbs do enter more deeply into the tissue, but the perception of pressure *per se* is minimal.

In the case that the tissue does not immediately soften under gentle pressure, it is worth staying there and just listening to the tissue for a minute or two, making sure that one's own hands are relaxed (most bodies will resist acupressure from uptight hands). In many cases the tissue does soften once the patient's body relaxes into the situation. In other cases, there will be a sense of movement in some direction other than the one initially envisioned, representing a twist or shear in the tissue. Sometimes a point is simply not open for business and other points or alternative assessments should be considered. More commonly, one realizes one's location has been slightly off and the tissue a few millimeters away is happy to respond.

In any case once the tissue and the touch are engaged, it becomes very easy to imagine that the Qi really is moving in the desired direction. As my teacher Tom Bisio said about this type of therapeutic method, don't bother asking yourself whether the experience is wishful thinking – it is. The point is that it frequently helps and can't possibly hurt, as you're pressing the point anyway. I keep an eye out for birth team members who have a well-developed meditation, prayer, bodywork, yoga/Qigong or martial arts practice – these people's wishful thinking seems particularly potent. Points that work particularly well with redirecting pressure (along with their apparent effects) include:

- LI-4 – moves Qi downward during labor, reduces pain.

- GB-21 – moves Qi downward during labor, pushing and lactation.

- PC-6 – moves Qi downward for nausea, hiccupping, belching, etc.

- SP-1 – moves Qi upward to slow postpartum hemorrhage (together with Western care of course). Immediate heavy pressure with a fingernail has appeared to slow blood flow markedly in a number of cases I have seen.

- GB-30 – moves Qi downward during labor, reduces pain. Pressed bilaterally with thumbs or palm roots, this point sends the Qi downward and reduces pain for any labor. With OP, it becomes a critically important comfort measure post transition, as the head pushing on the sacrum painfully stretches the sacrotuberous and sacrospinous ligaments during contractions. Pressing steadily with a fist into the point on the side that hurts (or straight into the sacrum, if it's bilateral) supports the ligaments enough that they stop screaming.

- Du-20 – raises Qi for fatigue, and to focus pushing energy on the perineum.

- KD-1 and LV-14 – see Box 5.4.

Box 5.4 Key Redirecting points: Kidney-1 and Liver-4.

KIDNEY-1

This point on the bottom of the foot has a very calming effect when stimulated with gentle to moderate pressure, with the middle finger or thumb (depending on Mom's position) while holding the outer sides of the foot steady with the rest of the hand. This grasp is extremely comforting, and a go-to to calm and root the spirit when there is anxiety or fear. A brilliant young colleague of mine teaches acupressure to expectant couples in her practice, and calls KD-1 "the Panic Button."

LIVER-14

Liver-14 is a point that I learned to needle inward and then angle down for retained placenta, from the expert Canadian obstetrical acupuncturist Jean Levesque in 2005. I never got around to needling the point for this purpose, partly because the condition doesn't occur terribly often so I didn't have occasion to, and partially because I don't love needling over the lungs in birth (the point lies in the space between the ribs at the bra strap line, directly below the nipple). However, in 2008, returning to the room of a patient my students had seen, I walked in on a doctor pulling on the umbilical cord with what looked like alarming force, while massaging the uterus to free up the placenta. I decided that acupressure was in order – stat! – and pressed strongly in and then down. There was an immediate, wet, sucking sound as the placenta released; the doctor and I looked at each other, equally surprised. Since that time I have used the technique a number of times and never seen it fail. Do remember that the point is quite tender, so pressure needs to start gently.

5.2.2.2 Thumb circles

Thumb circles can be thought of as a dynamic way to redirect Qi away from tight places. Rather than pressing into the tissue in one place, which can be painful, the practitioner makes small circles with the thumb or instrument: 1 cm to 1 in. in diameter, one to three circles per second. The movement can hover over one or more points, such as the points UB-31 to UB-34 in the sacrum directly behind the uterus; or can move along the edge of something such as the sacroiliac joint, shoulder blade or spine. The pressure needs to be carefully tuned to Mom's tolerance, using the same listening approach, but often the pressure feels great and the only limiting factor is thumb strength. In this case a massage tool may come in handy – anything with a ball or rounded end, and a solid place to grip. Knuckles or elbows can also work. In a pinch at home, the blunt handle end of a wooden spoon will do.

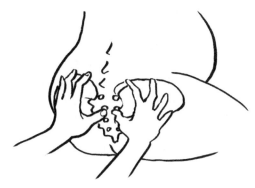

Figure 5.4 Sacral points.

Box 5.5 Sacral points.

The four acupuncture points on either side of the sacrum correspond with the holes in it, where nerves and blood vessels come through. Nearly any kind of moderate or strong pressure or massage on the sacrum both stimulates these points (which promotes contractile activity) and softens them (which helps the pelvic floor to release and the cervix to move forward). While you are in the neighborhood, it is also useful to press or make thumb circles at the outer edge of the sacrum (right where it meets the pelvis, you can feel a vertical line where the bones meet) and again outside that vertical line of bone. These points can be stimulated for 5 minutes every hour to hasten cervical ripening under time pressure, or anytime during labor as desired.

Other areas appropriate for thumb circles include:

- Around the edges of the scapula, (for acupuncturists, UB42-44), plus in its center (SI-11), to promote lactation.

- Along the paraspinal muscles that surround the vertebrae of the neck and back, to loosen the muscles and ease tension (circles with the palm root may also feel good here).

- Around the medial and lateral malleolus of the ankle and along the sole of the foot, to relax the patient and soften the pelvic floor.

5.2.3 Clearing heat

As discussed in Chapter 4, excess heat is just Yang Qi that is lodged in the body, heating it up rather than flowing through. Clearing heat from the body is thus a strong, targeted version of moving Qi. Due to the inherently nourishing nature of acupressure, the hand techniques discussed above are less effective at clearing heat than acupuncture. For those not licensed to use needles, a few options are presented: there are specific "heat points" on the hands and feet, used since 200 BCE to reduce heat, and these can be stimulated in various ways. Additionally, for those with appropriate licensure and/or legal freedom to use lancets, drawing a few drops of blood from selected acupoints can quickly lower fever (see Chapter 6).

Other important methods for cooling hot bodies include a spray bottle of water, a manual or electric fan, and oral ice chips and/or cold water as appropriate.

5.2.3.1 Hand heat points

One of the basics of acupuncture theory is that most points located where the fingers and toes meet the hands and feet have a property of quickly clearing excess heat from the body. These points are too small to be usefully stimulated by finger pressure. However, the heat-clearing points on the Pericardium and Heart channel can be strongly stimulated by grasping a comb such that it meets the palm at its upper crease – a highly effective comfort measure as well, particularly where there is heat or stagnation.

5.2.3.2 Foot heat points – Liver-2 and Stomach-44

Some of the body's strongest heat-clearing points are between the toes, just where the webbing joins the normal skin at the top of the foot. Among these, I have found LV-2 and ST-44 (the first–second and second–third toe spaces, respectively) to be extremely effective for clearing heat. I originally used the combination for mastitis, as both channels travel through the breast; I found that not only did fever drop, but the pain, redness and swelling was greatly improved, along with the headache, bitter taste and general feeling of unwellness associated with infection. I have subsequently had similar effects with intrapartum fever as well. These points can be stimulated by strong steady pressure with a comb or any other not-too-sharp object such as an auriculotherapy probe, or in a pinch a toothpick or the tine of a plastic fork. Pressure should last 1–2 minutes each, treating all eight points and repeating until the fever drops or other action is taken.

5.3 Birth Bodywork

As previously indicated, the term birth bodywork is used in this book to describe Tuina techniques that move or activate a body region rather than just a single channel – such as rocking the hips or warming the whole lower back with circular palm movements. Like acupressure, birth bodywork shines in its ability to combine nourishing and moving capabilities. All of the techniques below are quite flexible, and can be adjusted to be more nourishing or more moving according to Mom's needs in the moment.

5.3.1.1 The Handwich

The Handwich is one of the most powerful and versatile therapeutic methods in birth, despite its apparent simplicity. As will be seen below, it's worth using at every opportunity both because of its multiple benefits, and also because those benefits greatly increase with practitioner experience – so getting more practice is good for everybody.

At its grossest physical level, the Handwich is an excellent warming technique for patients with deficient Yang, or painful contractions that may be due to cold. Seated facing the side of a recipient – who may be seated or reclining – the practitioner simply centers one hand each on the lower back (the pinky should bump up against the top of the sacrum) and under the bump, as close as possible to the pubic symphysis. Explicit verbal permission should of course be obtained, and can be as simple as, "I'm going to put one hand on your back and the other on your lower abdomen, if that's okay?" Both practitioner and receiver usually feel considerable warmth quite quickly, as well as a sense of the hands being connected to each other through the lower abdomen and pelvic floor. In most cases there is a profound sense of calm and relaxation as Mom's Qi drops back its center, which is right between the hands. This sense of dropping and connecting with the pelvic floor almost always leads to Baby dropping and the cervix relaxing. Indeed, babies seem to love this technique and one can often feel them squiggle into the space that opens between the hands.

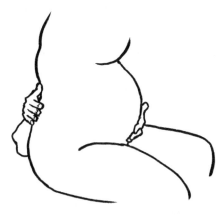

Figure 5.5 The Handwich.

At the subtlest level, once the hands feel connected to the belly and pelvic floor, remarkable insights often emerge as to the nature and location of any bony or soft tissue obstacles to progress. This is not magic or even special Qi manipulation. It is more like the way visually impaired people use sound to get a sense of the space around them – a skill that develops over time. With practice, it does begin to feel like a kind of sonar. Often after a few quiet moments it becomes plain as day that Baby is angled crookedly, or conversely that the head is fine and the cervix is just tight (a cue to use Belly Breathing). With practice there is usually a spontaneous desire to "unwind" the soft tissue, lifting or twisting the hands infinitesimally to free up kinks and resolve flow. Craniosacral therapists and other bodyworkers will find this type of subtle listening easiest, but it's a skill well worth cultivating for anyone serious about birth.

One caveat with the Handwich is that there are a few people – including most Yin-deficient patients – who just don't like the intimacy of it. If in any doubt, it's important always to step in slowly, starting from the back and the top, moving the hands down into position with decisive, predictable zig-zags, keeping an eye on the patient's face to make sure it's really okay. In the absence of a visual cue ask something like, "Is this okay?" and watch the face and body language of the answer. If it's not so clearly okay, then just smile, ask a question about Baby's movements or favorite place in the belly and move on to another comfort measure.

5.3.1.2 Round rubbing

Anyone who has ever rubbed gentle circles on the belly of a colicky baby, or the back of a cranky loved one, has practiced round rubbing. EAM principles aside, the steady slow rhythm of the circles and the warm human touch are inherently comforting. In terms of technique, four things are important:

- Therapeutic location and effect. Which channels or organs are stimulated determines the therapeutic effect of the technique. The two locations most useful in birth are on the back, with one big circle taking in both sets of paraspinal muscles (for acupuncturists, the inner and outer Bladder lines).

- Full-palm contact. Unless the recipient is tiny, round rubbing is performed with the whole surface of a flat palm. There is not much pressure between the hand and the back, just enough to keep the whole palm in solid contact.

- Good body mechanics. Care should be taken to position oneself and the recipient such that the movement is performed with maximum relaxation and minimum effort. This is easiest in the same position we used for the Handwich: recipient seated, practitioner facing their side. The movement works best pushing out over the top of the circle and pulling in at the bottom of the circle. The rate is slow but not sluggish (approximately 1–1.5 seconds per circle; regular cadence is important).

- Qi generation. Similar to making a glass sing by running a finger around the top edge, when we perform round rubbing at a good speed with good body mechanics and a good level of pressure, within a few circles there starts to be a feeling of something happening. It's not much – a little feeling of warmth, and a subtle sense of something flowing into the circle that we have made, like a whirlpool. The feeling is often quite pronounced for the recipient, and lasts for a few minutes after the movement has stopped.

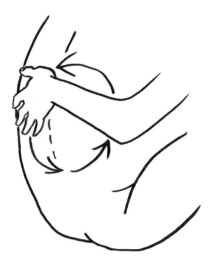

Figure 5.6 Round Rubbing.

Round rubbing can be used anytime during pregnancy, labor or postpartum to relax the back and nourish vital substances. Which substance it affects the most is determined by the location, speed and pressure of the circles: more pressure and speed produce more heat, warming Yang and activating Qi.

The two main uses for round rubbing in birth are:

- behind the diaphragm: to boost Blood and Qi in labor
- at the lower back (between the sacrum and the rib cage): to boost Yang and/or Yin in labor.

Round rubbing at the mid-back addresses the problem of Blood deficiency in several different ways. Most generally, this territory is directly behind the diaphragm. The round rubbing loosens the area, which allows for deeper, more relaxed breathing (important for these patients who tend to anxiety and dissociation). At the specific level of acupoints affected, Urinary Bladder 17 (UB-17) is referred to as "the influential point of Blood." It is used clinically to nourish not only the substance of Blood but also its functional capabilities such as softening the sinews (for us, the cervix and pelvic floor). UB-17 is located at the level of the seventh thoracic vertebra, at the high point of the paraspinal muscles about an inch out from the midline. UB-18, right below it, is a key point used to address the functions of the Liver – and indeed, the point is located directly behind the physical Liver organ. In EAM, the Liver has a function of "storing the Blood," and releasing it when needed. From a Western perspective, the liver holds some 15 percent of the body's blood supply within its extensive vascular networks at any given time. It is my clinical sense that in addition to freeing up the diaphragm (and partly as a result of it), the round rubbing decreases the twisting and tightening forces placed on the liver, allowing the blood to flow more freely through it and in effect increasing the flow volume of what's available to the rest of the body. I find that after 5–10 minutes of round rubbing, Blood-deficient patients are often markedly less pale as well as more relaxed and grounded.

Round rubbing on the lower back excels when a birthing person is both frightened and deficient – often as a next step after the Handwich. In EAM, the Kidneys function essentially to store and distribute the body's total supply of Yin and Yang. They also have a strong relationship with the emotion of fear (think: adrenals). Chronic or excessive fearfulness easily injures the Kidneys, and is often a sign that they are struggling. UB-23 (located deep in the lumbar curve) is a point commonly used to nourish the Kidneys, while the Kidneys themselves are located at the base of the ribcage. By rubbing in a circle around the entire lumbar curve, we nourish and relax the acupoint, organ and surrounding musculature. If Mom tends to cold or Yang deficiency, rub a little more briskly and with slightly more pressure to warm the area. For Yin deficiency use less pressure, and have an intention to communicate relaxation and ease with each stroke.

5.3.1.3 Yin footrubs

Any comfortable massage on the feet inherently nourishes the Yin and helps to relax the pelvic floor and cervix. To leverage this inherent therapeutic effect in birth, include the following techniques in whatever massage is given, taking constitution into account:

- breaking the Bread – boost Yin, relax the pelvic floor

- chafing – boost Yang or Yin as appropriate

- thumb circles all around the inner ankle – relax the Yin channels. (It's worth noting that the point used in some Western reflexology systems to address the uterus is near to Kidney-5, which is used in EAM to treat menstrual disorders.)

Breaking the Bread is a technique from Thai massage, whose system of energy flow includes lines along the soles of the feet, in the spaces between the metatarsal bones. Quite simply, the operator loosens up these spaces and stimulates the lines each in turn, by grasping the foot in both hands with fingertips meeting each other, then rotating the wrists outward. In this way the thumb sides of the hands push downward on the inside and outside of the foot, while the fingertips press upward, accentuating the metatarsal arch and pressing into space between the metatarsal bones. Start on the space between the fourth and fifth metatarsal, as close as possible to the heel bone without being on it, and move toward the toes in about five squeezes. Then continue onto the next metatarsal space (between third and fourth) and so on. Between the third and fourth metatarsals, pay extra attention to the Korean Uterus point, which lies on the sole of the foot at the base of the toes, between the two joints.

5.4 Moxibustion

Historical research suggests that moxibustion long predates the use of acupuncture needles, and was first performed by female shamans. It is extremely useful, prenatally and postpartum, for rebuilding depleted Yang and Qi as well as Blood.

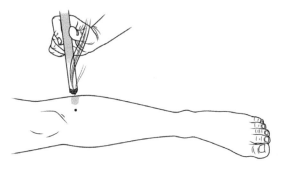

Figure 5.7 Pole moxibustion.

5.4.1 How to apply (or teach) pole moxa

To use pole moxa, you need:

- a moxa stick. These come in two kinds: smoky and smokeless. The smokeless burns somewhat hotter and makes much less smoke, but seems a little less effective. Either type can be easily obtained online or from a Chinese medical supply store

- a moxa extinguisher, or aluminum foil in which to wrap the pole after use to put out its fire (beware, it likes to smolder)

- an ashtray or bowl in which to drop ash

- a cup or bowl of water in case of stray ash

- Western or Eastern burn salve should also be kept on hand, in case ash drops and makes a small burn. In the United States I use *Ching Wan Hung* brand[5] with excellent results. Chinese medical supply houses or Japanese acupuncturists in any country will have a reliable reference for a preferred type.

Every 2–3 minutes, ash will build up on the tip of the pole. It's important to clear it frequently, but not by rapping the pole on the side of the ash receptacle. Rather, roll the pole gently against the side so that the ash is brushed off lightly and falls of its own accord. This prevents cracks in the pole, which can lead to chunks of still-burning ash falling off and burning the patient.

For UB-67 moxa (described in Appendix B), the moxa should be held steady near the toes. For most other uses, a "sparrow peck" technique should be used. As I learned this technique, the practitioner concentrates on the point and moves the tip of the moxa pole steadily toward it, with a feeling of pushing heat inward, holds the heat there for a moment, then backs off to a distance of perhaps 6 in. (15 cm). This pushing movement should take about 1–2 seconds, and be repeated rhythmically for the duration of the treatment. The fingers of the other hand should surround the point, in order to accurately gauge temperature and keep the heat level comfortable.

Important perinatal uses of moxibustion include:

- Bladder-67 (Reaching Yin) for breech presentation, transverse or oblique lie, or OP (see Appendix B)

- Stomach-36 (Leg Three Miles) to nourish Qi and Blood, and direct blood flow to the uterus. One session is 15 minutes of sparrow

---

5   www.itmonline.org/jintu/chingwan.htm

peck each side (this may need to be shorter during labor). Sessions should be repeated daily or as often as possible for small babies or oligohydramnios, though I have seen even one dose markedly increase amniotic fluid

- Kidney-1 (Bubbling Spring) to warm the whole body, for anyone who is cold, damp or Yang deficient.

- Bladder-17 – Geshu (Diaphragm Transport), to nourish the Blood and promote lactation. Bladder-17 is located on the mid-back, approximately 1.5 in. (4 cm) on either side of the spine – right in the middle of the paraspinal muscle bands – at the level of the space between T7 and T8. Moxa at Bladder-17 strongly nourishes the blood, which is deficient in nearly all moms prenatally and postpartum. The method is therefore useful for nearly anyone who does not have signs of heat or excess, and is particularly helpful when lactation is scanty.

Box 5.6 Moxibustion for intrauterine growth restriction (IUGR), Facebook post by a colleague.

PL, FACEBOOK "ACUMAMAS" GROUP, LATE 2018:

I'm 35 weeks Preggo with second baby. I have a 22-month little boy. My doctors are concerned about possible IUGR as baby is measuring small-for-date. I'm also toooootally exhausted and drained. I've been moxa-ing ST-36 and KD-3 every few days, which I do notice gives me a pep in my step. I've always been super conservative about herbs when pregnant/nursing (and just don't take them), but I'm feeling like this is a sitch that calls for them. Thinking about Ba Zhen San. But wondering if anyone out there had any other ideas! I have about 10 days until my next ultrasound that will access her growth/determine next steps

CC, FACEBOOK REPLY:

Hi PL – well and good to supplement blood if that's what's indicated, but anemia has to be pretty severe to cause IUGR and is not usually the issue in countries/families not suffering food insecurity. More common is that the trophoblast invasion in the first trimester has not fully transformed the uterine arteries so Baby isn't getting enough oxygen. In that circumstance often he sends out erythropoietin and your RBC count is higher than it should be (it's normal and even beneficial for the blood to thin out toward the end of pregnancy). So if you're frankly anemic then by all means do build blood but if not well below average for 35 weeks then my suggestion would be to skip the herbs and instead lie on your side for 15–30 minutes every 4 hours (side lying delivers most O2 to baby) and also moxa daily, just ST-36 (seems to increase blood flow to uterus).

PL, EMAIL, EARLY 2019:
Hey Claudia! Happy New Year! A quick update: my last ultrasound showed baby girl measuring at 22nd% (as opposed to 9th% three weeks prior). So I am out of the IUGR woods! I'm attributing it to the extra rest I was able to get over those weeks and the almost daily moxa at ST-36.

5.5 Movements and Breathing

These movements are all potentially useful during any birth, with constitutional type and therapeutic principle providing extra clues as to which ones to try first. It's great to teach the movements to parents at around 37 weeks, so that they can get used to them and decide which ones they like, while also loosening the pelvic floor and ripening the cervix.

5.5.1 Cat/Cow (hands and knees, and standing)

This small piece of yoga is widely known as a great way to bring awareness and blood flow to the lumbar curve of the back. From an EAM perspective, it alternates opening the Yin channels of the abdomen and the Yang channels of the back, strongly circulating the Qi with the breath and warming the whole system. The exercise is useful from labor preparation right through to postpartum recovery, for its multiple beneficial effects at the level of bone, flesh and spirit. Different aspects of the exercise can be emphasized to target its effects appropriately.

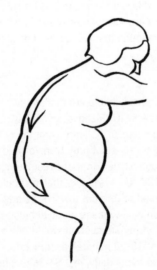

Figure 5.8 Cat.

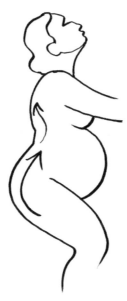

Figure 5.9 Cow.

In yoga class, Cat/Cow is usually taught down on hands and knees, or standing in a half-squat, with one's hands braced on the knees for support. During birth a modified standing position may work better for some, supported either by a partner's grip (wrist to wrist for stability) or by holding the doorknobs on either side of a sturdy door. In any of these positions, the movements are as follows:

1. Inhale deeply into the lower belly, and from there feel the breath (and Qi) pushing up through belly and diaphragm to fill the lungs, so that the sternum puffs up and out, carrying the neck and head up into a gracefully arched back, which does not at all compress the neck but rather lengthens it.

2. Just when the expansion has reached its absolute maximum, the tailbone tucks forward and the exhale begins, pulling the sacrum and spine into an outward curve. These two movements alternate.

3. Deepening the work: these points can be of help in coaching moms to use the exercise to create movement and space within themselves.

   a. On the inhale, look for a feeling of opening at the front of the spine that runs right up the center line with the big full in-breath.

   b. On the exhale, the tuck of the tailbone is really a pull up on the whole pelvic floor – as though trying simultaneously not to break wind or pee by pulling up on a string right in front of the tailbone. From there, the sacrum naturally tilts pulling the belly in and up as it empties. (This visualization brings awareness to the pelvic floor muscles, which need to be loosened to let Baby out and tightened to hold urine in.)

c. As the exhale continues, look for a very clear sensation of opening the *back* of the spine (just as the front opened before). This sensation travels up the back as the breath empties in front, and there should also be a feeling of pressing the back into a curve that already exists in space, the way one might wriggle backward in bed to be spooned by a sweetie. This feeling is strongest in the supported standing position – it's possible to relax deeply back into the "C" shape, imagining oneself as a hammock.

d. The next in-breath then becomes strongly activating, as it pulls good air into every little arteriole and capillary, picking up tension and cellular waste to be discharged on the next relaxing exhale.

e. During labor preparation and active labor – i.e. *at or after 37 weeks* – this big in-breath should also stretch down to the pelvic floor as though pushing it out with the inhaled air, as a complement and opposite to the pelvic floor raising as described in (b).

f. Patients before 37 weeks in general should *not* do the exercise in the supported standing position, as it tends to progress labor (the hands and knees position is fine). Once 37 weeks is reached, the exercise can be done safely.

Cat/Cow is an extraordinary exercise for birth, helping to move the Qi of the labor forward and smooth out challenges with bony structure, Qi and Blood, and even the emotions. It is key for opening the lower back, important for anyone who has a habitually closed/tight lumbus, and anyone who's had back problems and/or sciatica before or during pregnancy.

Cat/Cow on hands and knees is also a well-known go-to for encouraging OP babies to rotate (baby backs are heavier than their fronts due to spine and occiput, so in the hands and knees position gravity carries them around). During labor the supported standing position can be combined with a full or partial squat. In this position if moms can really focus inward, then leading the curve from the tailbone as described above can generate quite a large swing of the pelvis from front to back, encouraging fetal movement and potentially helping to resettle asynclitic babies and gather in little arms that may have strayed overhead, as well as encouraging large heads to find their way in and down. The movement is therefore extremely useful when a bony problem of some kind is suspected but it's not clear what it is. I know of no labor situation in which Cat/Cow is *not* helpful.

I also find that this exercise boosts the Qi of the whole labor, helping any deficiency presentation and also helping stagnant Qi to flow. It's particularly helpful with damp, which easily tends to stagnation and also to symptoms of Qi or Yang deficiency. I think of it any time contractions are sluggish or irregular, and it can also be useful in deepening the frequent/shallow contraction pattern typical of Yin deficiency.

The instruction to pull up on the pelvic floor may seem counterintuitive in labor, given that the desired direction of baby movement is downward. However, it's actually important! Most of us have no clear tactile sense of our pelvic floor, and therefore no ability to voluntarily relax it, even if we're told that relaxing it will help the baby descend and progress the labor. But with a baby head there to pull against, pulling up on the pelvic floor muscles serves to tire and therefore relax them, while also providing Mom with a conscious idea of exactly where to open up on the inhale (if the birthing person does yoga, tell them to think of it as a Duplex Lion Pose for the genitals).

On a spiritual and emotional level, the upward, activating nature of this exercise inherently focuses and raises the mood (try it and see!). This effect is extremely useful in energetically mitigating any "down" emotions – fear, anxiety, frustration, even grief about a previous labor or stillbirth. Think of it anytime Mom's attention is scattered by extraneous personnel or emotions. When using it to calm anxiety or fear, invite moms to inhale through their noses and exhale through their mouths – a simple calming technique that seems terribly underused. The physical movements of Cat/Cow are both inherently grounding to the Qi and also a useful vehicle for introducing the Handwich and/or Belly Breathing (see below).

5.5.2 Hula Hips (large and small)

Hula Hips is useful for all kinds of patients, including but by no means limited to those with back pain or sciatica. It's also in many daily Qigong sets to keep the Qi flowing and prevent Blood stasis from settling in. The exercise consists of two kinds of hip circles – large and small – which together serve to stretch and loosen the Belt channel that circles the waist. In the Qi map of the body, the Belt channel is the one channel that travels sideways rather than up and down: it circles us between the hips and waist and holds us together, like a rubber band around a bunch of pencils. Inhaling while the hips are forward of center, and exhaling while they are toward the back, strengthens the body's natural alternation of Qi flow up the Yin channels of the inner legs and belly, and down through the back and sacrum. A longer, more conscious inhale can help to focus on cervical ripening and dilatation, while deep, strong breathing in both directions serves to activate Yang and encourage contractions.

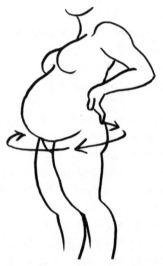

Figure 5.10 Large hip circles.

For the large hip circles, the movements are as follows:

1. (Very important!) Place the hands flat against the lower back to protect the back from strain. Hands should be as close to the center as shoulder flexibility comfortably allows, fingers pointing down. See that the feet are shoulder width apart, very slightly toed in, with a slight bend in the knees (see Figure 5.10).

2. Keeping the hips level (i.e. not bending the knees to tilt the pelvis) and the head as steady as possible, rotate the hips first out to the left, then forward, then to the right, then backward. When the hips go back, there's temptation to bend the knees, stick the bottom out and lean the torso forward to stay in balance. It's an unusual feeling to move one's center of gravity out away from the center line, but that's exactly what we're doing. So we to try to keep knees and hips mostly straight – the image to think of is oneself as a section of rope hanging from the ceiling, with the hips being pulled around in a circle but feet and head remaining stable, as though the rope is tied to something above and below.

3. Do this for 2–5 minutes, alternating directions. There will likely be sticky places, or one corner where the hips like to cheat and flatten out the circle. Slow down there, focusing the attention on body

sensations. This may raise feelings of frustration or anger, like the foul gas that rises from swampy underwater plants when dislodged. Encouragement to be patient and loving with whatever arises may be useful, as well as a reminder that sticky places in the hip circles today are the sticky places in labor tomorrow.

For the small hip circles, both the movements and the feeling are quite different. It is as though the large circles stretch the Belt channel, increasing its size to loosen it up, which then allows the small circles to increase the pelvis's freedom of movement within the Belt. For people with good body awareness and flexibility, it's usually possible just to say, "Rest your hands on your hipbones and, holding the rest of the body steady, rotate only the pelvis and sacrum – as though your tailbone has a very long pencil attached to it and you're drawing circles on the floor." However, many people – especially those who come to acupuncturists' offices with back pain – do not have an effective motor/sensory feedback loop in place, with this emotionally charged and often criticized area of the body. The instructions below can be useful for stepping these patients into the movement, and may need to be taken quite slowly, with each step constituting its own exercise, one exercise per session. In an otherwise healthy person these motor/sensory connections can be made quite quickly, if they're asked for on a daily basis.

Quite often, difficulty encountered in isolating and rotating the pelvis has a strong emotional component to it – commonly frustration and anger, occasionally anxiety or fear (particularly if there has been trauma). This may have some component of retained trauma, or it may simply reflect the frustration of trying to do something one's nervous system is not currently set up to do. It's important to go slowly and be gentle with these feelings.

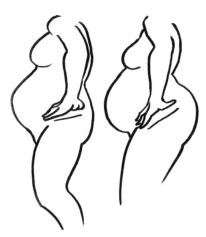

Figure 5.11 Small hip circles, Step 1: Swinging pelvis forward and back.

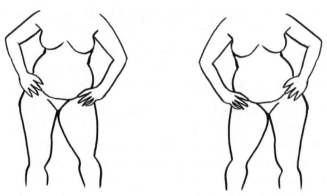

Figure 5.12 Small hip circles, Step 2: Swinging pelvis right and left.

Stepwise instruction in the small hip circles is as follows:

1. Teach the Cat/Cow movement, without so much emphasis on the breathing, tucking and the rest of the spine. Have moms press their hands into the top of their hipbones, so they can feel the pelvic movement clearly. You will likely also need a hand on the small of their back, encouraging them to flatten their Ming Men into your hand, then arch it away from you.

2. Once they've really got their pelvis swinging forward and back, the next thing to teach is swinging it side to side. The trick to this is that they need to start with some bend in their knees, then straighten the right while bending the left more, then reverse, and reverse again, etc. That's really all there is to it – every other movement is extraneous (and it's amazing how many extraneous movements people come up with when their pelvic area is stiff and doesn't like to move). Start with very small swings if necessary, let them stand behind you and feel what happens when you do it, and remember to keep the center line straight and the center of gravity centered – even though the pelvis is moving. If this is tricky, a search for belly dancing videos online may provide inspiration.

3. Once moms are getting front/back and side/side swings, it's time to increase their conscious control by coming back to a stable center position for a few seconds in the middle of each swing. Once they've got this, challenge them to make a plus sign with their pelvis – left, center, front, center, right, center, back, center, etc. This exercise requires considerable concentration – #4 is actually easier – but coming back to center is great for increasing motor/sensory feedback in the pelvic area. If this is too frustrating at first, go on to #4 and come

back the following session – it should be much easier (I also generally skip this step if Mom is in labor already).

4. Having taught "front/back" and "left/right" it's not too hard to combine those into a circle just by calling out "left, front, right, back." The trick is keeping the torso straight, so that the pelvis itself moves. If this is a problem, go back to #3. Making the circles smaller may also help.

5. Even more so than with the larger circles, there is a tendency to cheat, making the circle bigger in the corner where one's hip is loose, smaller where it's tight. Deepening the work in this exercise consists of focusing the attention inward – perhaps closing the eyes – and gently moving the hips into the tight places.

Teaching Hula Hips is a key component of labor preparation work and also very useful during latent phase. It's also a key diagnostic: if a patient struggles with the small circles, it's a sign that either the pelvis is locked up (likely with some history of physical or emotional pain) or the person is very much "in their head" and may have trouble fully inhabiting the area during labor.

5.5.3 Dancing

It would be difficult to overstate the value of dancing in labor – and quite difficult to teach in a book, too! This section is mainly a reminder not to leave this powerful medicine out of your labor toolbox, and an encouraging nudge to say that it only takes a little preparatory work to incorporate it (and a professional sense of what movements best stir the Qi in the pelvis). In particular, the pelvic freedom of African dance,[6] Latin dance[7] and belly dance[8] are perfect for labor. An extraordinary wealth of inspirational videos can be found on YouTube with the search terms "dance birth," "dance labor" and "dance labor with doctor." Here's an inventory of what I see as the key dance moves to open the pelvis and progress labor:

- "twerking" (aka Cat/Cow)[9]

- small pelvic circles (aka Hula Hips)

---

6   https://www.youtube.com/watch?v=dXUSAHTazxI
7   https://www.youtube.com/watch?v=tJPtE8t_GHY
8   https://www.youtube.com/watch?v=W3Dtjt9_c_o
9   This dance craze will likely have died out by the time the book is in print, but it features extraordinarily free and rapid movement forward and backward, in a manner that some American news commentators appear to have found sexually suggestive. This video shows a dolphin "twerking" its baby out https://www.youtube.com/watch?v=8M5cShzj9Ec

- stepping with side-to-side pelvic tilts. A staggered sequence of right–left–right–(hold), left–right–left–(hold) makes you look like you know what you're doing with very little practice! Just remember to do a little something with your arms

- shimmying (moves and relaxes stagnant Qi, stretches the pelvic floor)

- squats (performed with care)

- One-Hip Openers – these include movements such as stepping forward and toeing out with a bent knee, or stepping out and "twerking" the forward hip.

5.5.4 The Helper Hang

The Helper Hang is just slow dancing with a birth team member to allow a tired Mom to hang supported and relax (ideally, the team member is an intimate partner who can also provide a loving back and sacrum rub). Slow dancing is great in any labor to build oxytocin, and the hanging position is key for Qi deficiency, when the contractions need all the help they can get from relaxation and gravity.

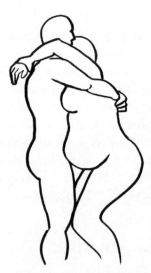

Figure 5.13 The Helper Hang.

5.5.5 Gentle bouncing

One other option, if dancing is just not tolerated either by Mom or by practitioner, is gentle whole-body bouncing. It looks a little foolish, but feels absolutely delightful: all that's needed is to get a little bounce going in the body by slightly bending and straightening the knees, quickly enough (two to four times per second) to get the internal and external tissue moving rhythmically (the arms may want to cradle the chest and/or bump for support; pulling up slightly on the bump also focuses the movement onto the pelvic floor). Start with a minute or so of bouncing while standing up relatively straight, to get the kinks out of the lumbus and thorax, then lean slightly to either side to loosen up the neck. There is no special need for coaching about the pelvic floor – located at the base of the torso, it is rhythmically stretched with each bounce no matter what the mind is thinking. However, patients may spontaneously focus the bouncing energy there, particularly if there's discomfort due to a stuck baby. By closing the eyes and going deep, Mom may be able to find just the angle and rhythm to loosen him up.

5.5.6 Hip Openers

"Hip Openers" designates a functional principle rather than a single exercise (in the terminology of this book, it's a "therapeutic approach"). The principle is well described in the website for the Miles Circuit,[10] as "anything that's upright and putting your pelvis in open, asymmetrical positions." "Open" refers to positions in which one or both legs are outwardly rotated, one leg is higher than the other and the body is moving toward that leg (with the knee staying at a greater than 90° angle, i.e. not going past the ankle). The baby's head descends asymmetrically through the pelvis, which opens to accommodate as best it can, necessarily on one side more than the other.

Done slowly, these stretches soften the bony and ligamentous articulations of the pelvis, which normally keep it rigid to support walking and running. Great pelvis-opening exercises include:

5.5.6.1 Stair-Crabbing

In this exercise, Mom lunges her way up the stairs, first standing at the left side of the step and lunging over her right foot two stairs up and over to the right, then climbing up the two steps (ideally sideways, as this further stretches the pelvis and pelvic floor), then angling back left to lunge over her left foot. This is a method of choice when Baby is not engaging or descending, suggestive of possible bony obstruction or tight pelvic floor.

---

10 www.milescircuit.com/the-circuit.html. This circuit, beautifully described and freely available online, is a gentle and restful way to optimize positioning in late pregnancy and early labor.

5.5.6.2 Sumo Walking

The Sumo Walk is performed with one helper on either side. This is partly for the physical support and partly because it works best when each step and squat is punctuated by a primitive guttural sound, something easier to do in a group than all alone. Steps are as follows:

1. Start with Mom in the middle, arms draped over helpers' far shoulders, or holding the near ones.

2. Everyone swings their right leg forward and steps out to the right, planting the foot with the toes pointing outwards and the first "Hunh."

3. Repeat with the left leg and a second "Hunh."

4. With feet wide and firmly planted, toes pointing out, everyone drops their tailbone as if to sit on a stool and bends the knees for a "Sumo Squat." This should be accompanied by a louder "Hoooh."

5.5.6.3 The Sumo Squat

The Sumo Squat is also useful performed on its own with support from the front, prenatally for strengthening and during labor for stretching. Support can be provided by a helper's grip, a door with sturdy handles or a towel slung round something strong (in this application the guttural roar can be omitted).

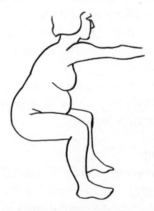

Figure 5.14 The Sumo Squat.

5.5.6.4 The Peanut Ball

The Peanut Ball is literally a peanut-shaped exercise ball[11] that can be used to separate the legs in side-lying position, wedging the pelvis open in a wide passive stretch. In a pinch, a similar stretch can be achieved with a stack of

---

11   https://www.baby-chick.com/what-is-a-peanut-ball

blankets, or a hospital food tray set 4–12 in. (10–30 cm) over the bed at knee level and padded with a towel or pillow.

5.5.7 Belly Breathing

A growing body of evidence suggests that regulating one's breathing can facilitate a shift from stress-oriented sympathetic nervous system activity to the parasympathetic "rest-and-digest" mode[12] (which also manages labor). In particular, slow breathing with a prolonged exhale appears to be particularly beneficial for stress reduction.[13] The rate should be comfortable – in through the nose for a slow count of two to four, out for four to eight (keeping the ratio at 1:2). The 2013 Listening to Mothers survey found that breathing was the comfort measure most commonly used by moms (48%).[14]

Ask moms to place their hands on the belly and feel the breath expand from deep inside as they breathe (or the Handwich can be very comforting if there's anxiety or fear). Once they are feeling the expansion well in their belly, invite them to imagine the breath expanding downward through the pelvic opening, so that their entire pelvic floor is gently massaged and softened with the in-and-out movement of the breath.

This exercise can benefit anyone, but is most important for:

- anxiety and/or fear

- Yin or Blood deficiency

- slow dilatation or descent.

I'm not aware of any contraindications for Belly Breathing. One important thing, however, is to make sure that regulating the breathing does not reduce oxygen intake. Specifically:

- If Mom is on an oxygen mask, reduce the inhale-to-exhale ratio to 1:1.5 rather than 2.

- If Mom is using nitrous oxide gas as a labor aid (quite common outside the United States and increasingly accepted here), the NO2 should be turned down and the oxygen up during regulated breathing.

---

12 Jerath, R., Crawford, M. W., Barnes, V. A., & Harden, K. (2015). Self-regulation of breathing as a primary treatment for anxiety. *Applied Psychophysiology and Biofeedback*, 40(2), 107–115.

13 Van Diest, I., Verstappen, K., Aubert, A. E., Widjaja, D., Vansteenwegen, D., & Vlemincx, E. (2014). Inhalation/exhalation ratio modulates the effect of slow breathing on heart rate variability and relaxation. *Applied Psychophysiology and Biofeedback*, 39(3–4), 171–180.

14 http://transform.childbirthconnection.org/wp-content/uploads/2013/06/LTM-III_Pregnancy-and-Birth.pdf

5.5.8 The hospital workout

One of the biggest problems with being stuck semi-reclining in bed is the lack of opportunities for moving the pelvis. Another is the tendency to slide downward, so that the fold of the bed folds Mom directly across the bump, stagnating Qi and slowing labor progress. A direct approach to both challenges is to teach the "hospital workout," which can usually be performed even with epidural analgesia on board. In essence, Mom walks on the ischial tuberosities as though they were little feet – which requires using the obliques and other muscles of the trunk to pick up first one side of the pelvis then the other – a movement within the pelvis similar to Stair-Crabbing. It can be taught in steps as follows:

1. Sit up with the back straight and the legs slightly lowered if possible.

2. Use the muscles along the side of the body to pick up the right hip, leaning slightly left if necessary, until the sitz bone comes up off the bed.

3. Move the right sitz bone forward then set it down, as though taking a small step.

4. Repeat the movement on the other side, walking forward and then backward on the bed until the buttocks are aligned with the fold in the mattress.

5. This movement can be repeated hourly, or any time that gravity has moved the buttocks forward.

This exercise should not be performed without first consulting the nurse. It will affect monitor readings, and may be inadvisable if membranes are ruptured, or if tubing is present such as an intrauterine pressure catheter or cook balloon (urinary catheters are usually okay as long as they are not kinked under Mom, but it is the nurse's judgment call to make).

5.6 Chapter Summary

Table 5.1 summarizes the basic therapeutic methods covered in this chapter, along with notes on their usage. In general, warming and activating methods are used for Qi- and Yang-deficient moms, while nourishing and grounding methods are for those who are Blood and Yin deficient. Methods that move stuck Qi are separated into gentle and strong, with the gentle ones most appropriate when Mom also shows signs of deficiency or trauma. Heat-clearing methods are to be used any time Mom feels hot or has a fever.

Table 5.1 Basic therapeutic methods and when to use them.

Category	Point/channel area	Method	When to use/Notes
Warming and activating	ST-36	Gentle pressure Moxibustion Chafing **down** shin	Fatigue **Anytime Baby needs more blood flow** *Warm with palms or thumbs*
	Lower back/ abdomen	**Handwich**	Anytime Mom is cold or frightened *Combine with Belly Breathing for fear* *Yin-deficient moms may not like it*
	LI-4	**Pulsing pressure**	**To strengthen Qi and contractions**
	Duyin	Pulsing pressure	To strengthen contractions
	Inner ankle (KD-3)	Vigorous chafing	Warms Yang for cold, edema, sluggish contractions
	Cat/Cow		Also gently moves, opens space
Nourishing and grounding	SP-6	Gentle pressure	Slow cervical ripening (deficient mom) Yin or Blood deficiency *Can also chafe Liver Gummy area*
	KD-1	Redirecting pressure	"Panic button" for fear, anxiety, rising Qi *Can also moxa to warm cold moms*
	UB-17	Moxa Round rubbing	Nourishes blood for resilience during birth and postpartum lactation
	Inner ankle (KD-3) or Liver Gummy area	**Slow gentle chafing**	**Nourishes Yin** to address anxiety, restlessness, lack of sleep
	Yin footrubs		
	Belly Breathing		Grounds, comforts; for fear, panic, rising Qi *Combine with Handwich*
Gently moving and softening	Hip rocking		**Right side down for occiput posterior**, alternate with Cat/Cow, Hip Openers *Keeps labor moving when Mom is exhausted or stuck in bed*
	Hula Hips		Great for cervical ripening and to progress labor *Use bouncing if Mom is too shy to dance*
	Dancing		
	Gentle bouncing		
	Peanut Ball		Opens hips in side-lying position

Strongly moving	Liver Gummies	Dredging	Anytime cervix is misbehaving – slow to ripen or dilate, rim/lip, edema *IMPORTANT to adjust pressure to Mom's tolerance* *If no change within the hour, check for cold or Yin/Blood deficiency*
	LI-4	**Strong pressure**	**Redirects Qi downward to relieve pain, progress labor**
	GB-21	Strong pressure	Directs Qi strongly downward to assist fetal descent **Avoid when there is blockage by bones or hard cervix** *Great for sluggish pushing with epidural*
	Liver-14	Strong pressure	Directs Qi down to help release placenta *Press into rib space, then down* *Start 15 minutes after birth*
	Stair-Crabbing		Strong pelvic movement, best for tight pelvic floor and/or suspected bony obstruction (Baby not engaging or descending)
	Sumo Squats Supported Squats		*Sumo Squats are also warm and activate – for fatigue, frustration, anger* *Supported Squats help fetal descent*
Heat clearing	Foot heat points (above toe webbing)	Poke 1–2 minutes with anything not too sharp	Anytime Mom feels hot or has fever Hand heat points also move Qi strongly as a comfort measure *Combine with fan, spray bottle, ice chips*
	Hand heat points (palm crease)	Grasp comb	

Bold = Four Core methods; shaded = also a comfort measure.

5.6.1 Key points to remember

1. Labor support is the art and science of being helpful during labor. It is taught in doula training programs, and to birth partners during prenatal classes.

2. EAM labor support is based on restoring and/or maintaining Yin–Yang balance by supporting the vital substances, interrupting pathological processes of insufficiency and stasis as they occur.

3. In general, Qi and Yang are supported by therapeutic methods that encourage movement and warmth, while Blood and Yin are supported by nourishing methods and those that encourage calm.

4. Acupressure, birth bodywork, moxibustion, movement and breathing all provide a variety of methods for accomplishing these therapeutic goals.

    a. Acupressure and birth bodywork in particular can combine principles of movement and nourishment, which tend to be mutually exclusive.

    b. Acupressure techniques range from gentle techniques that mostly nourish and warm, to strong pressure that mostly moves.

    c. Movement and breathing exercises have a range of beneficial effects from calming (Belly Breathing) to activating and moving (Cat/Cow).

5. This chapter provides approximately 20 therapeutic methods, constituting a "starter toolkit" for EAM labor support. Among these, the most important are:

    a. LI-4 strong pressure for comfort, or gentle pulsing to strengthen contractions

    b. SP-6 gentle pressure during contractions to nourish Yin and Blood and assist dilatation

    c. Liver Gummies – dredging along medial shin to move Qi and strongly promote dilatation

    d. hip rocking to support Qi and encourage progress.

6. Moxibustion is the most efficient way to add heat to the body. Used at ST-36, it appears to promote blood flow to the uterus and increase amniotic fluid.

7. Movements and breathing together can move large amounts of Qi, open the hips and activate Yang.

    a. Regulated breathing can also be extremely effective for anxiety.

Chapter 6

ADDITIONAL METHODS FOR PROBLEM-SOLVING IN BIRTH

Chapter Outline

— 6.1 Assessing and Assisting with Obstruction: Bone, Flesh, Spirit

— 6.2 Advanced Acupressure Methods

— 6.3 Additional Birth Bodywork

— 6.4 Auriculotherapy

— 6.5 Additional Miscellaneous Treatment Methods by Situation

— 6.6 Acupuncture

— 6.7 Summary Table

— 6.8 Key Points to Remember

This chapter builds on concepts and methods previously discussed, extending them to specific problems that arise in birth. The first section of this chapter introduces differential analysis by bone, flesh and spirit, providing a list of key methods for each level. Subsequent sections then proceed from the most familiar material to the most advanced. Section 6.2 describes a few additional points and point stimulation methods not covered in Chapter 5. Section 6.3 introduces a series of variations on hip rocking useful for specific situations, including hospital induction of labor and asynclitism or other bony obstruction. Section 6.4 describes both insertive and non-insertive techniques of auriculotherapy, which requires some additional training (requirements for certification or licensure will depend on region). Section 6.5 adds a number of miscellaneous therapeutic methods, including combinations of methods previously introduced. Section 6.6, the longest by far, is specifically for acupuncturists. It describes acupuncture techniques in detail, for specific therapeutic principles and points. All points introduced in this chapter are listed in Appendix A.

6.1 Assessing and Assisting with Obstruction: Bone, Flesh, Spirit

As discussed in Chapters 2 and 4, most dysfunctional labor can be described as obstructed flow of the baby out of the vagina. Restoring flow depends on understanding the nature of the obstruction. Specifically:

- Bony obstruction includes any true or functional cephalopelvic disproportion (CPD): the labor is not progressing due to the current interface of head and pelvis.

  - If contractions are strong (or augmented with oxytocin), then bony pain is typically quite severe, and may be atypically located – in the back, asymmetrically or moving around.

  - In an unmedicated labor, or with fatigue or deficiency, contractions may weaken, which obscures the characteristic pain symptoms.

- Obstruction at the level of flesh is the largest and most common category. It includes all lack of flow due to imbalance of the vital substances, such as:

  - Inadequate contractions due to insufficiency of Qi or Yang, or excess Yin dampness blocking the flow of Yang Qi.

  - Delayed cervical ripening and/or dilatation due to insufficiency of Yin or Blood, or Qi stagnation with underlying cold or emotional challenges.

- Obstruction at the level of the spirit is distinguished from the more ordinary, emotionally based Qi stagnation by the fact that ordinary treatments moving Qi don't help.

Table 6.1 identifies the most commonly occurring challenges for each of the three categories, and shows how they tend to present across time in latent phase, active phase, transition and pushing. Subsections 6.1.1 to 6.1.3 specify the therapeutic goals used to address these challenges, along with key methods for each goal. Methods previously described in Chapter 5 appear in bold type; the rest are introduced later in this chapter.

Table 6.1 Obstruction at the levels of bone, flesh and spirit.

	Bone	Key signs and approaches	Flesh	Key signs and approaches	Spirit	Approaches
Latent phase	Non-engagement due to: • Functional cephalopelvic disproportion (CPD) (swayback, OP) • True CPD (rare, usually flat pelvis)	Back pain, swayback posture Hip rocking, right side down, alternated with Cat/Cow, Hip Openers	Slow cervical ripening due to Qi stagnation; underlying factors include: • Yin and/or Blood insufficiency • Fear, anger, other emotions (also spirit) • Cold/insufficient Yang	• Yin and/or Blood insufficiency: dryness, impatience, anemia, oligohydramnios. Slow chafing inner ankle/Liver Gummy area; dim lights, quiet voices • Cold/damp/insufficient Yang: cold and/or edematous, polyhydramnios. Pulsing pressure on LI-4; vigorous chafing up inner ankle or down outer shin; bright lights, rotating personnel • Fear: KD-1 pressure, Handwich, Belly Breathing • Anger: Liver Gummies, movement especially Sumo Squats; Gripping Comb	Life journey challenges include: • Traumatic history or previous loss • Other unresolved grief • Problems with partner, parents, birth team, etc. • Not ready yet	Listen carefully for trauma, loss, relationship challenges; ask about baby preparations: • Create a safe space in which to relax, removing personnel if necessary • Remember Three Rs – relaxation (between contractions), rhythm, ritual: find what helps and encourage it • Fear/trauma: KD-1, Handwich, Belly Breathing
Active phase	Not usually a problem here, except: • Occiput posterior (back labor) • Asynclitism (labor stalls)	Hip rocking, right side down, alternated with Cat/Cow, Hip Openers, Hula Hips	Two basic problems: • Slow cervical dilatation (same factors as for slow ripening) • Contractions weak or irregular (Qi/Yang insufficiency)		Active phase is usually less sensitive to narrative challenges than latent and transition phases	
Transition	True or functional CPD signs include: • Persistent or sudden onset back pain • Severe pain that wanders or is asymmetrical • Ribside (fundal) pain	Vigorous hip rocking alternated with Cat/Cow, Hip Openers, Hula Hips, Sumo Hips & Supported Squats	Not usually a problem here, other than cervical lip and/ or cervical edema due to Qi stagnation	For cervical lip or edema, Liver Gummies are usually very effective	Emotional/spiritual challenges include: • Acceptance, allowing body to move beyond conscious control • Overcoming helplessness, fear, fatigue • "Problem person" may be present – partner, parent, doctor/nurse	• Anxiety, helplessness: round rubbing mid-backs verbal praise and encouragement • Very gentle hip rocking is often extremely soothing • Look for signs of overstimulation – darken room, quiet voices
Pushing	• Prolonged if transition is incomplete • Shoulder dystocia		• Prolonged by exhaustion/ Qi insufficiency (risk for postpartum hemorrhage)	Vigorous chafing up inner ankle and/or down outer shin; pulsing pressure on LI-4; Helper Hang	• Fear/pain of perineal tearing • Helplessness, fatigue • "Problem person"	

6.1.1 Treating bony obstruction

True or functional CPD is addressed primarily by moving the pelvis: changing its angle beneath the abdomen, changing its relation to gravity, and introducing rhythmic movement to encourage Baby to wriggle through. Key methods include:

- Cat/Cow
- "Hip Openers" including Stair-Crabbing and Sumo Squats
- Hip rocking (right side down if suspected occiput posterior (OP))
- Shaking the Apples
- Pelvic vibrating.

Acupressure or acupuncture to "soften the pelvic floor" and stretch pelvic ligaments may also be added. These include:

- sacrotuberous and sacrospinous ligament release
- dredging downward along the iliotibial band (GB channel on thigh)
- dredging outward beneath the clavicle
- connecting acupressure or needling **UB-60 to KD-3**.

6.1.2 Restoring balance and flow in the flesh

As previously discussed, labor flow may be impaired by insufficiency or stagnation of vital substances. The therapeutic goals summarized here build on those first introduced in Chapters 4, along with examples of a few key points. They include:

- activating Qi, used to counter fatigue and encourage blood flow to the uterus. Important subsets of activating Qi include:
  - promoting contractions, e.g. **LI-4**, Duyin
  - raising Qi, prenatally to address threatened miscarriage or premature cervical shortening; or intrapartum to address fatigue or brain fog: **Du-20**.
  - supporting uterine blood flow, any time there is concern regarding fetal well-being: **Moxibustion or warming on ST-36**; gentle pressure on the "Soojok uterus point," in the meaty flesh on the sole of the foot, between the bases of the third and fourth toes (see Figure A9).

- calming the uterus, used to reduce contractions that are premature or excessive, e.g. SP-4, KD-9

- clearing heat, to reduce fever, e.g. LV-2 and ST-44

- descending Qi, to redirect Qi downward when it is not descending as it should. Different points are selected depending on the dysfunction to be addressed. These include:

  - PC-6 and ST-31, to counter upward movement of digestive Qi such as nausea, vomiting, belching, hiccupping

  - LV-14, to address retained placenta

  - GB-21, to address headache or hypertension as well as assist fetal descent

  - KD-1, to descend rising panic and anxiety, grounding the spirit

  - the "emotional release points," known to acupuncturists as the back-shu points. These are most useful during prelabor or early labor treatments, but can also be of help when a labor has stalled for emotional reasons. They are described in detail in Appendix D.

- Nourishing Yin and Blood grounds and stabilizes Qi, as well as supporting cervical softening and dilatation, e.g. **SP-6 gentle pressure, round rubbing at UB-17.**

- Reducing pain: these are treatments primarily aimed at reducing Mom's discomfort, while also correctly identifying and addressing pain-inducing factors such as bony obstruction, cold, Blood/Yin deficiency and Qi stagnation due to emotional challenges, e.g. auricular birth basics and pain points; **LV-3 and GB-34.**

- Softening the cervix; softening the pelvic floor: these two goals overlap considerably, using gentle movements such as hip rocking, as well as acupoints that affect the tissues in question, e.g. **Liver Gummies**, GB-31 and 41.

- Warming the Yang: these therapies add heat to the body for moms who are cold or damp, e.g. **the Handwich, chafing the inner ankle.**

6.1.3 Treating spirit stuck, or not ready

As discussed in Chapter 4, obstruction at the level of spirit has three main presentations. Working with the "emotional release points" can be extremely useful for any of them prenatally and during early labor; see Appendix D. Specific approaches per presentation are as follows:

- Sticky or obstructive emotions, showing in slow labor onset, slow dilatation and/or clear signs of emotional distress, often in moms with a history of sexual or other trauma.

  - These can be addressed by shifting the narrative as well as strongly moving Qi, with **Liver Gummies** or exercises such as **Sumo Walking**.

- Emotional lockdown that only gets worse with strong Qi-moving methods such as Liver Gummies.

  - "Calming the spirit" is the therapeutic goal of softening this lockdown, typically with auricular acupressure, acupuncture, **pressure at KD-1**, **Belly Breathing** and the **Handwich** (if its intimacy is tolerated).

- "Spirit not ready" overlaps with the pattern of dissociation; both may occur without overt signs of emotional distress, typically at engagement or transition. Most common is a complete absence of normal labor initiation – pelvic floor softening, cervical ripening, etc. – as well as poor response to Western cervical ripening methods.

  - There can also be a simple refusal of the fetus to descend despite normal cervical behavior – as though the woman's body simply wills not to have the baby. I have seen this in cases of sexual trauma, and also when there is a "problem person" in the room – a family member or medical provider whom the body seems to perceive as threatening or annoying.

  - Spirit-calming points KD-1 and the Handwich with Belly Breathing can help root Mom back in her body; acupuncturists may consider points such as KD-1, HT-3 and Ren-17 to reconnect the Heart and Kidney.

Spiritual challenges tend to present at the two big turning points of labor: engagement, when the pelvic floor allows Baby to drop into the pelvis, and transition, when Mom's whole body allows him to turn and drop into the pelvic outlet. When they present without overt emotional distress, spiritual challenges are difficult to distinguish from CPD, and also from miscellaneous problems such as a short cord, or a due date set too early so that the body is actually just not ready to go into labor.

6.2 Advanced Acupressure Methods

This section describes use of a few additional points not covered in Chapter 5, along with three new techniques: connecting points, tapping and dredging.

6.2.1 Additional points
6.2.1.1 Duyin – pulsing pressure

This point is located on the "distal interphalangeal crease of the lower extremity second digit" – in other words, on the underside of the second toe, in the crease closest to the toe tip. It is one of acupuncture's "extra" points, not part of the regular channel numbering system. I don't know the origin of its use to strengthen contractions, but the effect is undeniable, and it is widely used for this purpose. In using the point to best therapeutic effect, two issues are important.

First, I find this point more effective at increasing the strength of contractions within a pattern that is already established, rather than initiating contractions. In other words, it strengthens the Qi of the contraction, rather than performing the Yang function of contraction initiation (for this I use tapping on UB-67).

Second, it's a symptomatic treatment that doesn't address the underlying constitutional or positional reason why contractions are weak. I therefore use the point mostly late in labor when contractions are slacking off due to fatigue.

I stimulate the point with the edge of my forefinger, holding the tip of the toe with my thumb on top. I stimulate with rapid gentle pulses, perhaps three per second, as the contraction ramps up, and keep the pulses going until it has mostly subsided. At that point I switch to supplementing Qi and/or Yang – this might be chafing or round rubbing at ST-36, or ankle chafing (Section 5.1.1.4). If it's late in labor but the contractions are slow or irregular as well as weak, then I tap on UB-67 to activate Yang when a contraction is due or at the 3-minute mark, whichever is sooner. Once the contraction has initiated, I then switch to Duyin.

Duyin should also be stimulated in the case of postpartum hemorrhage – immediately, together with a fingernail at SP-1 (Section 5.2.2), while instructing helpers to press LI-4 and/or stimulate the nipples. Contraction of the uterine muscle fibers is the main mechanism by which uterine bleeding is stopped. I have seen that quick application of these natural methods seems stop mild bleeding, and for severe bleeding seems to reduce blood loss in the time before oxytocin and misoprostol can be administered.

Duyin can be stimulated symptomatically for weak contractions at any time. However it is most appropriate for:

- weak contractions due to Qi deficiency late in labor (with ST-36 or ankle chafing)

- postpartum hemorrhage (with SP-1).

6.2.1.2 Inner Leg points – gentle pressure or massage

Located along the inner calf and thigh, along the territories of the Liver and Kidney channels, the Inner Leg points gently move Qi, softening the Liver channel and cervix. They are so-called "ashi" points, ashi being Chinese for "Oh, that's it!" Ashi points have no standard location but are tender points located by palpation, usually in a general region where the practitioner suspects trouble may be brewing. There are often stable two-way relationships between areas of tenderness and other trouble spots in the body. For example, Liver Gummies tend to be more exquisitely tender when there is a tight cervix or some other stagnation in the uterus, and releasing them tends to move stagnation and soften the cervix. The Inner Leg points can be thought of as larger, less-focused Liver Gummy points, gentler and more appropriate for patients with underlying deficiency or a history of sexual trauma.

In working with these points it is critically important to proceed from a deep awareness of the vulnerability of the area. Extreme tenderness of the points does tend to suggest that there has been a history of trauma, which makes it all the more important to use a careful, predictable, trustworthy touch. I think of using the points when the Liver Gummies are too tender to be useful, or when they have not helped progress. I palpate starting at the knee, with my four fingers spread about a half-inch apart along the inner surface of the calf. The fingers take turns pressing into the tissue gently, one or two at a time as though playing the piano; the hand proceeds steadily downward, gathering information about what's tight. It's also important to maintain eye contact to assess what's tender. This should feel pleasant, so that if nothing is especially tender nobody's time has been wasted, it was just a nice leg massage.

If there are tender areas on the lower leg, then the same method of downward sweeps with alternating pressure from the fingers should help to open flow in the channels, relieving the soreness and promoting dilatation. If the method seems helpful, then it may be appropriate to start the procedure higher up – always asking for permission first. Three downward sweeps seems to be most useful, starting first below the knee, then above the knee, then at the midpoint of the thigh, where there are almost always several very tender points.

6.2.1.3 ST-31 – Biguan, "Thigh Gate" – redirecting pressure

Stomach-31 is located at the level of the lower border of the pubic symphysis, in a palpable depression just outside the sartorius muscle – more or less on a straight line up from the outer edge of the kneecap to the point of the hipbone. Strong bilateral pressure on the point moves Qi downward while also softening the pelvic floor.

During the first and early second trimester I consider gentle pressure or shallow needling at ST-31 as a stronger way to redirect digestive Qi downward when PC-6 alone is not doing the trick. Pressed or needled more deeply during labor, it seems to relax the pelvic floor while also helping the Qi of the Stomach channel to move in its appropriate downward direction. Persistent nausea, hiccupping or belching during labor are relatively common, and indicate that the Qi of the Stomach channel is traveling "counterflow" upwards (an episode or two of vomiting during transition is no problem and does not need to be addressed). It is worth experimenting with combinations of ST-31, PC-6 and LI-4, as well as standing movements if possible, to see whether digestive order can be reinstated.

6.2.1.4 Waist points – redirecting pressure

These points are located at the high point of the hipbone, right where you might rest your hands while standing impatiently. This area lies along the course of the Belt channel, which circles the waist and helps to hold Baby in during pregnancy. Pressing slowly and deeply into these points can help the pelvic floor to release during labor. I think of it particularly for strong woman syndrome, and for labors that have started with membrane rupture and/or induction before Mom's whole body was fully ready.

The method works best from behind, with Mom seated or standing. First find the high point on both sides, then gently press in with index and third finger together, slowly increasing pressure inward. As you press, Mom should feel a growing heaviness in the pelvic floor – a perfect opportunity for Belly Breathing, with additional instructions to feel as though the pelvic floor is inflating like a balloon. The pressure is considerable, and on a pregnant person your fingers will go quite deep, but if you proceed slowly there will be no discomfort, only a deep, spreading sensation as the pelvic floor softens.

6.2.1.5 Sacrotuberous ligament release points – strong pressure

The sacrotuberous ligament connects the sacrum to the pelvis, attaching at the ischial spine and all along the edge of the sacrum. It is not easily accessible for bodywork, but well worth the trouble to find. Pressing deeply into the ligament stretches it, which in turn can create a few extra millimeters of space in the pelvis, where, during labor, a millimeter is a mile. This technique is important for any labor with a large baby or difficult transition, but is particularly important for OP as it creates space between the sacrum and the pelvis.

Stretching the ligaments prenatally is also a strong labor preparation treatment, best saved for 38 or 39 weeks unless you know for sure that cervical ripening is behind schedule. The technique absolutely requires practice: I suggest practicing on friends first, then using it routinely when appropriate for labor preparation, so that it is rock solid if needed in labor. Video is available on my website, Citkovitz.com.

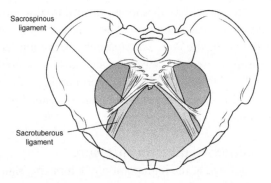

Figure 6.1 Sacrotuberous and sacrospinous ligaments

Due to the geometry of the pelvis, these ligaments are really only accessible when the hips are at a 90° angle. Easiest for the practitioner (and for practicing with clothed friends) is if Mom is on hands and knees. Perhaps more comfortable (but somewhat less effective) is with Mom lying on her side, knees bent to 90°. The method goes as follows:

- Pressing with your palm into the buttocks, find the ischial tuberosity (sitz bone) and place one finger on it.

- With the other hand, find the top of the tailbone where it meets the sacrum and draw an imaginary line between the two points (in my classes, students do this with rubber bands).

- Find the midpoint of the line and place your thumbs flat on the surface, so that they cross the line at perfect 90° angles, like cross-streets in a city with a regular grid (this angle is important in order to stretch the ligament properly; if you cross it at a different angle it will not stretch as well).

- Very slowly and steadily, lean your body weight into your thumbs, keeping them flat so that the ligament cannot scoot up along your thumb and avoid stretching. Before long, you should feel the ligament under your finger; the feeling should be something like feeling a pencil under a thick mattress pad. When practicing with friends, palpate the area above and below the ligament to reassure yourself that you feel it.

- At this point the ligaments will begin to release under your fingers. The skill here is to notice when that happens and take up the slack, moving inexorably inward as the ligament stretches and holding your ground in between releases, never giving up a millimeter.

- After about 5 minutes (or when your thumbs are tired) release the pressure as slowly and deliberately as you applied it; it should take some 30 seconds to withdraw.

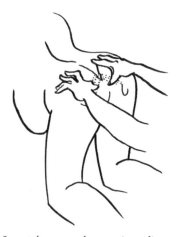

Figure 6.2 Sacrotuberous and sacrospinous ligament release

6.2.1.6 Sacrospinous ligament release – strong pressure

The sacrospinous ligaments lie deep to the sacrotuberous ligaments, running between the ischial spines and the edges of the coccyx (tailbone). The release for them is similar to that for the sacrotuberous ligaments, and should be done immediately afterward. It is slightly trickier, and also less important as the ligaments are smaller. It is worth doing if there is coccyx pain during the labor, or a history of previous injury. It can also be very useful postpartum if there is coccyx pain, but must be done with exquisite slowness in that case.

After performing the steps for the sacrotuberous ligament release, the sacrospinous release is as follows:

- Move your thumbs upwards and inwards along the imaginary line, until they cross it at about the ¾ point.

- Lean in slightly, bending your elbows, then rotate the elbows slowly down and in so that the whole hand begins to rotate – fingers outward, thumbs inward.

- Lean into this rotation with your thumbs, so that they spiral toward Mom's spine in the direction of her head. The goal is to trap the small sacrospinous ligaments up against the bottom surface of the larger, flatter sacrotuberous ligaments.

- In many cases, one side will be tighter and/or more tender than the other. Particularly after coccyx injury, this asymmetry can remain for decades, contributing to back pain and feelings of disorientation. Patients in regular clinical practice often report feeling remarkably straighter and more grounded after one or two of these treatments.

6.2.2 Tapping method

Tapping is a more focused, more specifically activating version of pulsing, used to strongly activate Yang or move stuck Qi in a given region. Depending on the size and location of the point, it can be done with a single fingertip or several bunched together.

The key skill of tapping is that the movement comes from the whole arm, allowing for an easy bounce in the wrist – the feeling should be like throwing a very small ball. It takes a little bit of practice to pull all five fingers together so that the tips and nails are even, but it is well worth it for the large, versatile treatment tool it makes (a "chicken hand," in Tuina terminology – unparalleled for tight, fatigued necks and shoulders). The technique also works well with just the forefinger and middle finger held together, both bent and cradling each other so that the fingertips are even and their force combines smoothly.

With its dynamic arm movement and sharp strike, tapping excels at activating Yang when labor has gotten sluggish due to damp, deficiency or fatigue. The most common uses of tapping in birth are:

6.2.2.1 Du-20 – Baihui (Hundred Meetings)

Du-20 is the highest point of the head. Tapped with two or five fingers, it is very helpful for cutting through damp or fatigue in a long labor. I also like to self-administer this technique when tired or foggy.

6.2.2.2 Urinary Bladder-67 – Zhiyin (Reaching Yin)

UB-67 is the same point on the fifth toenail that is warmed with moxa for breech babies. When tapped with one finger, using the fingernail or an auricular bead to focus pressure on the tiny point, the point has two quite specific effects that have a range of possible uses. First, Baby's heart rate usually shows a brief acceleration a few seconds after tapping begins. This is a positive sign if there is any concern about fetal well-being.

Second, if there is already contractile activity, then 5–20 seconds of tapping will usually stimulate a contraction on the spot. One contraction on demand is not so clinically useful, but combined with ankle chafing the method can help to start or reinstate a regular contraction pattern (see contraction wrangling under combined methods in Section 6.5).

6.2.2.3 Trapezius (GB-21) and Iliotibial band (GB-31)
These are both areas rather than single points. Both areas store tension and feel delicious when Qi is moved with five-finger tapping with just the right amount of force (err on the gentle side at first).

6.2.3 Dredging
As the name implies, dredging involves dragging a flat finger or palm root along a channel or bone edge, in order to free up restrictions in the tissue there (often with strong effects elsewhere in the body). It is more moving than thumb circles, and often less comfortable, although carefully listening to the tissue can improve the experience considerably. The applications of dredging below all help to soften the cervix or pelvic floor, particularly for Qi stagnation or strong woman syndrome; they can be used for labor preparation as well as during labor:

- Liver Gummies – the thumb pushes upward along the posterior edge of the shinbone, rubbing out any "gumdrops" found at the border of bone and tissue. The journey from just above the ankle to just below the knee should take 2–5 minutes per side, depending on severity and sensitivity, with level of pressure carefully titrated. As a go-to for moving Qi to promote dilatation, it can be repeated hourly (see also Section 5.4).

- Clavicle – the tip of the thumb pushes laterally along the inferior surface of the clavicle, from the sternum outwards until stopped by bone, going as deeply as tolerated to soften the pelvic floor. The process should take 1–3 minutes and can be repeated every 2 hours or as tolerated.

- Gall Bladder channel – the palm root pushes downward along the Gall Bladder channel (contiguous with the iliotibial band at the side of the thigh) from the hip to the knee. Most strongly indicated for athletes whose powerful central Qi is still holding the baby weight out of the pelvis, vigorous use of this technique can make a big change, though it is not comfortable.

6.2.4 Connecting points

In some cases, redirecting pressure works best when two acupoints are pressed simultaneously by the thumb and the second or third finger. The third finger is more sensitive and seems to connect better, perhaps because it has an acupoint right at the tip. A few commonly used connecting point combinations are:

- LV-3 and KD-1 – this combination strongly moves Qi downward, for situations like hypertension (alongside Western care). Debra Betts recommends it for retained placenta as well.

- PC-6 and TH-5 – this combination seems to be symptomatically useful for the shivering that sometimes happens at transition or with epidural analgesia.

- SP-9 and ST-36 – together with needle or tapping stimulation at Du-20, this combination seems to help clear the fogginess or lethargy sometimes experienced by damp patients.

- UB-60 KD-3 – this combination moves Qi downward and softens the sacroiliac joint to open space; it is also very helpful for back pain.

6.2.5 Mini protocols

Below are a few point combinations or combined methods that are used together often for a specific purpose. They are grouped here to provide a shorthand for use in Chapter 7.

6.2.5.1 Promote contractions

Technically, "promote contractions" should be considered as a subset of "warm Yang" and "boost Qi." It is a collection of acupoint locations and stimulation methods that have all been observed to help initiate or strengthen contractions. These include:

- UB-32 (pressure, jiggling or small circles with the thumbs, or acupuncture with manual or electrical stimulation).

- Duyin – this point on the second toe tends to strengthen rather than initiate contractions; it is also more convenient for acupressure than acupuncture.

- LI-4 – with light, pulsing pressure rather than the strong pressure used for pain, LI-4 boosts Qi and can strengthen contractions.

- UB-67 – needling or tapping acupressure.

6.2.5.2 Betts occiput posterior combination

A simple acupressure point combination to open space and encourage OP babies to turn is presented in Debra Betts' online resource and app.[1] UB-60 is commonly used in acupuncture clinics to relax spasms in the lower back and free up the sacrum; together with SP-6 it seems to create more space in the pelvis for OP babies to wiggle and turn the right way around, which UB-67 encourages them to do. The stimulation is as follows (all points are stimulated on both sides):

1. 5 minutes – thumb pressure on UB-60, located in the hollow directly behind the ankle bone. This works best when the fingers reach around the Achilles tendon to give the thumbs something to brace against.

2. 5 minutes – thumb or finger pressure on SP-6. Spleen-6 is located on the inner leg, a hand's breadth up from the ankle bone in a depression behind the shin bone. Practitioners with large hands or tired thumbs can just slide the middle fingers up from where they were bracing, apply pressure with the middle finger and brace with the rest of the hand. Otherwise the hands can reverse their orientation and brace on the outside of the leg to press the inside.

3. 5 minutes – pressure on UB-67, located at the outer corner of the pinky toe. This small point is difficult to stimulate effectively with a fingertip. If available, an auricular ear seed placed on the point makes it easy to stimulate. Otherwise the toe can be grasped with the thumb underneath and the index finger on top, using the very tip of the finger (right before the nail, which should be short).

6.2.6 Other point stimulation methods
6.2.6.1 Pricking method

Regulations differ by region regarding who is and is not allowed to use a lancet of the type used for diabetic fingertip testing. Use of these lancets at acupuncture points to release a few drops of blood is one of the best ways to quickly cool the body and/or reduce blood pressure. All that is required is alcohol swabs, gloves and a (non-safety) lancet. With gloved hands, the point should be cleaned with one swab, then a fresh swab opened and kept ready. Blood should then be pressed toward the point with one hand, before pricking with the other. Two to four drops of blood should be expressed and

---

1   Dr. Betts' excellent app with videos is available at the Apple Store. Free printed guides for practitioner and birth team are available for download at: https://acupuncture.rhizome. net.nz/download-booklet

wiped with the swab, after which no further manipulation is needed. Fresh swabs can be used to remove blood until bleeding stops on its own. The following points are most useful for clearing heat during labor:

- Ear Apex venules – just below the highest visible point of the ear, look for small red venules and prick if apparent. If none is seen, use other points instead. This method is also extremely helpful to most hypertensive patients.

- Ba Feng (Eight Winds), at the webbing between the toes. Start with the great toe of both feet; this may be enough. These points are most strongly indicated when there are risk factors for infection such as ruptured membranes.

- Du-14 – Da Zhui (Great Hammer), at the base of the neck, in the depression between C-7 and T-1. This point is particularly indicated when the fever onset was after placement of epidural, together with pressure or needling at LI-4.

6.3 Additional Birth Bodywork

All of the new birth bodywork methods introduced in this section are essentially variations of hip rocking. The first is just a deeper look at the original technique, emphasizing its information gathering capabilities. Then follow three other variations useful in situations such as labor induction and bony obstruction.

6.3.1 Hip rocking (with deep listening)

The learning curve for hip rocking is not steep – the technique is pretty easy to pick up for most – but it can keep climbing indefinitely. Like the Handwich, over time the sight and feel of the wave form as it moves through the body becomes a kind of sonar, pointing out places that resist the flow and bounce out of sync. With minimal effort the bounce of the wave can be focused on the resistant places, almost always with positive results. After more than 20 years I have not yet discovered a limit to the depth of information exchange that can happen between my hands and a mom's body. Steps for entering into this conversation are below:[2]

---

2 Practitioners interested in this way of working may want to look into a movement education system called the Trager approach, which does not explicitly claim roots in Tuina but excels at restoring flow. https://www.tragerapproach.us

1. Begin with an easy rocking rhythm at the hips.

2. Once the rhythm has started, *listen*. The wave impulses tend to return to the hand slowly and smoothly if the tissue carries it all the way up the body, and abruptly if there is an interruption of flow in the bones and/or soft tissue.

3. Once you've started a conversation, keep asking questions. I try to use this method like sonar once a steady rhythm is established, directing the wave impulses not just forward but in wide sweeping arcs to the left, right and center, looking for obstacles. You don't need to force this curiosity – it is natural and will develop on its own, just as you naturally ask good clarifying questions when interested in somebody's story.

4. If the purpose of a treatment is labor preparation, or to assist cervical ripening in someone who's being induced with an unripe cervix, it's particularly good to focus as much as possible of the tissue bounce at the pelvic floor, and "listen" carefully to what comes back. In doing so we are rhythmically stretching cells, which induces them to cyclically release and uptake prostaglandins (including synthetic ones left there by doctors), which then makes the tissue stretchier.

The utility of hip rocking is by no means confined to birth: it is a key intervention for any patient complaints involving back pain and/or Qi stagnation anywhere. It is particularly useful for prevention as well as acute treatment of painful periods, and assists fertility in any situation where Qi stagnation or reduced Blood flow is part of the problem. For labor preparation, hip rocking is terrific to soften the pelvic floor, and should therefore be used in moderation during the second and third trimester. That said, the method is magic for pregnancy-induced sciatica, so unless Mom has signs of Qi sagging or a history of early cervical shortening, it's fine to do 3–5 minutes on each side, but not much more until week 37 (it's also fine to rock the hips before 20 weeks, when the fetus doesn't weigh much).

6.3.1.1 Leg swinging

Leg swinging is a complementary variant of hip rocking that works with a seated or reclining patient. I use it frequently in the office during labor preparation as well. It is also indispensable as an adjunct therapy for hospital inductions that keep the patient in bed, such as balloon stretching of the cervix and some topical prostaglandin applications. Like hip rocking, but from a different angle, leg swinging jiggles and stretches the soft tissue around and within the pelvis, softening the pelvic floor and helping to propagate the secretion and uptake of prostaglandins in the cervical ripening cycle.

During hospital inductions I tend to cycle each hour with approximately 20 minutes of each (if size of the birth team allows), then 20 minutes of rest.

Leg swinging works with the same kind of wave form propagation as hip rocking, only instead of a forward displacement of the hip, the wave is a rhythmic rotation of the leg inward then outward, with the femur as the center of the rotation. With the patient lying supine or reclining (the legs should be on a relatively level plane), push on the thigh as though pushing a child on a swing, with the intention to rotate the femur inward. The leg will swing back on its own, quickly or slowly depending on the range of motion and tightness of the underlying tissues. The Yang channels run down the outside of the leg, so we always start leg swinging at the top of the thigh and move gradually down the leg to the level of the ankle, finding a comfortable rhythm as we go. The flow of a patient's Qi can easily be assessed by looking down: if the wave carries through to the ankle, then the foot sways gracefully a half-beat behind the leg. With Qi stagnation the thigh may move, but the foot rotates stiffly back and forth like a windshield wiper. With practice, many patients who initially present with this stiffness can effectively be loosened up by leg swinging – and it is an approach I also use for sciatica and any gynecological Qi stagnation.

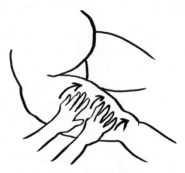

Figure 6.3 Leg swinging (inward).

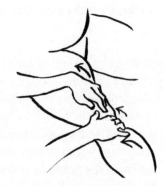

Figure 6.4 Leg swinging (outward).

Once a comfortable rhythm has been found swinging the leg inward to open the Yang channels, the movement can be performed in reverse, swinging the leg outward to open up the Yin channels. The full technique consists of cycles down the outside of the leg (rolling the leg inward) and back up the inside (rolling the leg outward), 30–60 seconds per side with the number of repetitions depending entirely on patient preference (most find it extremely comfortable). With practice, it becomes possible to feel areas of tightness and direct the waveform there, as with hip rocking. Acupuncturists may also enjoy focusing the waveform selectively along the Liver channel (to focus on the cervix) or the Kidney channel (to focus on the pelvic floor lower back). This is achieved simply by using the fingertips to initiate the movement, right along the channel, rather than the relaxed flat fingers one would naturally use.

6.3.1.2 Pelvic vibrating

Pelvic vibrating is another variant of hip rocking for use in seated or reclining patients; like leg swinging, it introduces a waveform from yet another angle, and complements hip rocking well. In particular its movement is much smaller and more specific to the bones of the pelvis. When there is body obstruction its tiny jiggles can be extremely useful to break up the experience of pain and open extra millimeters of space.

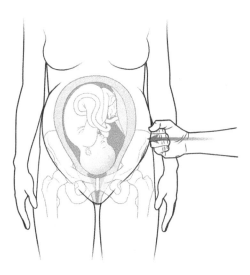

Figure 6.5 Pelvic vibrating.

The method is deceptively simple, and correct body mechanics are critical to a good effect. Steps for practitioners are as follows:

1. Find the Mom's "iliac crest," the part of the hipbone that pokes out to the side on slender people, right below the waist.

2. Align your body sideways to Mom's, seated or standing such that when your (dominant side) elbow hangs straight down from your shoulder it is at about the level of their hipbone.

3. Make a loose fist, bend your elbow and contact the iliac crest with your knuckles – specifically with the place on your fingers just distal to the knuckles, where a line drawn from your elbow through the center of your wrist would go.

4. With your feet well grounded, your elbow bent less than 90°, and your other hand touching Mom's leg to provide more normal therapeutic contact, begin to vibrate the pelvis by making tiny, rapid jiggles in the pelvis. Speed and regularity is critical, and the size is absolutely as small as you can make it. Our pelvises are not accustomed to being moved in this way, and even the tiniest movement feels gigantic.

6.3.1.3 Shaking the Apples (two techniques)

"Shaking the Apples" is a term I learned from a midwife to describe something I was already doing: extreme hip rocking in circles rather than straight lines, to jostle a stuck baby out of a bad alignment so that he can find a better one. A similar effect can be obtained from a different angle with seated or reclined patients, by moving the femur sharply back and forth along its axis (this requires a fairly specific grasp and technique). Both techniques should be practiced on several diverse (but non-pregnant) pelvises in order to get a feel for the techniques and the range of possible responses.

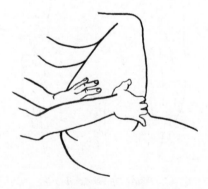

Figure 6.6 Shaking the Apples.

The hip-circling technique is done in the following steps:

1. With Mom in lateral recumbent position, find a comfortable hip rocking rhythm.

2. While rocking, move the top hand (the one closer to Mom's head) onto the iliac crest so that the front of the hipbone (the anterior superior iliac spine, or ASIS) is cupped quite stably in the fingers (this is now the top/front hand).

3. With the bottom/rear hand, increase the amplitude of the rock by pushing the top hip forward into the top/front hand.

4. The top/front hand then carries the hip in a circular motion forward, down and then back, pulling back into the bottom/rear hand, which continues the circle back and up.

5. This change of trajectory will slow the rocking rhythm down somewhat, but should not lose it – keep this big circle going for three to six cycles in order to make room for Baby to shift.

The femur-shaking technique is as follows:

1. With Mom seated (this is best) or partially reclining, you sit or kneel in a stable position so that Mom's knee is at about your chest level, the femur and kneecap pointing directly toward your sternum.

2. Grasp the knee from below, with the fingers wrapped around the tibia and calf right below the knee, and one thumb at each of the "eyes" of the knee on either side of the patellar tendon.

3. From this position, keeping your body well grounded, shake the femur forward and backward directly along its axis, three to six times at about two shakes per second. The amplitude of the movement will be about an inch or less, depending on the tightness of Mom's tissues.

6.4 Auriculotherapy

"Auriculotherapy" designates use of pressure points on the ear to improve well-being. It does not specify a method of stimulation; commonly used methods include small acupuncture needles, semi-permanent tacks (used in the US military for acute pain relief[3]), and electrical point detection and stimulation. The main method discussed this book is acupressure using small seeds on sticky plasters; however, acupuncturists are invited to substitute needles and/or electrical stimulation as appropriate.

Regulations regarding use of penetrating and non-penetrating auricular methods differ by region and should be checked, but in general there are few restrictions on the use of ear seeds. Auriculotherapy should not be performed without some training, but there are several online options. The brief, inexpensive online "Ear Cure" training includes a downloadable booklet and is absolutely sufficient to support the use of ear seeds as described in this chapter.[4] For those wishing to use auriculotherapy for differential analysis and problem-solving, I can recommend the comprehensive online course by Dr. Terry Oleson.[5]

Below I describe two sets of points that the Acuteam uses in nearly all births, followed by a few other single-point techniques. Unless otherwise specified, seeds should be placed on both sides, and stimulated hourly with strong pressure, lasting 5–15 seconds per seed, for total stimulation time of about 1 minute per ear. The pressure will be slightly uncomfortable, in order to stimulate an endorphin response.

6.4.1 Birth basics ear seeds

As the title implies, this set of five ear seeds is a "basic" treatment useful for almost any parturient. Note that Qi stagnation is already addressed within the five-seed protocol. The combination is suitable for labor preparation, any time from week 37 on, or during labor. My mnemonic for remembering them (in the order they should be needled) is "Sometimes U Should Leave Early" – Sympathetic, Uterus, Shenmen, Liver, Endocrine. Place seeds on both sides if possible. See Appendix A, Figure A10 for auricular point locations.

---

3 These "ASP" needles work extremely well for pain management during birth; however they are not easily removed, so permission must be obtained from the primary provider. Also, care must be taken to use the titanium rather than steel needles, against the possibility that neurological symptoms develop, requiring magnetic resonance imaging (MRI).

4 https://www.miridiatech.com/shop/en/all-products/auriculotherapy/auriculotherapy-training.html

5 https://quantumuniversity.com/courses/auriculotherapy-training

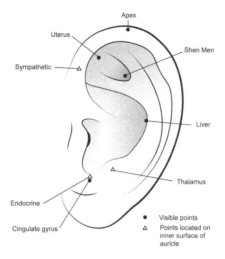

Figure 6.7 Auriculotherapy points.

6.4.2 Pain points

Cingulate Gyrus and Thalamus are the two key points of the Battlefield Acupuncture protocol, used in the US military for pain relief during troop transport and rehabilitation. Acupuncturists may want to carry the tiny titanium ASP needles that can be embedded in these points for more powerful pain relief.[6] Otherwise strong stimulation on ear seeds or tacks can work well. Regular ear needles are not recommended during labor as they easily fall out of these points and don't tape down all that well.

6.4.3 Individual ear points

The following points may also be added to the birth basics treatment:

- Bladder and Sciatica points for back labor (OP).

- The Constipation point is useful for any labor with Qi stagnation and/or digestive disruptions.

- Constipation and Sciatica points can be threaded for pain.

- Point Zero – consider this point to "turn up the volume" on a treatment when there is some response but there's room for improvement.

---

6   The ASP needles take some practice to insert without undue discomfort, but it's worth it. Note that titanium must be used, as a stainless steel needle would be unsafe in the unlikely but not unheard of event of neurological symptoms after birth that require MRI scanning.

- Spine points – when there is mid- or upper-back pain during labor, it can be very useful to locate tender points on the antihelix as it maps to the spine. Place two or three seeds each on the front and back of the tender area, for stronger pinching effect.

6.5 Additional Miscellaneous Treatment Methods by Situation

This section covers therapeutic methods that are called for by situation or symptom, rather than in relation to a given constitutional diagnosis or treatment principle. Some examples are retained placenta, or postpartum hemorrhage, which present across constitutional types.

6.5.1 Irregular contractions with ripe cervix – contraction wrangling

This extremely gentle form of labor induction or augmentation only works when the cervix is mostly ripe and the fetal head is in place, but contractions are irregular. If there is no contractile activity at all, then stronger stimulation with needles or electrical stimulation is more likely to be effective.

Alternate 4 minutes of vigorous ankle chafing with 20–40 seconds of sharp tapping on UB-67; this can be thought of as "CPR for the contractions." The ankle chafing imbues the system with Yang Qi, which the tapping then activates. This method is very useful for Yang- or Qi-deficient moms and those whose flow of Yang Qi is blocked by damp; it can be part of a labor preparation treatment, during hospital induction or during active phase if contractions should "space out" or become irregular. Repeat the process described above 5–10 times, or until the contractions seem stronger or begin to initiate spontaneously on schedule, then hold off for half an hour and see whether the contraction rhythm has "taken." Repeat that cycle as needed to keep contractions moving.

6.5.2 Ineffective pushing with epidural analgesia

In this very specific situation, two acupressure points are extremely useful. The first is GB-21, which has been discussed for its ability to descend Qi, and definitely helps in this context.

The second point that helps focus scattered Qi downward with epidural is –ironically enough – Du-20. Whether needled forward or stimulated with gentle pulsing pressure, the point's location at the opposite end of the Du channel from the perineum appears to focus energy there.

6.5.3 Occiput posterior – "opening the back door"

Strong pressure on the sacrum can also be extremely helpful in managing pain from an OP baby after transition. This is not UB-32 *per se*: the reason the pressure is helpful in this situation is that the enormous baby occiput is pressing hard on the sacrum, which stretches the ligaments that stabilize the sacrum against the pelvis (sacrotuberous and sacrospinous, we'll meet them later) farther than they've ever been stretched in their whole little lives.

If Baby is OP before transition, I try to create space in the pelvis and use gravity and position to encourage her to turn. However if she persists in OP position, or turns OP after transition, then I trust that she is doing so because the pelvis will not allow her out in an anterior position. I therefore "open the back door" using the Betts OP combination of Bladder-60 and 67 and Spleen-6, with needles or acupressure, and stretch the sacrotuberous and sacrospinous ligaments (see Section 6.2.1 above).

6.5.4 Postpartum hemorrhage – SP-1 (plus contraction points)

Spleen-1 is located at the medial, proximal corner of the great toenail, and it is classically indicated for dysfunctional uterine bleeding. In office visits it is treated with direct moxa – little threads of fuzz from the moxa leaves that heat the small area strongly. However, in practice, whenever I see more than an ounce of blood after delivery I immediately jam my thumbnail into the point, and I train all my students to do the same, while also stimulating Duyin (the underside of the distal interphalangeal crease in the second toe) or LI-4. In several instances when the Acuteam has used these points, doctors or nurses have remarked on the sudden decrease in the rate of bleeding.

6.5.5 Prelabor rupture of membranes (PROM) – Check OP; hip rocking, right side down

If the membranes rupture releasing prostaglandin-rich amniotic fluid, but labor does not start, then something is not quite right. Most commonly, this is OP; otherwise, the cervix may not yet be ripe. Rocking the hips with the right side down is almost always the appropriate method for addressing OP (see Section 7.1.2.1). It is also a strong method for ripening the cervix by rhythmically stretching the tissues as they are bathed in amniotic fluid. See also Appendix D.

6.5.6 Send Qi and Blood to the uterus – warming ST-36 and/or Soojok uterus point

Based on long experience with moxibustion on ST-36 for low fluids and IUGR – my own and others' – I feel quite confident that it increases blood flow to the uterus. During labor, I use my palm to warm or chafe the point anytime I am concerned about Mom's Qi or Baby's oxygen supply. On the fetal heart rate monitor, flat tracings often seem to perk up somewhat when the point is warmed, and in some situations decelerations become shorter or less persistent.

Another point that seems to improve heart rate tracings is located on the sole of the foot, in the meaty flesh between the bases of the third and fourth toes (see Figure A9). The Acuteam calls it "the Soojok point," because it is the one point any of us knows in the entire Soojok system of Korean acupuncture – the one that points to the uterus. We learned it years ago from a Russian student who had been an obstetrician back home, and had also studied some Korean acupuncture. There was a deeply deficient mom all alone in Room 4, being induced for IUGR at 34 weeks with a terribly flat tracing. Mom's pulse and Baby's were both quite slow, and Mom's was deep and weak as well. Though only 26, she had clearly had a hard life both in China and New York. It was a busy day on the unit, so although she had not progressed past 5 cm all day and was not given oxytocin due to the unfavorable heart tracing, she was not rushed to C-section as more urgent cases went first. My assessment was that the prognosis for vaginal delivery was poor, and that she would jump to the front of the line as soon as the baby's heart rate decelerated from fatigue. After we made our rounds I steered the students toward other cases more likely to end with them assisting at a vaginal birth, but Elena refused to leave this mom; for hours she sat at the foot of the bed, warming and gently massaging these points with her thumbs. To everyone's surprise including mine, the lackadaisical contraction pattern picked up a little, and the heart rate variability increased slightly – but only when Elena's thumbs were in place. After about 3 hours Mom had progressed to 8 cm, though contractions had not been strong, and at the 7-hour mark, she pushed out a tiny baby girl with Elena by her side.

6.6 Acupuncture

The purpose of this section is not to teach acupuncture to those not licensed to perform it, nor to review the locations and actions of familiar points. Rather, it is to share the points and point combinations most commonly used in labor by the Acuteam, adding my commentary or notes on usage and technique as appropriate. Points are grouped by treatment principle.

It is hoped that acupuncturists will not feel limited by this core toolkit, but will bring their own unique methods and capabilities to every birth. The points are presented by therapeutic principle, with a few points appearing more than once with different stimulation methods, or in combination with other points. The therapeutic principles themselves have been adapted from more conventional East Asian medicine (EAM) treatment principles for the purposes of this book.

6.6.1 Promoting contractions

6.6.1.1 SP-6, LI-4, UB-32 – "acupuncture induction"

This point combination (with strong manual or electrical stimulation on UB-32) is the acupuncture equivalent of Pitocin or Syntocinon. No birth acupuncturist I know questions whether electrical or strong manual stimulation at this combination of points can initiate contractions. The question is only whether promoting contractions is the most appropriate therapeutic direction to take for a given birthing person. In many cases, moderate or gentle stimulation provides a better result, helping ripen the cervix to prepare for a more effective active phase. For this reason and others, I avoid use of the term "induction" for prelabor acupuncture treatments.

Remembering the cervical ripening cycle from Chapter 3, everyone tends to initiate labor according to their own constitutional strengths and weaknesses. Qi- and Yang-deficient moms tend to drop early as their central Qi is overcome by the baby weight, and cervical ripening follows (unless the Yang is so deficient that hormonal activity is impaired). Damp patients also tend to run past their due date with ripe cervixes but no contractions. For these situations, contractions are the weak part of the cycle; this treatment is perfect for strengthening it – like bringing a Yang match to a Yin pile of wood.

By contrast, moms whose labors are delayed for other reasons – position, Yin or Blood deficiency, Qi stagnation – may need the Belt channel softening and cervical ripening more than they need contractions. Exactly what EAM does well is to differentiate the underlying constitutional and other factors impeding the course of labor and work with them specifically, rather than applying a generic point prescription. Under time pressure (e.g. ruptured membranes, incipient induction) and having first ruled out OP, this combination can be very useful to help create appropriate hormonal conditions labor initiation, without inducing *per se*. One final note is that, in my experience, if contractile activity is present but not regular then contraction wrangling may well be sufficient to consolidate and strengthen the rhythm.

TECHNIQUE

LI-4 works best for birth when needled slightly proximal to its normal location, at a tender point that should be palpable at about the most proximal place where the thumb fits between the first and second metacarpal bones. For promoting contractions the stimulation should be strong supplementation, such as the "setting the mountain on fire" method[7] in which the needle is rotated clockwise nine times each at superficial, middle and deep levels. For Yin- or Blood-deficient patients, a moderate or gentle supplementation method is preferable.

In the context of this treatment, SP-6 should be supplemented in Yin- or Blood-deficient patients, and reduced if there is Qi stagnation without deficiency.

For manual stimulation of UB-32, best results are achieved when the needle directly enters the sacral foramen under the point, meaning a 3 in. needle for most pregnant patients and longer if they are heavy. The points are easiest to find with the patient seated at the table and leaning forward onto it. Needling right into the foramen requires practice, as well as careful palpation with the non-needling hand to find exactly the angle at which the point feels wide open. Some patients just have tricky shaped foramina that do not easily admit the needle; when this is the case, it is important to acknowledge this, and not just apply manual or electrical stimulation as though the needle has reached the point, when it has not. If time is of the essence, alternate plans should be made such as contraction wrangling if there is contractile activity and electrical stimulation on SP-6 and LI-4 if there is not.

For electrical stimulation of UB-32, UB-31, 33 and 34 should be palpated to assess which has the best combination of tissue reactivity and feeling of open space to needle into. The selected point should then be joined to the ipsilateral UB-32, each pair on its own side.

Box 6.1 A few words about electrical stimulation (E-stim).

Basic training in E-stim is outside the scope of this book. It is assumed that practitioners are using small portable machines such as the Ito ES-130.[8] On these and similar devices, there is no difference between the red and the black leads as there is on higher-end machines. I am assuming that practitioners

---

7 Xinnong, C. (1987). *Chinese Acupuncture and Moxibustion*. Beijing: Foreign Languages Press.

8 ITO Physiotherapy and Rehabilitation. (2019). General Catalogue for Electrotherapy. Retrieved July 4, 2019, from www.itocoltd.com/products/es-130

who use phased devices or ion pumping cords can make their own therapeutic decisions regarding polarity. A few other points:

— Frequency: I use continuous frequency at 2 Hz for its calming effects. If Mom is damp, tired, or lethargic, then 10 Hz is a better choice.

— Crossing the midline: I am sometimes questioned regarding the use of E-stim between bilateral SP-6 or SP-4 points. Some acupuncturists have been trained not to cross the midline with electricity and are hesitant to do so. What's important to understand is that "midline" is really a didactic shorthand for the three functional areas that could actually suffer damage from electrical current: spinal cord, heart and brain. Electricity will take the shortest possible path, so electricity between points on the leg will skitter across the inferior surface of the perineum, which is perfectly safe as long as Baby's head is not yet in the vaginal canal. In order to avoid sending electrical current across the heart, LI-4 points should not be connected to each other, or to contralateral Spleen points (ipsilateral connections are fine). The sacral foramina are below the spinal cord, but by convention they are still connected only ipsilaterally.

6.6.1.2 Duyin

Duyin is located at the distal interphalangeal crease of the second toe. My experience with this point is that needling tends to increase the reactivity of the uterus, making contractions stronger but not necessarily more regular, and that the effect seems to last about a half hour. Based on the idea of Qi governing strength of contractions, as well as the point's proximity to the Jing-Well point of the Stomach channel, I have assumed that its mechanism of action is to activate Qi rather than supplement it. This is consistent with its behavior as a short-term stimulant for contractions in the moment rather than a constitutional solution going forward.

Recommended stimulation for sustainable action with Qi deficiency during labor is therefore acupressure with the side of the finger in pulses before and during the contraction, with a switch to chafing up the Kidney channel or down the Stomach channel between contractions. An ear seed may be applied to focus the effect of the pressure.

Needling the point works best once pushing has started, or to cut through damp in a robust patient. Retention of ear tacks or ear needles (in stirrups) provides strong stimulation.

6.6.1.3 Bladder-67

Bladder-67 is well known for its use with moxibustion for breech presentation. When needled, it appears to promote both contractile activity and fetal movements for 10–20 minutes depending on Mom's Qi. For this reason, I needle it to encourage a change in fetal positioning (together with SP-6 and UB-60, as suggested by Debra Betts).

6.6.2 Raising and activating Qi

Raising Qi is critical for prenatal care, to prevent and address threatened miscarriage and premature labor. Counterintuitively, it is often important during labor as well. This could be compared to the way people lift their center of gravity in order to press down on something, or raise a hammer to drive in a nail. In this way, a weak raising function can actually engender weak descent.

6.6.2.1 Du-20

As the highest point in the body, Du-20 is naturally the preeminent point for raising Qi. It is additionally useful in labor both because it calms anxiety and also because, being on the opposite end of the Du vessel, it appears to focus Qi on the perineum. I needle it routinely, along with pressure on GB-21, to help first-time moms figure out their pushing. This is particularly helpful with epidural on board.

I seldom needle Du-20 in a posterior direction against channel flow, as some practitioners do, to direct the Qi downward. As discussed above, upward and downward movement engender each other, and I prefer to use the point to do what it does best. A ½ in. needle is most stable, threaded under the thick scalp tissue nearly to the handle.

6.6.2.2 Du-20 and Stomach-13

I learned this combination in acupuncture school from Kiiko Matsumoto. Officially in the notes it is indicated for "visceroptosis" or organ prolapse. However, I also have a strong memory of ST-13 being referred to colloquially as the "boob lift point." I use the combination to strongly raise Qi for any threatened miscarriage, cervical shortening or prematurity. I use it preventatively for any patient with Qi deficiency during pregnancy. I also needle it during any treatment for musculoskeletal pain before 36 weeks, on the grounds that if baby weight is sagging onto the bones and joints, it must not be fully supported by the Qi.

For this indication Du-20 is threaded forward and ST-13 is threaded laterally under the collarbone with a small-gauge 1 in. needle and gentle supplementing stimulation. The mental image is of pulling gently upward on the Stomach channel, particularly the horizontal piece from ST-30 to 31 as representing the pelvic floor. This can be thought of as the direct inverse of downward pressure on GB-21.

6.6.2.3 Du-20 and Spleen-9

This combination excels for raising clear Yang while descending damp turbidity. When a labor is sluggish due to damp, these points can be extremely helpful either as part of a "time-out" treatment or with SP-9 threaded downward with a 1 in. medium-gauge needle and taped.

6.6.2.4 Stomach-36

To strongly activate Qi during labor, I use the "setting the mountain on fire" technique from the classic *Chinese Acupuncture and Moxibustion* text previously referenced. The technique for this is as follows:

1. Insert a 1.5 in. medium-gauge needle as painlessly as possible and obtain Qi at a shallow level (approximately 0.5 in.)

2. Lift/thrust and rotate the needle to supplement nine times. The thumb should be moving forward on the insertion as the breath and intention moves out the arm and into the point; use right ST-36 if right-handed and left for left.

3. Retaining a strong sense of Qi on the needle, push it slowly to a medium depth (approximately 1 in.). Repeat the nine thrusts.

4. Repeat at 1.5 in.

5. Repeat the whole operation three times or until the patient feels a spreading warm sensation.

6.6.3 Softening the sinews

In labor, points that soften sinews can usefully be mapped along two axes: whether their action focuses more on the pelvic floor or cervix, and whether their nature is more moving or more supplementing. As previously discussed, Blood deficiency in most cases is at least a contributing factor to tightness of the cervix and pelvic floor. It is therefore advisable to start with more nourishing points and techniques and proceed to more moving ones if necessary.

6.6.3.1 Spleen-6

SP-6 is nourishing in nature and strongly promotes cervical ripening and dilatation. When needled or pressed it not only treats pain, but also seems to help convert the force of the contraction from pain (i.e. stuck Qi) into dilatation (i.e. flowing Qi). Accordingly, it is not the most useful point when a Qi/Yang-deficient or damp labor is trying to establish itself and the contractions are not yet strong or stable.

A variety of techniques can be used to elicit SP-6's many capabilities (see entries under other principles below).

- Most nourishing to promote dilatation (but not strongly effective for pain) is acupressure with each contraction rather than needling.

- For cervical ripening under time pressure, the two SP-6 points can be connected with E-stim at 2 Hz.

- To stimulate contractions under time pressure when needling UB-32 is not practicable, SP-6 can be connected with E-stim to LI-4. It is critical that both points be *on the same side*; I usually use the right side as contractions most commonly initiate in the right uterine horn.

- According to Jean Levesque, the posterior aspect of SP-6 (i.e. focusing on it as a Kidney point) is useful to drain damp. I seldom use it this way (preferring SP-9) but I do use the posterior location when I want to boost Yin as well as promote cervical ripening.

6.6.3.2 Liver-8

Liver 8 has some similar effects to SP-6, and can be substituted in patients whose ankles are so swollen that needling into them is not preferred. It nourishes Blood more strongly and seems more effective for pain of the type that is disproportionate to contractions, due to Blood deficiency or sexual trauma. It is also very effective for slow dilatation due to these causes. However it does not promote contractions, and seems less useful for cervical ripening than SP-6. Its effects appear more systemic and less specific to the cervix, and I therefore think of it as an excellent complement to the Gallbladder points used for softening the pelvic floor, to address mild Liver Qi stagnation with Blood deficiency. LV-8 can also be thought of as a softer version of Liver-3, more nourishing and less moving.

- For cervical ripening, I use a 1.5 in. or 2 in. medium-gauge needle, obliquely upwards along the channel with a strong Qi sensation and intention of connecting with the cervix along the large planes of fascia that run up the inner leg. The needle can be taped in this position and usually tolerates some movement (e.g. some walking but not squats). It should be retained for 15–40 minutes depending on the degrees of stagnation and deficiency.

- For pain, I find a tender area on the Liver channel below the knee joint and needle obliquely downward along the channel with a 1 in. medium-gauge needle, with gentle stimulation and an intention of drawing tightness out of the thigh and genitals to soften the channel. The needle can be taped in this position and usually tolerates some movement.

6.6.3.3 Liver-3

Liver-3 excels in labor for moving Qi while still nourishing the Liver somewhat (versus Liver 2, which is most moving in nature).

- Needled through to KD-1, it strongly descends Qi. With a 1 in. or 1.5 in. needle I obtain Qi at LV-3, then bring my other middle finger to KD-1 and "call" the Qi with it. Once there is a warm sensation of Qi at KD-1, I direct the needle downwards until Qi is obtained at KD-1 or there is an additional warm sensation in the listening hand. (If you feel physical pressure from the needle at KD-1, you've gone too far; draw back slightly and rotate the needle to obtain Qi.)

- Combined with GB-34, LV-3 can be very helpful for any labor pain felt other than OP. A small-gauge 1 in. needle inserted obliquely toward Liver-2 can be taped in this position and usually tolerates some movement.

6.6.3.4 Liver-2 and Liver-5

Liver 2 and 5 are the most moving of the Liver points I use in labor; I reserve them for when "extreme softening" is needed. From Jean Levesque I learned to use Liver-2 to reduce cervical edema, and it excels for this. I had been using Liver-5, and I find the combination extremely useful any time the cervix is misbehaving despite adequate contractions. This includes dilatation with slow effacement, effacement with slow dilatation, asymmetrical dilation, cervical lip or any time the cervix is tough in consistency but progress is urgently needed. As discussed previously, it is best to start with gentler methods unless time is of the essence. This is particularly important when there is significant Yin or Blood deficiency underlying the tight cervix, and gentler methods such as chafing up the Liver Gummy area are likely to work better anyway.

- For cervical edema, needle Liver-2 with a ½ in. small-gauge needle and stimulate strongly for 5 minutes.

- To dilate the cervix urgently, run E-stim between Liver-2 and Liver-5 at 2 Hz, alternating with 30 Hz (if Mom is anxious, use continuous at 2 Hz).

6.6.3.5 Inner Leg points

Over the years, I have found that nearly every laboring patient has extremely tender points on the Liver and/or Kidney channel above the knee. These points seem to move Qi strongly and soften the pelvic floor, and usually respond best to acupuncture. Acupressure can work, but is somewhat socially awkward and can be painful without an accomplished listening touch. These points are most useful for bedridden patients with slow progress due to Qi stagnation or strong woman syndrome.

- Insert a 2 in. or 3 in., medium- or large-gauge needle slightly upward along the channel, obtaining Qi as gently as possible and stimulating softly, with an intention of moving Qi smoothly up the channel through any blockage.

- The method can be very helpful if stagnation is due to sexual trauma, but great sensitivity is needed both in palpating and also hedging the treatment against likely emotional release, with auricular and other spirit-calming points, and Belly Breathing before and after insertion.

6.6.3.6 Gallbladder-41, Gallbladder-34 and Gallbladder-31

These Gallbladder points all help to soften the pelvic floor. Each has slightly different capabilities and useful combinations. GB-34 is often thought of first, as it softens the sinews and appears to spread the pubic symphysis, allowing a few extra millimeters for big babies. GB-41 is equally important for its property of opening Dai Mai (although the other two are on the course of the vessel and also help to soften it; I most often use GB-34 and 41 together). GB-31 is a larger point, gentler and more nourishing than the other two. It combines well with GB-34 and Liver-8 or Inner Leg points as a gentle way to soften the pelvic floor when it is tight due to Blood deficiency and/or sexual trauma.

6.6.4 Descending Qi

A wide variety of points are used to descend Qi in different ways. The descending action of Liver-3 needled through to KD-1 was discussed in Section 6.6.2. Lung-7 and LI-4 can also be used to descend Qi in labor, much as they are used for constipation. GB-20, 21 and 31 can be used together with Liver-3 through to Kidney-1 and LI-4 for emergent hypertension (though of course as an adjunct to Western care if possible). The points' actions and associated techniques are as follows:

6.6.4.1 Lung-7

As the body gears up for active phase, the pulse becomes more superficial. Holly Guzman, a formidable women's health practitioner in northern California, taught me to assess and treat Lung-7 as part of labor preparation. I see this treatment in the same spirit as opening the top of a tube so that water can drain out of the bottom, a principle frequently used to treat constipation. Depending somewhat on the patient's constitution, I thread the point proximally with a small- or medium-gauge ½ or 1 in. needle and strong *de qi*.

6.6.4.2 Large Intestine-4

LI-4's descending action can be used to strengthen Qi-deficient pushing, or to strengthen a treatment for hypertension. For use in labor it should be located proximal to the orthodox point, with a moderate-gauge 1 in. needle and strong supplementing stimulation.

6.6.4.3 Gallbladder-20

GB-20 relaxes the muscles of the neck, allowing excess Qi and Blood to drain from the head. It is commonly paired with GB-21 as a powerful treatment for hypertension. For this function it is needled with a 1 in. medium-gauge needle, obliquely toward UB-10 if there is marked neck tension.

6.6.4.4 Gallbladder-21

GB-21's powerful descending function is apparent from its name, "shoulder spring." In some Qigong practice, it is visualized as a waterfall flowing straight down from the shoulders to KD-1, carrying down any Qi that is pathologically rising or stuck. I am reluctant to needle it during the chaos of labor and use acupressure instead. That said, needling is stronger and may be used for emergent hypertension in conjunction with Western care or if such care is not available. In low-chaos situations it can be needled with a medium-gauge 1 in. needle downward and slightly laterally, such that the entire length of the needle would remain safely in the trapezius if fully inserted. For chaotic situations, small patients and those with a history of asthma or other breathing disorders, I prefer ½ in. needles inserted directly downward, or ear tacks.

6.6.4.5 Gallbladder-31

GB-31, like GB-20, is a "wind" point, meaning that its tendency is to relax and descend chaotic Qi. It does not have a strong descending function unless combined with other points.

6.6.4.6 Liver-3 through to Kidney-1

This combination works wonders to descend Liver Yang and root it in Kidney water. Get Qi at Liver-3, then find the Qi at Kidney-1 with the fingers of the non-needling hand (I use the third finger). Send the needle straight down toward it, until you just barely feel a sense of heaviness in the Kidney-1 hand. If you feel the needle itself through the sole of the foot, you've gone too far.

6.6.5 Reducing pain

It's important that a strategy for reducing pain with acupuncture be undertaken in relation to differential analysis. As previously stated, worse-than-ordinary pain is usually caused either by bone-on-bone pressure, or by constitutional factors such as cold, Blood or Yin deficiency, or Qi stagnation due to fear and/or trauma. Identification and resolution of those other factors, if present, is the most potent pain relief. Among the points and combinations below, some help to shift bony obstruction or other root causes of pain, while others simply address the discomfort.

6.6.5.1 Spleen-6 and Spleen-8

Among its many other capabilities, SP-6 helps to reduce pain when needled with strong stimulation and retained. A 1 in. small-gauge needle is inserted at a slight oblique downward angle, then the handle bent upwards and taped. If not inserted too deeply, these needles will be reasonably comfortable for walking and movement and can be retained as long as the pulse stays strong. For patients stuck in bed, SP-8 can be added to increase pain reduction but does not tolerate much movement.

6.6.5.2 Bladder-60, Bladder-67 and Spleen-6

This combination, recommended by Debra Betts for shifting OP position, is highly effective in my experience and should be used (in conjunction with hip rocking and right-side lying) any time contractions hurt in the back. It is also useful for shifting asynclitism. UB-60 can be used for ordinary lumbar or thoracic pain in labor as well.

- UB-60 – during labor pain this point can be needled with a medium-gauge 1 in. needle obliquely down the channel with strong stimulation, then taped. It tolerates movement well.

- UB-67 – for this indication the point can be stimulated with an ear tack or needled upward along the channel with an auricular needle.

- The technique for SP-6 is as described above.

6.6.5.3 Liver-3 and Gallbladder-34

This combination is effective for reducing the soft tissue pain of a typical labor, softening the sinews and nourishing any underlying Blood deficiency as well as moving Qi. The combination appears also to marginally increase flex at the sacroiliac joints and pubic symphysis, perhaps allowing an extra millimeter for big babies. GB-34 can be needled normally, or threaded downward with a small-gauge 1 in. needle and taped to tolerate some movement.

6.6.6 Calming the spirit

Most acupuncturists have their own repertoire of calming points and should feel free to use them. Below are notes on the ones most commonly used.

6.6.6.1 Yintang

In the movie *The Business of Being Born* there is the briefest shot of a laboring patient sporting a pale blue ear needle at Yintang that I inserted. Threaded downward with a small-gauge ½ in. needle, the point is convenient and tolerates movement well. I think of it particularly for difficult inductions and transitions, telling moms that the purpose of this "third eye" point is to help see past the current slog to the joyful moment in the near future when they get to meet their newest family member.

6.6.6.2 Heart-3

I learned to use Heart-3 in labor from Jean Levesque. As a He-Sea point it is very stabilizing, a godsend for working with Blood-deficient patients. It is also extremely useful to have a spirit-calming point that is not painful to needle. With a small-gauge ½ or 1 in. needle inserted in the largish depression on the Heart channel proximal to the medial epicondyle (i.e. slightly above its orthodox location), this point can be taped and tolerates movement well.

6.6.6.3 Nap and Dilate (666)

This simple point combination nourishes Yin and Blood and calms the spirit, reducing anxiety and encouraging sleep anytime a break is in order. In addition to descending Qi, PC-6 calms the spirit. KD-6 and SP-6 together draw Qi down to the lower extremities and strongly nourish Yin and Blood. No special technique is required.

6.6.7 Calming the uterus

It is not uncommon for moms to experience mild, fleeting contractile activity before 37 weeks, particularly during summer when dehydration makes muscle fibers more prone to activation. These incidents need to be observed with caution, and are a severe cause for concern if they become stronger or more regular.

Spleen-4 is the point that I have always used to quiet the uterus. While I was doing a study of acupuncture during labor in 2005, I remember reading a research report from Russia in the 1970s (a time when there was a great deal of acupuncture research). As I remember it, the doctor had thought that electrical stimulation at SP-4 might enhance labor, presumably because of its relationship to Chong Mai, the Conception Vessel. He found instead that the labor stopped dead in its tracks and went to Cesarean section, which led him to use that treatment the next time he saw a patient with threatened miscarriage – with excellent results. If I use E-stim, I use 2 Hz, which in itself appears to be quite a calming frequency. I suggest starting with just the needles, which together with calming ear seeds, is often enough that the frightening electrical gadget is not necessary.

Debra Betts, who did her PhD thesis on threatened miscarriage, uses Kidney-9 to calm the uterus. Well known in Western circles as the "pretty baby point" for its use in prenatal care, KD-9 does not have an agreed-upon mechanism of action for quieting contractions. Anecdotally, however, Debra herself and the midwives that she teaches have found the point highly effective.

6.6.8 Clearing heat

In general I find bleeding more powerful than needling to clear heat. If bleeding is impracticable, strong reduction of needles at LV-2, SP-10 and LI-11 can clear heat from the Blood and uterus.

6.7 Summary Table

Table 6.2 is a complete inventory of the therapeutic methods introduced both in this chapter and also in Chapter 5. For ease of reference, basic methods from Chapter 5 are rendered in bold type , and section numbers are provided for all methods.

Table 6.2 Inventory of EAM therapeutic methods for birth.

Function	Point/ channel area	Stimulation method	When to use/*Notes*
Activate Qi	UB-67	Moxibustion	Encourages fetal movement
		Needle	Encourages fetal movement Initiates contractions
		Tapping – fingernail or ear seed	Initiates contraction, fetal movement
	ST-36	Gentle pressure Moxibustion Chafing down shin	Fatigue Any time Baby needs more blood flow *Warm with palms or thumbs*
	Inner ankle (KD-3)	Vigorous chafing	Warms Yang for cold, edema, sluggish contractions
	Cat/Cow		Also gently moves, opens space
	SP-9 and ST-36	Connecting pressure Needle	Clears fogginess, lethargy with damp moms *Use with Du-20*
	SP-6	Gentle pressure	Slow cervical ripening (deficient mom) Yin or Blood deficiency **Can also chafe Liver Gummy area**
Calm the spirit (see also Nourish Yin/Blood)	KD-1	Redirecting pressure	"Panic Button" for fear, anxiety, rising Qi *Can also use moxa to warm cold moms*
	Ear birth basics	Needles or seeds	Sympathetic, Uterus, Shenmen, Liver, Endocrine – calm spirit, reduce pain, soften cervix
	Yintang	Needle	"Third eye" to see past difficult labor
	HT-3	Needle obliquely upward and tape	Slightly above orthodox location
	SP-6, PC-6, KD-6	Needle – "Nap and Dilate protocol"	Reduces anxiety, replenishes Yin by encouraging sleep
Clear heat	Hand heat points	Grasp comb	Also comfort measure, helps Qi stagnation
	Ear Apex	Pricking method	Red venules near top of ear, three or more drops of blood with needle or lancet
	Ba Feng (foot heat points)	Toothpick or fork tine Pricking method Needles	Above toe webbing – use first to second toe only, unless fever is severe Add ST-44 for mastitis
	Du-14 (C7-T1 space)	Pricking method Needle in and out	For post-epidural fever with no sweat, combine with LI-4
	LV-2, SP-10, LI-11	Needle, reducing method	Intrapartum fever
Descend Qi	UB-60	Pressure or needle	Moves Qi downward, opens sacroiliac joint,
	UB-60 to KD-3	Connecting pressure or needle	treats back pain, occipital headache or tension Use to open space in occiput posterior
	GB-21	Strong pressure	Directs Qi strongly downward to assist fetal descent *Avoid when there is blockage by bones or hard cervix* *Great for sluggish pushing with epidural*

	Liver-14	Strong pressure inward then downward	Directs Qi down to help release placenta *Press into rib space, then down* *Start 15 minutes after birth*
	LV-3 to KD-1	Connecting pressure or needle	Strongly descends Qi for hypertension, panic, severe Qi stagnation
	ST-31	Pressure Needle	In labor, to descend digestive Qi (nausea, hiccups, belching, etc.) and relax pelvic floor During pregnancy, for intractable nausea
	LU-7	Needle – thread proximally, strong de Qi	Descends Qi to initiate labor *Use when labor needs to start but LU pulse is not floating*
	GB-20	Needle Redirecting pressure	For neck tension: needle toward UB-10 or steady pressure For hypertension: with GB-21 and GB-31, needle or pressure
	Helper Hang	Mom supported by partner or helper	Great for exhaustion or to encourage relaxation/acceptance
Nourish Yin and Blood, Stabilize Qi	KD-1	Redirecting pressure	"Panic Button" for fear, anxiety, rising Qi *Can also use moxa to warm cold moms*
	UB-17	Moxa Round rubbing	Nourishes blood for resilience during birth and postpartum lactation
	Inner ankle (KD-3)	**Slow gentle chafing**	**Nourishes Yin** to address anxiety, restlessness, lack of sleep
	Footrubs	Anything that feels good – thumb, circles, etc.	
	Belly Breathing		Grounds, comforts; for fear, panic, rising Qi *(combine with Handwich)*
	Inner Leg points	Gentle pressure Massage	
	SP-4	Needle	I have found this point reliable to calm premature contractions
	KD-9	Needle	Debra Betts uses this to calm premature contractions
	PC-6 and TE-5	Connecting pressure	Relieves shivering at transition Shivering/itching with epidural
Open space	**Sumo Squats** **Supported Squats**		*Sumo Squats also warm move – for fatigue, frustration, anger* *Supported Squats help fetal descent*
	Hip rocking		**Right side down for occiput posterior**, alternate with Cat/Cow, Hip Openers *Keeps labor moving when Mom is exhausted or stuck in bed*
	Pelvic vibrating		Reduces bony obstruction pain Encourages realignment
	Shaking the Apples		Strongly encourages realignment
	Hospital workout		Encourages realignment Circulates Qi, restores healthy posture in bed

Promote contractions	LI-4	Pulsing pressure	To strengthen Qi and contractions
	Duyin	Pulsing pressure Ear tack	To strengthen contractions
	UB-67	Needle	Encourages fetal movement Initiates contractions
		Tapping (fingernail or ear seed)	Initiates contraction, fetal movement
	Contractions Combination	Needles at LI-4, SP-6, sacral points (strong manual or electrical stimulation), birth basics ear seeds *Most appropriate when cervix is ripe; otherwise modify or use with caution*	
Raise Qi	Du-20	Two- or five-finger tapping	Clears the mind – for fatigue, dampness, brain fog (Mom or practitioner)
		Redirecting pressure	During pushing, to focus Qi on perineum (especially with epidural)
		Moxibustion	**With practice**, to raise Qi for threatened miscarriage or cervical shortening
	ST-13	Thread needle laterally	With Du-20 to prevent or address early cervical shortening
	SP-9	Redirecting pressure	With Du-20 for mental fogginess, to drain dampness downward and raise clear Qi
Reduce pain	Auricular pain points	Needle or seeds Spine points: thread needle or place seeds front and back Electrical stimulation	Cingulate gyrus, Thalamus For occiput posterior: Bladder, Constipation, Sciatica points For back pain: Spine points by palpation E-stim: sympathetic to endocrine
	LI-4	Strong pressure	Redirects Qi downward to relieve pain, progress labor
	LV-3	Needle Pressure (with KD-1)	With strong pressure – moves Qi and relieves stagnation/pain With gentle pressure – nourishes Blood and Yin, descends Qi
	LV-8	Needle Gentle pressure	Nourishes blood, promotes resilience during birth Promotes cervical ripening
	SP-6, SP-8	Needle	SP-6 can be taped down for mobility SP-8 is strong for pain but does not tolerate much movement
	LV-3, GB-34	Needle	Reduces non-bony pain, especially with tightness
	Also consider:	Grasping a comb – with Qi stagnation, heat Handwich – with fear or cold Hip rocking – when tired or stuck in bed Liver Gummies – with Qi stagnation Pressure at GB-30 or sacrum – for back pain Round rubbing mid-back – with blood deficiency SP-6 pressure – with Yin deficiency	

Soften cervix and/ or pelvic floor	Liver Gummies	Dredging upward	Anytime cervix is misbehaving – slow to ripen or dilate, rim/lip, edema *IMPORTANT to adjust pressure to Mom's tolerance* *If no change within the hour, check for cold or Yin/Blood deficiency*
	SP-6	Gentle pressure	Slow cervical ripening (deficient mom) Yin or Blood deficiency ***Can also chafe Liver Gummy area***
	Ear birth basics	Needles or seeds	Sympathetic, Uterus, Shenmen, Liver, Endocrine Add Spleen, Kidney or other organs as constitutionally appropriate
	Hula Hips		**Great for cervical ripening and to progress**
	Dancing		**labor** *(use bouncing if Mom is too shy to dance)*
	Gentle bouncing		
	Waist points	Redirecting pressure	Labor prep or labor to soften pelvic floor, especially prelabor rupture, not ready or strong woman syndrome *Combine with Belly Breathing, inflate pelvic floor downward with breath*
	Sacrotuberous and sacrospinous ligament release	Strong pressure	OP late in labor, to open "back door" Labor prep, 38 weeks or after
	LV-2 and LV-5	Needle E-stim Strong pressure	For cervix that is misbehaving due to stagnation – edema, slow ripening or dilatation (also consider cold)
	Inner Leg points	Gentle pressure Massage	Also nourishes Yin and Blood
	Below clavicle	Dredging outward	Before/during labor to soften the pelvic floor and cervix Strong woman syndrome
	Gallbladder channel	Dredging downward along iliotibial band	
	GB-31, GB-34 and GB-41	Needling	Usually two in combination to soften pelvic floor GB-31 is gentlest, most nourishing
	Lower back/ abdomen	Leg swinging	Best for hospital induction with unripe cervix
Warm Yang	**Lower back/ abdomen**	**Handwich**	Anytime Mom is cold or frightened Also softens cervix and pelvic floor Useful for locating body obstruction
	Inner ankle (KD-3)	Vigorous chafing	Warms Yang for cold, edema, sluggish contractions
	Cat/Cow		Also gently moves, opens space
Additional or compound therapies	Occiput posterior	5 minutes pressure each: UB-60, SP-6, UB-67 (or needles) Hip rocking, right side down (change to left if pain gets worse) Alternate with standing Hula Hips, Hip Openers	
	Postpartum Bleeding	Select from among: SP-1 – strong pressure with fingernail LI-4 or Duyin – pulsing pressure to promote contractions Nipple stimulation to promote contractions	

	Increase uterine Qi/ Blood flow	ST-36 – chafe or warm with palm Foot Uterus point – warm or gentle pulses with thumb	
	Nap and Dilate	SP-6 PC-6 KD-6	Reduces anxiety, replenishes Yin by encouraging sleep

Bold = core methods; shaded = comfort measure.

6.8 Key Points to Remember

- Once comfortable with basic labor support, practitioners can think about anticipating and working with problems in labor as they arise.

- In order to sort out what may be causing problems at any given time, it can be helpful to perform two simple sorting processes as shown in Table 6.1: phase of labor, and apparent nature of the problem.

  - Is the labor in latent phase, active phase, transition or pushing? Even for birth novices, this should be relatively clear.

  - Does the nature of the problem appear to be bony obstruction, challenges with dilation/contractions, or something of an emotional or spiritual nature?

- Bone-, flesh- and spirit-level obstructions are characterized as follows:

  - Bony obstruction, characterized by severe pain in non-standard location, resolved by movement.

  - Flesh, characterized by signs of insufficiency and/or obstruction of Yin, Yang, Qi or Blood.

  - Spirit, may present with or without overt emotional/narrative challenges.

- Within each combination of labor stage and obstruction type, the possibilities for what can be happening are relatively manageable. They can be addressed using the therapeutic principles and methods listed in Table 6.2.

DIFFERENTIAL ANALYSIS OF PROLONGED LABOR

A big piece of my PhD research was on how clinical knowledge can be transmitted through practice manuals. The executive summary is (1) present the material in an orderly list; and (2) don't list specific things practitioners should do, e.g. needling specific points. Instead, give them functions to fulfill, questions to ask or options to try. That's what I've done for this chapter, which is a practice manual for problem-solving in labor. It lists the events of birth in their usual approximate order from engagement and cervical ripening to transition and pushing, allowing practitioners to identify where problems are and consider possible approaches based on analysis of signs and symptoms. The list is numbered from 1 to 9 and organized in triangular form, with the ordinary landmarks of labor in the center, and possible challenges at each of the corners.

If the labor is going well, then the labor support cycle described in Chapter 5 should be all that's needed: support comfort, flow and balance, and learn more and reevaluate what's working as the labor unfolds. This chapter builds on that "learn more" step of the cycle through differential analysis, the process of clinical problem-solving by first looking at the possible causes of a difficulty encountered, then differentiating those causes by their other signs and symptoms. The 'Labor Triangle' below shows 9 key landmarks or challenges in labor. The challenges are the 3 'acute angles' of the triangle and practitioners should be on the alert for them at all times; the landmarks proceed more orderly from top to bottom. Each chapter section contains differential analysis and therapeutic options, as well as cross-references to other sections (e.g 'go to 3').

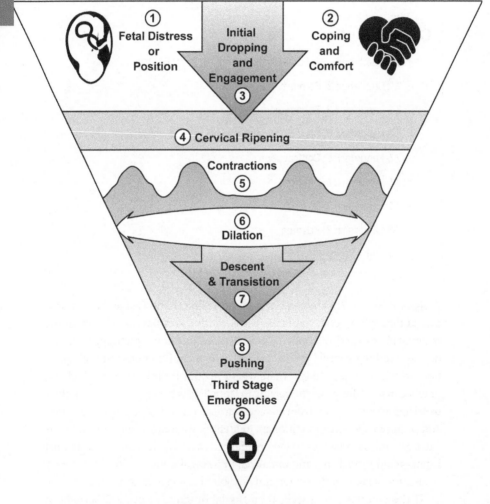

Figure 7.1 The labor triangle.

7.1 Challenges 1A, Fetal Distress; and 1B, Bony Obstruction

These two distinct situations are presented together because they are often considered together. Decelerations or "decels" – dips in the fetal heart rate that are taken as a warning sign for potential fetal distress – can also indicate that Baby's head is being compressed by a bone-against-bone impasse. A full discussion of fetal heart rate monitoring is outside of the scope of this book (though its relationship to East Asian medicine is a fascinating topic). The essentials needed for basic problem-solving are presented below.

7.1.1 Challenge 1A, fetal distress

Frustratingly, many potential signs of fetal distress can also present without serious problems, leading to surgical intervention in some cases where fetal health was not in fact compromised, though it appeared to be in danger. Potential signs of fetal distress include:

- Fetal heart rate decelerations, a change in baseline rate or a rate that is out of the "safe" range of 120–160 (bradycardia or tachycardia).

- Any of the above accompanied by vaginal bleeding (this suggests premature detachment of the placenta and calls for emergency delivery).

- Passing of meconium.

Table 7.1A Main presentations and therapeutic goals for fetal distress

1A: Main Presentations and Therapeutic Goals for Fetal Distress			
Tissue level	Bone	Flesh	Other
Presentations	Early decelerations before full dilation: likely asynclitism or malpresentation (Early decels with full dilatation usually suggest incipient delivery, no action required)	Fetal heart rate may be • slow in yang deficiency • highly variable in blood deficiency • rapid in yin or qi deficiency	Significant vaginal bleeding: *emergency – possible placental abruption, call for help* Passage of meconium – general sign of possible fetal distress, the thicker the more concerning
Therapeutic goals:	Move and encourage realignment	Identify and address possible insufficiencies	Support uterine blood flow
Key Therapeutic Methods:	**Vigorous hip rocking Cat/Cow Miles Circuit** Shaking the Apples	**Bradycardia, decels: warm or chafe ST-36 Tachycardia: SP-6 gentle pressure If fever: spray bottle and fan**, hand and/ or foot heat points, ear apex	**ST-36 (outer shin), Warm or chafe** Soo-jok uterus point: gentle pressure

Possible causes of distress or disrupted heart rate are as follows:

- Cord compression, resulting in V-shaped ("variable") decelerations occurring before or after contractions. This may be benign and resolve with position change, or it can be life-threatening if the cord is wrapped or kinked in such a way that it worsens as Baby descends. Our approach is to explore which positions and movements seem to produce positive change.

- Fever, resulting in tachycardia or baseline shift up: this may be a sign of infection, a side effect of epidural analgesia or simply the result of being in labor. Our approach is to clear heat. (Acupuncturists may also choose to "release the exterior" with SI-3 and/or TH-5 if there is an absence of sweating.)

- Head compression, resulting in "early" decelerations, meaning that the lowest point of the "decel" coincides directly with the vertex of the contraction. When presenting after transition, these mean that Baby is getting ready to be born! At any other time, they suggest that the head is pressing into something it shouldn't – either the sacrum or pelvis (as in asynclitism, occiput posterior (OP) or true cephalopelvic disproportion (CPD)). This pressure is usually accompanied by severe pain, which is not well covered by epidural. Our approach is to move Mom and pelvis, with the direction depending on the type and location of pain.

- Everything else, and the unknown: baby fatigue and/or illness can result in bradycardia, baseline shift down, late decelerations and/or passage of meconium. Unfortunately, meconium in the amniotic fluid can cause problems, even if the initial cause was benign. "Late" decelerations regularly occur after the peak of a contraction; if they persist despite oxygen and position change, they are an indication for Cesarean section. Placental insufficiency, cord wrap (around the neck, torso or legs), short cord and other unknown problems such as malpresentation or congenital defects can all have the same signs. In any of these cases, our approach is to warm points thought to guide Qi and Blood flow to the uterus.

One other important sign to be on the alert for is vaginal bleeding. Small amounts of pale or brownish blood may be present in vaginal mucus released during cervical ripening, and are benign. However significant amounts of bright red blood may indicate premature separation (abruption) of the placenta and warrant immediate medical attention.

Box 7.1 Challenge 1A, fetal distress: Differential analysis and assistance.

1. Significant vaginal bleeding – *call for medical help!*

2. Tachycardia:

    a. If fever, clear heat: hand points, foot heat points, spray mist and fan, ice chips.

    b. If no fever, warm ST-36 and/or foot Uterus point.

3. Bradycardia: warm ST-36 and/or foot Uterus point.

4. Early decelerations:

    a. After transition, likely benign, suggesting head is in place to push.

    b. Before transition, or with excessive pain: assume bony obstruction (go to 1B).

5. Decelerations late, variable or not sure: assume cord compression and change position, tracking carefully what's better or worse:

    a. Hip rocking – left side down, right side down.

    b. Reclining – pelvic vibrating.

    c. Standing or seated upright – Cat/Cow.

    d. Also warm ST-36 and/or foot Uterus point.

7.1.2 Challenge 1B, bony obstruction

Bony obstruction comprises true CPD as well as all the possibilities for functional CPD that present during labor: OP, asynclitism, malpresentation or any situation where the force of the contractions presses Baby's head against the pelvis and/or sacrum rather than against the cervix and out into the world.

Table 7.1B Main presentations and therapeutic goals for bony obstruction.

1B: Main Presentations and Therapeutic Goals for Bony Obstruction

General Signs:
- Persistent or sudden onset back pain
- Severe pain that wanders or is asymmetrical
- Ribside (fundal) pain

Type of bony obstruction	Presentation at engagement	Presentation during active phase	Presentation at transition
Occiput Posterior (OP)	Slow to engage Possible back pain Possible prelabor rupture of membranes Distinctive bump shape on observation or palpation	Back and/or sacral pain Distinctive bump shape on observation or palpation	Severe sacral pain relieved by counterpressure May occur suddenly at transition
Therapeutic goals:	Encourage rotation (usually right)	Open space Encourage rotation (usually right)	Loosen sacrotuberous and sacrospinous ligaments for OP delivery
Asynclitism	n/a	Labor may stall after 6 cm (typical of deficient moms) Extreme, bursting pain in front and back, will break through epidural (typical with strong moms and/or oytocin augmentation)	
Therapeutic goals:		Strongly move and encourage realignment	
True cephalopelvic disproportion (CPD)	Engagement does not occur – pelvis may be flat or simply small relative to fetus (e.g. underage)	Dilatation may arrest after 6 cm Descent may arrest after zero station	Unproductive pushing Swelling of fetal scalp (caput) Swelling of vulva
Therapeutic goals:	Treat as functional CPD until action is taken by primary care		
Functional CPD (Malposition, malpresentation)	Engagement does not occur – fetal head may be extended or arms up	Labor may be sluggish, pain may be severe or break through epidural	Various – unusual pain, sluggish progress, variable decelerations
Therapeutic goals:	Strongly move and encourage realignment		
OP Asynclitism – presents at late active phase True CPD – presents at engagement, transition Functional CPD	Two basic problems: • Slow cervical dilatation (same factors as ripening) • Contractions weak or irregular (Qi/Yang insufficiency)	Active phase is usually less sensitive to narrative challenges than latent and transition phases	Active phase is usually less sensitive to narrative challenges than latent and transition phases

Common signs of bony obstruction include:

- Unusual pain: any pain that is not located front and center is concerning, particularly if it is severe, or not covered by epidural. Locations and associated causes include:

  - In the back – this suggests OP.

  - In both front and back, with an extreme, bursting quality – this is typical of asynclitism (though the pain quality may be hard to differentiate from normal labor in Blood-deficient or first-time moms).

  - In one or the other inguinal groove, or wandering around the pelvis – this baby is lost, either wedged against the pubic ramus or seeking a way out through a pubic arch that is too narrow.

  - In the ribside or fundus (top of the uterus) – this is a concerning sign of bony obstruction, where the uterus presses painfully against Baby feet that just can't move down any more. I have most often seen it with true CPD.

- Labor is sluggish or contractions are irregular, with no signs of imbalance at the flesh or spirit levels. Common presentations and associated causes include:

  - Contractions may peter out in active phase or transition, with no signs of any fatigue or flesh/spirit problems.

- Less commonly, the cervical exam may be eccentric. A head station that is higher or lower than usual for its level of ripeness or dilatation, or a cervix that does not move anteriorly as it should, can be a flag for an unusual interface of head and pelvis:

  - The cervix is soft but the head is high. This suggests that the soft tissues are ripening appropriately, but the head is not pressing into the cervix due to true or functional CPD. This presentation is common in pharmaceutical inductions.

  - The cervix softens but remains posterior, suggesting that the head is not descending properly, likely because the pubic arch is narrow.

  - Less commonly, in asynclitism the side of Baby's head may jut downward below zero station before the cervix is well dilated.

As discussed in Chapter 3, OP is one of the more common reasons for non-engagement at term. When the baby's large occiput is positioned in back by the mother's spine, the angle of approach does not favor entering the pelvis, and Baby's head tends to butt into Mom's sacrum instead. This can cause back pain and quite commonly leads to prelabor rupture of membranes. Before labor has started, the situation is typically caused by Mom's postural habits (reclining with one's feet up, for example, encourages the baby to rotate backward). Baby may also be pushed OP by the shape of the pelvis during labor, whether he entered OP or occiput anterior (OA). In these cases the OP position will persist, and attempts to turn after transition may be counterproductive.

7.1.2.1 Occiput posterior

OP is usually not difficult to spot, once you know what you're looking for. Among the evaluation methods below, I generally start with the visual assessment, then use palpation to check myself. However, if I'm uncertain, I'll ask Mom if she has a clear sense of where her baby likes to hang out, and where she feels "kicks and wiggles." All of the support methods described here are quite benign before labor onset: they only function to encourage Baby into the right orientation, so if you're mistaken and Baby's position has righted already, they won't have any effect (other than perhaps helping the cervix to ripen).

On visual inspection, an OP bump simply looks funny (see Figure 3.5). Relative to a regular bump – where the baby's back faces outward, usually at a slight angle to the right or left, and makes a smooth curve from the buttocks down to the upper back – an OP bump usually has too much of it sticking out up high. This is the baby's knees you are seeing, and they are usually right in the center (which is not a common place for babies to hang out otherwise). If you're not quite sure what you're seeing (e.g. if Mom is overweight or there's a lot of fluid), then you can ask her to lie back briefly. It's important that this be brief – 30 seconds or less – because in pregnancy the weight of the baby on the inferior vena cava can cause problems. When Mom is lying back in an OP pregnancy, you can usually see a marked drop-off below the knees so that the navel, which should be pushed out convex by the baby's back, instead has an abnormal concave look to it.

When you palpate for OP you're just using your hands to check for the curve of the baby's back. Your first step (after asking permission and washing your hands) is to gently feel for the top of the bump – which should be the buttocks – right below the ribcage on the right or left of center. Remember, if the biggest protuberance of the bump is high and in the center, that's already a tipoff it's OP – most OA babies prefer to keep their backs angled left or right rather than directly forward. Your next step after finding the buttocks or knees is to check whether you can feel the back. Simply slide your hand down along where the back should be, and if instead of a smooth curve you feel a drop-off, that's clear confirmation of OP. You can then try palpating Mom's sides, between her hips and ribs to see if you can feel the baby's shoulders – this may tell you whether the baby is on the right or left, which is useful (though not strictly necessary) in encouraging the baby to come around to the front.

With OP before engagement, there may or may not be back pain. At this point, a hands-and-knees position (or rocking with the right side down) is usually sufficient to encourage rotation. This should be alternated with Cat/Cow to encourage engagement. The Miles Circuit[1] is also an excellent resource for encouraging rotation and engagement; it is a sequence of supported rest positions alternating with Hip Openers such as Stair-Crabbing (Section 5.5.6.1), which softens the hips and pelvic floor, and encourages optimal fetal positioning. It is freely available on the website below.

After engagement, shifting position is more challenging as Baby has less space to turn. If there are contractions, they will be painful in the back and may be "coupled" – two contractions close together, followed by a longer space. Some combination of the Miles Circuit or other Hip Openers, plus acupuncture or pressure at points such as UB-67, UB-60 and SP-6, are generally needed to open space for Baby to turn. Then movements such as hip rocking or Cat/Cow to encourage rotation may be successful.

After transition, OP back pain is severe, usually located at or next to the sacrum and relieved by strong counterpressure. The pain may be persistent, or may appear suddenly after transition, indicating that Baby has turned OP after descending normally. Like all bony obstruction pain, this will break through epidural analgesia. At this point I consider that positional change is no longer likely, and shift my efforts from encouraging rotation to "opening the back door" for OP delivery – using acupuncture and/or pressure to soften the pelvic ligaments, particularly the sacrotuberous and sacrospinous ligaments, which connect the pelvis and sacrum (see Figure 6.1).

Box 7.2 Challenge 1B, bony obstruction: Active differential analysis and assistance.

1. Pain in back – likely OP:

   a. If severe, reduce with counterpressure on sacrum or GB-30 on painful side, also pressure on UB-60.

   b. If before transition, Cat/Cow on hands and knees *or* hip rocking right side down; reassess in 15 minutes.

---

1   www.milescircuit.com

       i. If pain resolves – resume labor support.

       ii. If pain worsens with right-side rocking – immediately turn to left side down.

   c. If after transition or unresolved after 15 minutes – "open the back door."

       i. Seeds or tacks on UB-67, needle UB-60/SP-6. *Or*

       ii. Pressure on UB-60 (5 minutes); SP-6 (5 minutes); then UB-67 (ear seeds or fingernail pressure, 5 minutes). *Then*

       iii. Sacrotuberous and sacrospinous ligament release.

       iv. Alternate with Cat/Cow if tolerated.

2. Any other pain that is excessively severe, bursting, wandering, asymmetrical or fundal – true or functional CPD.

   a. Shaking the Apples or vigorous hip rocking; reassess in 10 minutes.

   b. If no change, try approaches below, reassess after 20 minutes:

       i. Alternate Hula Hips, Cat/Cow and Shaking the Apples with opposite side down.

       ii. If pain is in one inguinal groove, consider pelvic shaking from the femur on that side.

       iii. Consider Blood/Yin deficiency, fear/trauma as possible obstacles to coping (go to Item 2).

       iv. Treat as for OP (above).

       v. Soften pelvic floor: dredge GB channel or needles at GB-34, GB-41, ST-31.

       vi. Consider knee–chest "reset" (consult primary care practitioner).

Other than OP, which announces itself relatively clearly, most bony obstruction can only be surmised from the type of pain, or by a skilled vaginal exam. With experience, the Handwich can be helpful in palpating where the obstruction seems to be, and the hip rocking family of interventions can be useful in shaking the pelvis in a place and at an angle that can free it. Shaking the Apples in particular is extremely useful for asynclitism. If pain is clearly on the pubic ramus of one side, then shaking that side of the pelvis via the femur can be extremely helpful in nudging Baby toward the center. If the pain does not respond to treatment for bony obstruction, it is also worth considering flesh- and spirit-level problems such as Yin/Blood deficiency, fear and trauma.

7.2 Challenge 2, Comfort and Coping

Sometimes a labor powers ahead without permission, but my experience in hospital birth is that if latent phase contractions are not well within limits of copability, then the active phase will not want to kick in without medication. Fatigue, persistent nausea, hiccupping or belching can also make labor difficult and even traumatic. It is therefore critical that attention be maintained throughout to Mom's physical and emotional state and energy reserves.[2]

In general, effective contractions that progress the cervix are far better tolerated than contractions where the force is diverted into other tissues. In addition to being inherently undesirable, pain or distress that appears disproportionate to the size of the contraction often points to an underlying positional, constitutional or emotional issue that needs work before the labor can progress. These issues include:

- Contractions pressing bone against bone (this is bony obstruction – go to 1B).

- Contractions pressing the head into an unwilling cervix. The typical presentation of this pain is that labor appears to be ramping up in intensity, but a vaginal exam shows little progress. Underlying causes may be Qi stagnation or Blood or Yin insufficiency.

- More rarely, ineffective contractions where the uterus fights itself by contracting unevenly, or with an initiation site other than the fundus. As with squeezing a toothpaste tube, pressure initiated at the far end is most effective; contractions like this appear as smooth waves on the monitor. By contrast, contractions that look "spiky" indicate stagnation of Qi in Mom's abdomen (as she fights with pain) or within the uterus itself. Typically there is a history either of stagnation due to cold (e.g. painful periods that improve with warmth) or of surgery such as myomectomy, dilation and curettage (D&C) or previous Cesarean section.

- If vigorous methods for treating physical pain aren't working, consider the possibility that gentler methods more geared to calming the spirit are in order.

---

2   Although no great fan of epidural, I have been known to counsel Blood-deficient women struggling to endure mild contractions at 3 cm that requesting an epidural is like ordering a pizza on a rainy night: better not to wait until the need is urgent.

Table 7.2 Main presentations and therapeutic goals for comfort and coping.

2: Main Presentations and Therapeutic Goals for Comfort and Coping				
Level	Bone	Flesh	Spirit	Other
Presentations	Painful contractions: bony obstruction (go to 1B)	Painful contractions: • Qi stagnation • Yin/Blood insufficiency • Cold	Contractions hard to manage: • Spirit stuck (e.g. trauma, previous loss) • Spirit not ready (e.g. underage, inadequate birth education) • Emotional distress (fear, anger, anxiety, etc.)	Nausea, GI distress, hypertension: Redirect Qi downward Itching/shivering: • Ground the Qi • Warm as appropriate Fever, feeling hot: Clear heat
Therapeutic goals:		Restore flow in Liver/Yin channels Identify and address cold or insufficiency	Create safe space: • Find rest and safety between contractions • Breathe through contractions Move and/or redirect Qi to address emotion	
Key methods:	• Hip rocking (right side down unless that increases pain) • Strong pressure at GB-30 or sacral points • Shaking the Apples • Ear Bladder, Sciatica points • UB-60 and KD-3, pressure or needles	First line for pain: • LI-4 pressure, rocking, Belly Breathing, Handwich • LV-3 and KD-1 • Ear birth basics, Pain points Constitutional measures for pain: • Cold – heating pads or Handwich • Qi stagnation – movement e.g. rocking, Sumo Squat E-stim for pain: • Uterus to Zero, 2 Hz	• Fear, anxiety – KD-1, Handwich, Heart Area support or needle HT-3 • Low resilience, Blood deficiency – Handwich, round rubbing mid-back • Grief, disappointment – pressure or round rub emotional release points, needle LU-3 • Disappointment with change of birth plan – listen, reframe around East Asian medicine possibilities	Nausea: • Pressure at PC-6, direct downward LV-3 to KD-1 • Needle ST-31

Because the perception and management of discomfort is so personal, objective differential analysis is impractical. A real-time "action differential analysis" is preferable, learning from what does and doesn't work.

Constitutionally appropriate comfort measures should keep pain manageable. If they do not, consider bony obstruction (go to 1B). If unsure of constitution, first-line comfort measures include:

- BB Ears, Pain points

- LI-4 with contractions

- Hip rocking

- Handwich with Belly Breathing

- Doula squeeze

- Liver-3 and Kidey-1 – best for fear, panic

- electrical stimulation between the Uterus and Zero points can be very helpful, but should be saved for transition, as the effect cannot be counted on to last for an entire labor.

If the above approaches don't resolve discomfort, consider:

- Blood insufficiency – nourish Blood with round rubbing and soften the cervix with gentle Liver Gummies.

- Yin insufficiency – nourish Yin with ankle chafing and/or the Nap and Dilate protocol, and soften the cervix with gentle Liver Gummies.

- Cold – ask about cold feet and bottom, hating winter and history of dysmenorrhea. Warm with Handwich or heating pads.

- Disappointment with elements of birth plan, including comfort measures and birth team performance. In this situation, it can be useful to reframe the experience around what East Asian medicine (EAM) can do, explaining some of the basic concepts and taking the emphasis off previous expectations.

In an OP birth, extra discomfort should be anticipated. The following measures may help:

- Bladder-32, Gallbladder-30 – strong counterpressure

- Ear Bladder, Sciatica and Constipation points

- Bladder-60 and Kidney-3 – pressure or needles

Persistent nausea, vomiting, hiccupping or belching are seen as Qi moving the wrong way up the Stomach channel (episodic vomiting at transition is quite normal).

- All of these usually respond to pressure at PC-6.

- If persistent, consider:

  - connecting pressure at Liv-3 and KD-1

  - needling at ST-31 to draw Qi down the channel.

The most commonly seen types of emotional distress are considered below, along with treatment methods that tend to be effective. However, these are only starting points; all reproductive health practitioners will have built their own systems for recognizing and addressing distress:

- fear: KD-1 pressure, Handwich; HT-3

- anxiety: Handwich, KD-1 pressure; SP-6

- unresolved grief (e.g. recent bereavement, previous stillbirth): round rubbing at upper back (between shoulder blades) and pressure at LI-4; needling at LU-3 and 7, and pressure at LI-4

- strong or unresolved anger (including with members of the birth team): Liver Gummies; GB-21

- history of trauma including sexual trauma: KD-1, Handwich (as tolerated!); gentle pressure at SP-6; HT-3, SP-6, KD-6.

7.3 Landmark 3, Engagement

By week 38 or 39, there is usually a visible shift in how Baby is carried. Mom's back usually flattens out (i.e. becomes less arched) as the pelvic floor relaxes and the baby moves down into the pelvic opening. If Baby has been putting pressure on Mom's stomach and/or lungs (as is often the case), this often eases up, while urination becomes even more frequent. Also notable visually is a backward shift in the center of gravity and a change of walking gait, as weight transfers from the bump (out in front of her) to inside the pelvis (closer to her back and bottom). This process is known as engagement, described in Section 3.1.2. Engagement may occur as early as 36 weeks (particularly in first births and those with Qi deficiency). It is a promising sign when it does happen, but not necessarily pathological when it doesn't – particularly in those who have given birth before, and also those of African heritage, for whom Baby tends to descend later. As seen in Figure 3.14, the cervical ripening cycle depends on the pelvic floor and cervix being stretched by baby weight, and tissue softening tends to encourage fetal descent. In the absence of vaginal exam results, engagement can therefore be taken as a sign that the cervix is ripening.

If there is no time pressure, then a high head station is part of the clinical picture but not necessarily a problem to be solved. During a hospital induction, however, or with a looming due date, differential analysis should be conducted along the lines below:

- bone-related problems: OP (go to Section 7.2.2, bony obstruction), or CPD (true or functional)

- soft tissue problems: tight Belt channel, strong central Qi

- spirit challenges: spirit stuck or not ready

- indeterminate obstruction: short cord.

Table 7.3 Main presentations and therapeutic goals for engagement.

3: Main Presentations and Therapeutic Goals for Engagement				
	Bone	Flesh	Spirit	Other
Presentations	True cephalopelvic disproportion (CPD) Functional CPD: occiput posterior (OP), swayback, fetal presentation, etc.	Tight Belt channel Strong central Qi	Spirit stuck Spirit not ready Emotional distress (fear, anger, anxiety, etc.) All may present with or without tight Belt channel	Indeterminate obstruction, cord short or wrapped: no symptoms other than non-engagement May see decelerations if labor is induced
Therapeutic goals:	Move and encourage engagement	Move Qi and redirect downward Relax pelvic floor	Create safe space: Find rest and safety between contractions Breathe through contractions Move and/or redirect Qi to address emotion	Keep trying positional change; cord wrap or malpresentation may resolve
Key methods:	Hip rocking (right side down unless that increases pain) Cat/Cow, Hula Hips Shaking the Apples	Hip rocking Pressure on Waist points, GB-21, UB-60, SP-6 Dredging GB channel Needling ST-31, UB-60, 67, LU-7	Pressure at KD-1, Inner Elbow points Round rubbing or sequential pressure on emotional release areas Ear birth basics Needling by diagnosis; KD-1/HT-3, LU-7, etc.	Hip rocking (right side down unless that increases pain) Pressure on Waist points, GB-21, UB-60, SP-6 Dredging GB channel Cat/Cow, Hula Hips ear birth basics

7.3.1 True or functional CPD

It is not common that the head is genuinely too big to descend into the pelvis, but it does happen, most often with flat or platypelloid pelvis (see Section 3.1). True CPD can also occur in couples where the genetic father is much taller than the person carrying the baby, in teenage moms and in those who grew up under nutritional or other stress such that their own growth was less than the genetic potential. One reason I strongly recommend stretching the sacrotuberous ligaments as part of labor preparation treatments is that, in doing so, the practitioner get a sense of Mom's pelvic shape and size.

More common is what might be termed functional CPD, where the pelvis is not too small for the head in absolute terms, but acts as though it is, for one of several reasons. For example, if Baby's head is extended back rather than flexed forward, or asynclitically cocked to one side, then even the small head will be functionally too large to pass through the pelvis. Another common cause of functional CPD is where Mom's back is arched and tight due to the baby weight pulling forward on it. This swayback posture rotates the pelvis forward, which in turn swings the baby out away from the spine (which then worsens the pull on the back, keeping it all the more arched and tight). Acupuncturists will note that moms with a history of back pain are prone to this presentation, as are those with Yin or Yang deficiency. Diastasis recti (where the belly muscles pull apart) is also common in this situation.

Helping the back to relax and reduce its curvature is critical to labor preparation. In acupuncture, the space between the second and third lumbar vertebrae is called "Ming Men," or Life Gate; it is at the body's center of gravity, and learning to relax and "open" (i.e. flatten out) its curvature with the breath is important in many martial arts traditions. It is also where the catheter is inserted for epidural analgesia. Opening Ming Men creates an open pathway for gravity to drop the baby into the pelvis, while closing it literally blocks the way down, sending the baby weight forward.

7.3.1.1 Assessment and assistance for CPD

The sacrotuberous ligament release is not a precise method of assessing the pelvis, but it gives us an idea of the terrain. If the pelvis is long and narrow, we can be less aggressive in trying to resolve OP, as it's more likely that Baby will need to descend that way. Conversely, if the pelvis seems quite short from front to back, that's an indication to increase frequency and strength of labor preparation treatments, as the bigger Baby gets, the more realistic the possibility of true CPD. Thus, whether there is true CPD, or if the back is just arched and tight, the first step in labor preparation either way is to relax the back and help Mom open Ming Men. A key concept here is that it's the rare baby who is bigger than the pelvic opening in absolute terms: much more common is some combination of functional CPD and a relatively bigger baby having a relatively harder time finding just the right angle to enter. Therefore, at this early stage *I treat all suspected CPD as functional CPD*, on the grounds that it may help and won't hurt.

The treatment goal for functional CPD due to swayback and other causes is to relax, open and "enliven" Ming Men. The lumbar area is not mapped very precisely in our brains, meaning that many people have very little conscious awareness of the area to relax or move it, so that must be awakened. Bodywork and home exercises are thus key. Acupuncture, moxibustion and heating methods can also be extremely helpful in helping the back to relax and open, particularly in winter or if there is a history of back pain or injury. In particular, Cat/Cow and Hip Openers such as the Miles Circuit encourage Baby to drop into the pelvis by repeatedly opening the true pelvic space and aligning it with gravity. If this simple mechanical process does not work, then consider soft tissue or spirit challenges.

7.3.2 Tight Belt channel, strong central Qi

In some cases, there is no true or functional CPD, but the baby declines to drop prenatally, or even during active labor. As discussed in Chapters 4 and 6, this presentation is common for strong women with high-stress jobs, those with a history of sexual or other trauma and also those who just like their control. In most cases, particularly when there is traumatic history, the Yin channels of the inner thighs will also be quite tight. Liver Gummies are usually quite effective in helping to soften the Yin channels, but close attention must be paid to pressure – too much pressure will cause further tightening, particularly for trauma survivors.

As discussed in Chapter 3, the onset of labor can be seen as the direct result of Baby's weight exceeding the strength of Mom's Qi to hold it up. In patients with Qi deficiency, we try to guard against this happening too soon, but for physical and spiritual athletes who have trained their central channels to soar upward against gravity, the baby weight may not be a sufficient drag on the pelvic floor to stretch it and initiate cervical ripening. Most moms appear pretty weary by 39 or 40 weeks, with Baby's weight visibly taxing their strength, and a general sense of "losing it" with household and personal chores, particularly if there are older siblings to care for. When a 40-week pregnant patient twinkles into your office and asks you how *you* are doing, rather than making a beeline for the restroom or sagging into a chair, you can positively identify this clinical picture of core strength not yet letting go.

7.3.2.1 Assessment and assistance for tight Belt channel and/or strong central Qi

It is not urgent to distinguish between tight Belt due to stress and strong central Qi, as they often co-occur in busy working people, and treatment principles overlap. Direct questions like "How's your stress level?" and "How's it going getting everything ready?" will usually elicit whether stress is a primary or secondary contributor to the situation.

Exercises and lifestyle measures useful for releasing the pelvic floor include:

- acupressure at ST-31, GB-31 and the Waist points (Section 6.2.1)

- Belly Breathing (Section 5.5.7), gentle bouncing (Section 5.5.5), dancing, with as much shimmying as possible

- sex (as long as membranes are intact) and orgasm

Acupressure and birth bodywork measures include:

- strong steady pressure on KD-1 and the Waist points (GB-26), 5 minutes each

- the Handwich, particularly if there is anxiety or cold.

Auriculotherapy:

- Birth basics plus the Diaphragm point are useful to relax the pelvic floor.

- With needles, E-stim at 2 Hz may be run from Sympathetic to Diaphragm to calm and relax the pelvic floor.

Needling:

- GB-41, GB-34 and KD-1 are key points; ST-31 may also help to release the pelvic floor. In a lateral recumbent office treatment the GB points may be balanced with TH5 and LV-3 through to KD-1 (which also strongly descends Qi). Gentle hip rocking can be performed during needle retention, or more vigorously before and after.

- A seated treatment could include: Du-20 (going posteriorly); GB-21 (carefully, with shallow insertion); LI-4; GB-26, 31, GB-34 and GB-41; LV-3–KD-1 and SP-6. The Handwich can be performed during needle retention.

- When time is of the essence, E-stim at 2 Hz may be run between bilateral points GB-34 and SP-6 during a seated treatment, or from GB to 34-41 and Liv3–SP-6 in a lateral recumbent treatment.

Other:

- Throughout of the scope of this book, passive shimmying with a Rebozo,[3] vibrating massagers, and orgasms can all be extraordinarily effective for relaxing the Belt channel and central Qi.

7.3.3 Indeterminate obstruction: Spirit stuck, or short cord

It sometimes happens that the head stays up high, with no particular indications of any bony or soft tissue problems.

7.3.3.1 Assessment and assistance for indeterminate obstruction

It is not usually possible to make a positive determination of what causes a persistent reluctance to engage, once bony obstruction and tight soft tissue (plus or minus overt emotional challenges) have been probed without positive findings. As a point of differentiation, short cords may stall the labor at any point up to delivery, while spiritual and emotional disruptions tend to occur before engagement, early in active phase when contractions ramp up, or around transition.

Debra Betts reports unequivocal statements from the midwives she has trained that GB-21 acupressure normally works quite well to assist descent – except when the cord is short. This is my experience as well. As with actual versus functional CPD, I make a policy of treating as though the problem is a resolvable one. This means addressing the spirit when bone and soft tissue approaches have not worked, even if there aren't any overt signs of emotional challenge, and circling back to look for possible bone or soft tissue problems. I may have missed something in my assessment, and if not, then the treatment will help Mom to stay comfortable as long as possible.

In terms of therapeutic methods, there is an important distinction to draw between releasing a tight Dai Mai in a stressed-out person, and inviting the deep emotional and spiritual release that allows Baby to descend. The deeper and more subtle the emotional blockage, the gentler and quieter the release needs to be – versus release of a physical tightness based in stress, where vigorous movement such as shimmying is in order. If deep ambivalence or emotional blockage is suspected, try these deeper, gentler techniques first, then proceed to more physical release if there's no change – and vice versa.

---

3   This long Mexican shawl is used for a variety of purposes including birth, postpartum recovery and child-carrying. Many doulas use them; an excellent guidebook in languages including English, Russian and German is available at https://rebozo.nl/shop

Exercise, acupressure and birth bodywork approaches to calm the spirit and assist descent include:

- strong bilateral pressure downward on GB-21

- Handwich with Belly Breathing

- simultaneous pressure and/or needling on PC-6 and ST-31

- KD-1 acupressure (just gently holding the point provides a "pull" downward, versus GB-21's "push").

Auriculotherapy and needling approaches to calm the spirit and facilitate delivery include:

- birth basics plus Sympathetic and Zero (consider mild electrical stimulation between Sympathetic and Zero at 2 Hz)

- Du-20 (needled transversely), Du-24 and Yintang

- for acupuncturists – reconnecting Heart and Kidney: KD-6 and KD-10, PC-5 and HT-3 or comparable points (substitute LU-3 and LU-7 if there is a history of pregnancy loss or other grief).

7.4 Landmark 4, Cervical Ripening

Appropriate softening of the cervix at term leads to dilatation and effacement of the cervix, and depends on sufficiency and harmonious interplay of multiple factors. As discussed in Chapter 3 and seen in Figure 3.14, estrogen must be high and progesterone must drop appropriately, while relaxing increases and tissue stretch initiates a cascade of local prostaglandin secretion. In EAM terms, Yin and Yang must be sufficient and interacting appropriately to support the hormonal changes that soften the cervix, while abundant Blood and Yin are also necessary for the cervix to willingly shorten and open. Cervical unwillingness is expressed by pain and lack of progress in varying degrees. The cervix may also resist effacement and dilatation if Qi flow is stagnated by emotions, or by the presence of cold in the uterus.

Some differential analysis is therefore possible based on the Bishop Score findings. A complete lack of softening is usually indicative of Yin or Yang deficiency, or some blockage of their interaction that interrupts the normal hormonal flows. If there is some softening but dilatation and/or effacement are reluctant, then Qi stagnation is most likely, and underlying factors of blood deficiency, cold and stress or other emotional and spiritual causes need to be differentiated. Head station has been discussed above. *If the head is still unengaged, that in itself may be sufficient cause for lack of cervical ripening, so careful differential analysis should also be conducted to identify and address possible factors keeping the head high.* The final element of the Bishop Score is movement of the cervix forward in the vagina, which indicates that the fetal head and/or forewaters are appropriately curving down and forward through the pelvis. It's uncommon that this forward movement lags behind the other components of cervical ripening, but when it does it usually indicates either tight muscles and ligaments around the sacrum and coccyx, or else a pelvis that is narrow in front and will not allow much forward movement.

Table 7.4 Main presentations and therapeutic goals for cervical ripening.

4: Main Presentations and Therapeutic Goals for Cervical Ripening				
Level	Bone	Flesh	Spirit	Other
Presentations, goals and methods for no initial softening of cervix	If not engaged, also consider 3	Yin insufficiency – nourish and ground: SP-6 pressure, Yin footrubs Yang insufficiency, Yang blocked by damp or cold: warm and activate Yang: heating pads or Handwich, Cat/Cow	Heart Qi not descending: • Pressure at chest center, top of fundus, KD-1 • Needle RN-17, 15, KD-1, HT-3	Also promote hormonal activity: ear birth basics; romantic movies, orgasm, etc.
Presentations, goals and methods for soft cervix not moving anteriorly	Occiput posterior (OP), true or functional cephalopelvic disproportion (CPD) – go to 3	Tight Dai Mai, strong central Qi – go to 3 Tight lumbosacral area – move Qi – thumb circles on sacral points and coccyx; hip rocking	Not usually a spirit problem	Indeterminate obstruction – keep moving
Presentations, goals and methods for cervix slow to efface/dilate (latent phase)	Bony obstruction (go to 1B)	Cold – warm Yang: heating pads/Handwich, Cat/Cow Qi stagnation – move Qi: Liver Gummies, dancing Yin or Blood deficiency – nourish and ground: SP-6 gentle pressure, Yin footrubs plus gentle Liver Gummies	Tight Liver/Yin channels due to stress, trauma or history of previous injury – nourish and ground, calm spirit: KD-1 or SP-6 pressure, Handwich as tolerated	For all spirit challenges, delineate safe space

7.4.1 Cervix not softening

Even in multiparas who tend to hold their babies high until the last minute, some softening of cervical tissue should be palpable on vaginal examination by 38 weeks if not before. A firm cervix after this time can be taken as an indication that the EAM causes and conditions for Western hormonal activation are not in place. These may be Yin or Yang deficiency, or blockage of hormonal function by damp or other factors (such as occurs in polycystic ovarian syndrome). As seen in the discussion of non-engagement above, a traumatic history may also interfere with Qi flow between the heart and reproductive system, preventing progress.

With appropriate differential analysis, prelabor office visits can be very successful in setting the hormones back on the right track. However, if the window for home birth opens and closes, then hospital induction starts with application of topical prostaglandins to soften the cervix, obscuring this key symptom of hormonal insufficiency. In this instance, aggressive treatment with Liver Gummies to soften the Liver channel, and hip rocking to stretch the soft tissue and promote uptake of the topical prostaglandins can be of help, along with differential analysis of underlying constitutional causes as described below.

7.4.1.1 Assessment and assistance for cervix not softening

In many of the cases where the cervix does not soften at all, there has been use of assisted reproductive technology, suggesting underlying hormonal and/or constitutional challenges. Common presentations for differential analysis and assistance are as follows:

- Yin is insufficient; Yang is either insufficient or blocked by damp – these can be recognized and addressed as discussed in Chapter 4.

- Not descending due to trauma – *KD-1 acupressure* is the simplest way to assist descent when trauma is suspected. EAM practitioners may recognize the pattern of Heart and Kidney not communicating and treat according to their habit. In the hospital I needle contralateral HT-3 and KD-3, plus Ren-17, the latter two threaded downward and HT-3 threaded with channel flow. These can be taped and retained. In an office visit I treat these points bilaterally, adding Ren-15 and Ren-4.

If you're not sure about your differential analysis, then the following basic treatment principles and methods are always a step in the right direction. They also make a good core treatment to which more specific points or methods can then be added.

- Acupressure or acupuncture: SP-6, LI-4, UB-32 to soften and activate.

- Auriculotherapy: birth basics.

- Electrical stimulation: SP-6 to SP-6; Sympathetic to Endocrine (especially useful if there is anxiety; one side only). Mild stimulation at 2 Hz.

- Handwich, plus any other core repertory bodywork that is constitutionally appropriate and/or feels good.

7.4.2 Cervix not moving anteriorly

This is not a common presentation. As discussed in Chapter 3, it is normal for pelvic floor and cervical softening to happen in tandem, as the baby's head and/or forewaters drop into the forward-curving space of the pelvis, naturally lowering Mom's center of gravity, opening the lumbus and moving the cervix forward.[4]

If the cervix softens but does not move anteriorly, and Baby remains high, then this is still a problem of initial dropping, but with hormonal factors ruled out by the softening cervix. Remaining possibilities are:

- OP

- true or functional CPD

- tight Dai Mai/strong central Qi

- short cord/spirit not ready.

In some cases, the problem may be tightness of the lumbosacral area and/or coccyx. These can be released manually with thumb circles and hip rocking, or by local and distal needling.

7.4.3 Cervix not effacing and/or dilating (latent phase)

Cervical ripening and contractile activity tend to progress roughly in tandem. Effacement and dilatation tend to precede contractions in Qi- or Yang-deficient moms, and contractions sometimes progress more quickly than cervical ripening in those with deficient Yin or Blood. Absence or irregularity of palpable contractions in latent phase is not necessarily pathological, as long as the cervix ripens and dilates. The evaluation and intervention approaches below cover the situation where the contractions are becoming regular and there is significant discomfort that lasts more than 30 seconds, but the cervix is not yet shortening and/or opening.

Cervical effacement and dilatation are reported as separate parameters in the vaginal exam, and may advance at different speeds. In general, effacement needs to precede dilatation, as a long cervix cannot open much. By the time the cervix has dilated 3–4 cm, 70 percent is typical. "Cervical lip," is when the anterior or (occasionally) lateral aspect of the cervix remains thick, even as the rest of the cervix has thinned and retracted entirely. Conversely, the entire cervix may thin out, but with little dilatation. In my experience, radical mismatch between effacement and dilatation is a clear sign of Qi stagnation

---

4   My colleague Yi-Li Wu cites at least one source for which "Ming Men opening" prior to birth referred not to the lower back but to the cervix itself.

in the Liver channel, and usually resolves easily with Liver Gummies or other treatment to move stagnation in the channel. Slow progress of both effacement and dilatation may result from simple Qi stagnation, or from underlying factors such as Yin or Blood deficiency.

7.4.3.1 Evaluation and differential analysis for cervix not effacing and/or dilating

- Effacement and dilatation are only directly assessed through vaginal exam. Appropriate effacement and dilatation can usually be assumed if the labor is increasing in intensity hour by hour.

- If the cervix is not effacing and/or dilating, this is Liver Qi stagnation with possible underlying factors. These include:

  - Constitutional predisposition to Qi stagnation: look for full stagnation signs such as full pulse, robust build, history of menstrual pain/premenstrual syndrome or higher than usual drama quotient in the labor room or life story.

  - Yin or Blood deficiency: look for deficiency flags such as age, anemia, poor nutritional history, hard work, pallor, slenderness and pulse that is not appropriately full and large for pregnancy. Distinguish Yin and Blood based on physical and emotional presentation. In early labor, Blood deficiency tends to present with helplessness and low "copability" relative to contraction size, while Yin deficiency is more impatient and resists assistance or touching.

  - Cold cervix due to constitutional Yang deficiency or current viral infection. Look for current feelings of cold, or constitutional history of chilliness and/or painful periods better with warmth.

  - Local tightness/trauma to the Liver channel. Inquire delicately about history of sexual trauma, or history of previous injury to cervix, e.g. LEEP,[5] termination of pregnancy or other surgical procedures.

---

5   Loop electrosurgical excision procedure, meaning removal of abnormal cells from the cervix using a small wire loop. Scarring may cause difficult or asymmetrical dilatation, or (rarely) early cervical shortening.

7.4.3.2 Assistance for cervix not effacing and/or dilating

- For cold cervix, first ensure the room is warm and/or there are plenty of covers, then use local warming techniques:

  - Heating pads front and back are best. If not available, use hands.

  - If there is no change with 30–60 minutes of warming, then alternate moving/softening approaches below, 30 60 minutes each, as comfortable.

- Choose techniques from the moving/softening section of the toolbox.

  - Liver Gummies are key for full stagnation; the birth team should rub them out vigorously every 30 minutes, alternating with active dancing/moving.

  - With deficiency, cold or trauma, Gummies should be rubbed out quite slowly and gently, as tolerated. If there is discomfort with contractions, use steady pressure on SP-6 during contractions then return to Liver Gummies.

  - Slow, gentle round rubbing behind the diaphragm is key for Blood deficiency and trauma; footrubs and SP-6 pressure for Yin deficiency.

  - Hip rocking is helpful for everyone, particularly for for deficient moms, and for active people stuck in bed.

7.5 Landmark 5, Contractions

As discussed in Chapter 3, when Baby has dropped and the cervix is ripening, this indicates that the "first gear" of labor has kicked in. Prostaglandins in their binding sites have made tissues stretchier, and tissue stretch is stimulating increased prostaglandin secretion. Once sufficient prostaglandin binding has taken place, binding sites for oxytocin should open, enabling uterine tissue to behave like heart tissue by propagating contraction waves electrically from cell to cell. These start irregularly at first, as disparate sites in the uterus initiate separate signals. But as the Yang Qi of the uterus consolidates (with help from the Belt channel), the contraction pattern should become regular and gain strength. Contractile effectiveness does not depend on individual muscle fibers pulling harder, but rather on increased recruitment of muscle fibers, and better coordination of their effort.

In EAM, Yang and Qi together (aka Yang Qi) are responsible for recruiting and coordinating muscle fibers. Yang initiates the contractile activity, so when it is insufficient or blocked (by damp, cold or malposition) contractions will be absent, irregular and/or slow. Qi coordinates the contractions, so when it is scattered by fear or pain, or depleted by the stresses of pregnancy and labor, contractions will be small, short and ineffective. On the contraction monitor, rather than a smooth wave shape, they may show up as spiky looking (this is usually pain) or just oddly shaped.

Table 7.5 Main presentations and therapeutic goals for contractions.

5: Main Presentations and Therapeutic Goals for Contractions			
Level	Bone	Flesh		Other
Presentations, goals and methods for absent or inadequate contractions	True cephalopelvic disproportion (CPD) Functional CPD: occiput posterior (OP), swayback, fetal presentation, etc.	Insufficient Yang – warm Yang: heating pads or Handwich, ankle chafing Insufficient Qi – activate Qi: chafing Stomach line, movement, encouragement Damp – warm, activate and prevent stagnation: all above methods, with movement and frequent change		If ripe cervix with some contractile activity, contraction wrangling: 4 minutes ankle chaffing, 45 seconds tapping UB-67 If ripe cervix but no contractile activity, consider strong manual or electrical stimulation at sacral points
Presentations, goals and methods for stalled contractions	Bony obstruction (go to 1B)	Fatigue – encourage rest: Yin footrubs, Nap and Dilate protocol If sleep is not possible then more aggressive pain management, e.g. auricular E-stim or Western analgesia	Spirit not ready (go to 2)	Indeterminate obstruction – keep moving

7.5.1 Evaluating adequacy of contractions

- At home, duration and intensity of sensation are usually the most reliable indices of contraction effectiveness. The primary birth helper should time contractions for both interval and duration. Additionally, intensity should be graded as easy, moderate and strong. The key criterion for "strong" is that Mom should not be able to talk through them. Focusing inward and becoming "non-distractable" is a very positive sign of intensity. Duration should be estimated from beginning to end of the "strong" period.

- If in doubt regarding actual contraction intensity, it is useful to practice palpating contractions. Find an area of uterus that does not have a baby head or behind in it, and hold that during a contraction. The traditional mnemonic is that mild contractions feel like your nose, moderate ones feel like your chin and strong effective ones feel like your forehead. With practice, this actually becomes quite easy to assess.

- In the hospital, the contraction monitor is relatively reliable for frequency and duration of contractions, with some false negatives caused by missed signals with thick adipose tissue or side-lying position. It is not particularly reliable for strength, usually over-reporting strength in tight bellies and under-reporting in slack ones. It is thus useful to keep a watchful eye on regularity and duration and regularity as the most reliable indices of Yang and Qi (respectively) flowing through the labor.

7.5.2 Differential analysis and assistance with absent, irregular or inadequate contractions

Adequate contractions in active phase are 2–5 minutes apart, last about a minute, and are of at least moderate intensity. In order to effectively differentiate and assist with inadequate contractions, it is important first to rule out OP position and functional CPD due to swayback (go to 3). These are both common causes of absent, irregular or inadequate contractions, due to the head not providing appropriate pressure on the cervix (true CPD and malpresentation should also be kept in mind, as they cannot practicably be ruled out).

- Once OP and functional CPD due to swayback have been ruled out, the constitution should be assessed for Yang/Qi insufficiency, and for damp.

  - For insufficient Yang, heating pads and ankle chafing are key.

  - For insufficient Qi, Stomach line chafing is key, along with movement and encouragement from family.

  - For damp, all of the above may be of help, along with as much movement as possible to keep Qi flowing; change methods every 10–20 minutes to reduce stagnation.

- Absent of any constitutional conditions that would explain the lack of contractions, CPD or unusual issues of position/presentation are more likely, and should be discussed with the primary birth care providers if possible. Vigorous targeted movements such as hip rocking and Shaking the Apples are in order.

- In addition to the constitutionally based treatments above, the following situational treatments may be used to increase contractile activity if time is of the essence:

  - If there is some contractile activity, contraction wrangling can often help to establish a regular contraction pattern. I generally apply the technique for 20–30 minutes, then withdraw for 20 minutes and reassess, repeating if the pattern has improved but needs more help.

  - If there is no contractile activity at all, strong manual or electrical stimulation at the sacral points may jump-start the process.

7.5.3 Contractions as the pulse of the labor

Acupuncturists will find that contraction patterns on a tocometer screen strongly resemble the pulse images they studied in school. For non-acupuncture birth professionals, differential analysis of contraction frequency, regularity, duration and strength can provide a very clear picture of constitutional vulnerabilities even before they manifest in labor dysfunction, as follows:

- Slow, regular contractions indicate that Yang is insufficient and/or blocked by damp.

- If contractions become irregular during active phase, this is a concerning sign that Yang Qi is not flowing adequately through the labor due to bony obstruction.

  - Consider OP, asynclitism, severe deficiency, trauma or excessive pain.

- Rapid, small contractions suggest Yin deficiency (they are also a common side effect of cervical ripening agents, particularly topical prostaglandins).

  - Yin governs quiescence, so when it is constitutionally insufficient (or depleted by lack of sleep, as is common in laboring women) the uterus is unable to fully relax between contractions.

- Coupled contractions: these appear in pairs, where a second contraction wave begins before the first has subsided. They represent an extreme disruption of the uterus's Yin settling function, and appear most commonly with cervical ripening meds and when the uterus is being physically irritated.

- Irritation may occur with OP (the uterus is being pinched between the sacrum and the baby head), and with low fluids or ruptured membranes (the uterus is contracting onto baby shoulders and knees rather than a watery cushion).

- Weak contractions: these indicate insufficiency of Qi, due to constitution or fatigue.

- Short contractions with Pitocin. These appear on the tocometer as "spikes" up and quickly down again, indicating a moderate to high intensity of contraction but with no "shoulders," as the peak lasts 20 seconds or less.

  - These are a concerning sign that the uterus is becoming exhausted, and should be considered as an indication of risk for postpartum hemorrhage.

- "Spiky-looking" contractions on the tocometer. These generally indicate pain, and often improve quickly with acupuncture and/or LI-4 pressure.

  - The more irregularly shaped the contraction, the less Yang Qi is flowing through the labor and the less progressive the contraction is. Consider bony obstruction (go to 1B) and other causes for difficulty coping (go to 2).

  - Occasionally, this pattern is caused by incoordination of contractions within the uterus, usually with a surgical history, e.g. Cesarean section or myomectomy.

    » In these cases the spikiness should be taken as a concerning sign of potential for rupture, the spikier and the less relaxation between contractions, the more concerning.

7.5.4 Evaluation and assistance for stalled contractions

Once contractions have become strong and regular during active phase, they should remain so. Loss of a good contraction pattern is a concerning sign suggestive of bony obstruction, or new onset fatigue or trauma reaction. Constitutional approaches are usually *not* sufficient to address contractions that become weak or irregular during the course of active phase, after initially being adequate. In general, any constitutional difficulties sufficient to disrupt active phase will already have shown themselves during latent phase. Differential analysis is as follows:

- Consider bony obstruction (go to 1B).

- Consider spirit stuck or not ready (go to 2).

- If fatigue from lack of sleep or a long labor is sufficient to disrupt the contraction pattern then a change of plan may be necessary. If the head is still above zero station and the cervix is not yet fully dilated, then it is unlikely that a fatigued person will be able to power through without a nap, particularly if this is their first birth. Calming methods including *Yin footrubs* and the Nap and Dilate protocol are in order.

- If sleep is not an option due to pain, this may be the point at which to discuss a more aggressive pain management plan, including auricular E-stim and/or Western analgesic methods.

Contractions may slow down or reduce in size at transition. *This is a common phenomenon, and is not pathological.*

- At home, it is usually clear from Mom's increased focus that deep work is being done inside and contractions are backing off to facilitate it. However, in the hospital it is easy to assume that something is wrong and needs fixing.

- If the clinical picture is otherwise consistent with the possibility of transition, allow 30 minutes or so before intervening. After this time, incomplete transition due to asynclitism or other causes should be considered as a possibility (go to 7).

7.6 Landmark 6, Dilatation

In order to assess a problem with dilatation, contractions need to be adequate – on their own. If oxytocin is in use, then the head must also be engaged (−2 or −1) before a problem with dilatation *per se* can be attributed.

7.6.1 Evaluation and differential analysis of slow dilatation

Differential analysis and assistance for this situation includes some of the same bony problems and constitutional disharmonies that cause difficulties with engagement (Section 7.4) and cervical ripening in latent phase (Section 7.5). These include:

- OP.

- constitutional predisposition to Qi stagnation

- Yin or Blood deficiency

- cold cervix due to constitutional Yang deficiency or current viral infection

- tight Dai Mai or strong central Qi

- short cord

Possible new onset problems include:

- Asynclitism (go to 1B).

- New onset emotional difficulties: fear, frustration, unskillful cervical exams and/or difficulty with family members are all capable of slowing or even reversing progress. These can be recognized situationally and addressed using the comfort and coping approaches in Challenge 2.

Table 7.6 Main presentations and therapeutic goals for dilatation.

6: Main Presentations and Therapeutic Goals for Dilatation				
Level	Bone	Flesh	Spirit	Other
Presentations, goals and methods for slow dilatation	OP (go to 3) Asynclitism (go to 1B)	Cold, Qi stagnation, Yin or Blood deficiency – go to 4 Tight Dai Mai or strong central Qi – go to 3	New onset emotional difficulties or stressors – go to 2	Indeterminate obstruction – keep moving
Presentations, goals and methods for cervical lip or edema	n/a	Local Qi stagnation – strongly move Qi: Liver Gummies, needling, E-stim or strong pressure at LV-2, LV-5	n/a	n/a

Therapeutic goals and methods most effective to assist dilatation during active phase based on constitution are identical to those presented in Section 7.4. For asynclitism before transition, vigorous hip rocking and Shaking the Apples are usually sufficient, alternating with Cat/Cow. Resolution of asynclitism usually results in an improved contraction pattern with less pain. New onset emotional difficulties can be addressed with the clearing sequence: create a safe space, address the distress and calm the spirit.

7.6.2 Cervical lip and cervical edema

Cervical lip and cervical edema are treated similarly, though they are quite different presentations. Both present toward the end of labor and respond well to Liver Gummies and other EAM methods.

It is also fairly common that a cervical "lip" or "rim" remains as an obstacle to descent. An anterior lip is the most common, and is generally the result of laboring supine. It is often soft and easily reduced by the practitioner, and does not have any particular constitutional indication. If the lip is thick or tough in character, is located asymmetrically or posteriorly and/or resists manual reduction, this is a clear sign of stagnation in the Liver channel and can be addressed with Liver Gummies, which almost always resolve the problem in short order. If they don't, this may indicate a problem with descent of the head (which should be addressed as a problem with transition). Conversely, the lip may be particularly tough or develop cervical edema.

Cervical edema occurs when the cervix swells, typically as a result of pushing before full dilatation. (The urge to push is sometimes very strong as early as 5 cm, and is usually a sign of liver stagnation. In hospitals it is often medicated away with epidural, but I find it is usually managed quite well with hip rocking or a Rebozo shimmy. The shaking somehow seems to break up the urge.) Once it has occurred, cervical edema can be very hard to manage, as the swollen cervix both impedes progress and also swells more in relation to increased pressure. One of the many reasons I am grateful to Jean Levesque is his insight that cervical edema responds well to strong stimulation at LV-2. This can be strong acupressure, an ear tack, needling at LV-2 and LV-3, or even electrical stimulation between LV-2 and LV-5.

7.7 Landmark 7, Descent and Transition

Once the head is engaged, there are no bony obstacles to descent until the ischial spines at the mid-pelvis. Reluctance of the head to descend to zero station therefore most commonly relates to insufficiency of contractions or tightness in the cervix and pelvic floor (discussed in the sections above). If sluggish contractions and/or slow dilatation have already presented in active phase, then slow descent of the head makes perfect sense, and can be assisted using the same approaches and modalities. Particularly in slow first labors where cervical ripening meds or augmentation have been deployed, it is not uncommon that the cervix finally arrives at full dilation with the head still at −1 station, and there is a need to "labor down." A rest period of 30–60 minutes provides an opportunity to recharge the Qi, allowing contractions more time to descend the fetal head before transition and pushing.

Table 7.7 Main presentations and therapeutic goals for descent and transition.

Landmark 7: Main Presentations and Therapeutic Goals for Descent and Transition				
Level	Bone	Flesh	Spirit	Other
Presentations, goals and methods for arrest of descent before transition	Occiput posterior (go to 3) Asynclitism, true or functional cephalopelvic disproportion (CPD) (go to 1B)	Tight Dai Mai or strong central Qi – go to 3	New onset emotional difficulties or stressors – go to 2	Indeterminate obstruction – keep moving
Presentations, goals and methods for stalled transition	Bony obstruction (go to 1B)	Fatigue: • If time allows, encourage rest: Yin footrubs, Nap and Dilate protocol • If no time, activate Qi: chafe, warm moxa or needle ST-36, tapping Du-20	Narrative challenges may include fear, insecurity, grieving for past, or relationship with current birth team: listen carefully and provide appropriate support	Indeterminate obstruction – keep moving Sluggish baby – support uterine blood flow: warm or chafe ST-36, foot Uterus point gentle pressure, tapping UB-67 Insufficient movement – Activate Qi: Cat/Cow, hip rocking, hospital workout

7.7.1 Arrest of descent before transition

In the less-common circumstance that the contractions are clearly adequate and the cervix dilates fully – but then progress arrests above the mid-pelvis – the arrest is a concerning sign. Possible causes for arrest of descent before zero station include:

- short or wrapped cord
- true or functional CPD: the fetal head may be large, or held at an inappropriate angle (e.g. military or face presentation), or there may be a compound presentation
- new onset emotional difficulties
- tight Dai Mai or strong central Qi.

This is a similar set of factors to those that disrupt transition, with evaluation and assistance for both discussed below.

7.7.2 Transition

As discussed in Chapter 3, Transition is the pivotal point at which Baby, having (optimally) entered the pelvis with the occiput transverse or obliquely forward, now turns direct OA to fit between the ischial spines at the mid-pelvis and the ischial tuberosities on the way out. By the end of transition, Baby is below the pelvic midpoint (usually +2 station), with the occiput facing anteriorly and the cervix fully dilated – all ready for Baby to slide out under the pubic arch in the second stage.

In general the larger the baby is in relation to the pelvis, the more closely she has to stick to this plan, if she is to successfully turn and dive through the curved space of the pelvis. Smaller babies have more wiggle room, which they occasionally use to paint themselves into corners, as with asynclitism. Emotional or traumatic factors may also obstruct progress, and if suspected should be explored through delicate questioning and close observation at this sensitive time. Absent of any indication of traumatic past or ambivalence about the future, movement and position change are the primary methods of addressing a stalled transition.

7.7.3 Stalled transition

In order to understand stalled transition, it is necessary to consider how normal transition is evaluated. Although the endpoint of transition is clear, its beginning is not well defined and signs may be difficult to spot, particularly when there is an epidural on board. Depending on the physical relationship of a woman's cervix to her pelvis, the fetal head may reach the ischial spines and be forced to begin turning as early as 7 cm. Conversely, the circumstances of labor may be such that she arrives at full dilatation with the head as high as −1 station (this presentation is particularly common when the labor has been initiated with cervical ripening medications and augmented with oxytocin).

In an unmedicated labor, transition in process can usually be recognized by one or more of the following signs:

- New onset vomiting, as the small intestine is perturbed by the gross movements of the fetus next door.

- Increase of intensity *between* contractions, so that the "non-distractible" quality persists throughout.

- The contractions themselves may *decrease* in intensity, or may space out; often there is a quiet stretch for 5–6 minutes while Baby turns, then a series of powerful contractions stimulated by the lower head station.

- Mom's attention seems (appropriately) directed inward to her physical experience; movement will often appear spontaneous and instinctive.

- Verbal communication stops being meaningful (particularly non-native languages).

- A strong feeling of rectal pressure develops, together with a powerful urge to push.

In births with an epidural, there may be vomiting and occasionally there is an increased sense of focus during transition. However, more commonly the end of transition appears to come abruptly out of nowhere, with a sudden strong sense of pressure (which is not covered by the epidural). Moms may begin pushing instinctively, which can be seen on the contraction monitor as small, sharp increases in pressure on the contraction monitor.

Other transition-related signs that appear on the monitor include:

- When Baby is descending rapidly, the fetal heart may disappear from the monitor strip at the peak of each contraction, indicating movement out of range of the monitor and then back again. The nurse may need to move the monitor downward several times.

- When transition is completed, "early" decelerations of the fetal heart occurring right with each contraction usually signal that the baby's head is being pressed into position.

- Before full dilatation, in some cases early decelerations may indicate that the fetal head is bumping against the ischial spines, or being compressed due to asynclitism.

7.7.3.1 Differential analysis of stalled transition

A smooth transition relies on an alert, unencumbered baby finding a path out of the pelvis that is large enough for his head.[6] It also requires that Mom reach deep within herself and find the strength of purpose to endure a level of intensity she has likely never felt before, a process of active acceptance.

It is common for contractions to slow or space out during transition. However, if the labor remains in a sluggish state for more than an hour, then transition may have stalled. Possible reasons include:

- True or functional CPD: this is usually accompanied by bony obstruction pain, as well as marked decelerations (go to 1B).

---

6   This is one reason that stillbirth is extremely painful physically, over and above the emotional difficulty.

- True or functional short cord: the presentation is similar to CPD, but the decelerations will usually be more marked, and there will usually be less pain. In the absence of oxytocin, contractions will often reduce considerably.

- Sluggish baby: parenteral pain medications, fatigue, low oxygen or other impairments may present Baby from maneuvering appropriately.

- Insufficient movement: this is the maternal complement of a sluggish baby, and is all too common in hospital birth. In a more natural state, Baby's and Mom's movements inform each other through the dance of labor. Epidural analgesia cuts that feedback loop entirely, while parenteral pain medications, fatigue, disempowerment and imprisonment in bed all conspire to reduce it.

- Mother and/or baby need a rest: as a general rule during labor, if Mom can sleep she should sleep, unless there is a specific reason for time pressure. In long labors it is not at all uncommon for the body to demand rest before the effort of pushing, and, indeed, in many cases the act of fully relinquishing control over the events in one's body requires going into a state of deep sleep, meditation or concentration.

- There is something spiritually or emotionally in the way: as discussed above, transition can be a pivotal moment of tremendous emotional intensity, and it takes courage to face it. New moms often describe their worst fears and insecurities rising up, and indeed utterances such as "I can't do this" are not uncommon. In most cases, some combination of emotional discharge, encouragement from loved ones and reminders that they are about to meet a new family member provide sufficient revitalization. However, it is sometimes the case that the labor will just not move until some kind of emotional obstacle is addressed. This may be a person present in the room who needs to leave,[7] a ghost from the past such as a memory of stillbirth or sexual trauma, or a feeling of not yet being ready to be a mom.

7.7.3.2 Assisting with stalled transition

Broadly speaking, there are two approaches to assisting a stalled transition: more movement and more stillness. Stillness – specifically the Handwich – is my approach of choice for initial information gathering. True and functional CPD both manifest with identifiable areas of pain where the baby's head is

---

7   I have been this person.

pressing, and it is often possible to discern through careful listening what direction of movement might possibly relieve the pressure. Hip rocking, Shaking the Apples, pelvic vibrating and pelvic shaking from the femur are all orders of magnitude more effective at helping Baby to find a clear pathway through when preceded by careful palpation.

If no particular insights arise from this quiet listening – or if Mom is not interested in sitting still for it – then hip rocking followed by Shaking the Apples is most likely to dislodge an asynclitic head, while a head butting into one of the pubic rami can often be moved to a better angle by pelvic shaking from the femur on that side (followed by hip rocking with that side up).

In all of the above situations, shaking of the pelvis should be followed by Cat/Cow if possible (standing, hands and knees, or seated). If you are quite sure by the pain symptoms that you are dealing with bony obstruction, but two rounds of shaking and Cat/Cow have not resolved it, then it may be worth suggesting a "reset," in which Mom starts Cat/Cow on hands and knees, then lowers her chest by bending her arms so that her weight rests on the forearms instead. Three to five full breaths in this position are usually sufficient to reduce downward pressure on Baby so that, if he is indeed wedged in a bad situation, he can try a better approach.

If transition is stalled but there is no telltale pain to indicate a bony problem, then the remaining possibilities are true or functional short cord, maternal fatigue, lack of movement and/or fetal sluggishness, and spiritual or emotional challenges. In the hospital, short or wrapped cord may announce itself with persistent decelerations, in which case your efforts should go to preparing Mom for Cesarean section. Otherwise, the possibilities of fatigue and emotional challenges should be explored in a trauma-sensitive manner, as discussed in Chapter 4. Frustration and Qi stagnation due to lack of movement in the hospital can best be addressed by positional change, or the hospital workout.

7.7.4 Late-breaking OP

It sometimes happens that, after descending in a perfectly unremarkable manner, the fetus turns to OP rather than the more usual OA position for birth. This may indicate a narrow pubic arch lacking space to deliver OA, or (as one of my friends assures me based on her experience with her son) a mischievous free spirit meeting the world on its own terms. As discussed in 1B, I do not waste any effort trying to turn a late OP; instead, I "open the back door." As discussed in Chapter 6, this technique is highly effective for stretching the ligaments but requires quite some practice to be able to do quickly on demand. Luckily it is also an excellent labor preparation treatment, which provides ample practice.

7.8 Pushing

For hospital and research record-keeping, the <u>second stage of labor</u> is considered to start at the moment of full cervical dilatation. However as discussed above, in many cases transition is only just starting at 10 cm, and needs another hour or more to complete. It is my team's experience at the hospital that generally if the patient has had two or more sessions of birth bodywork and/or acupuncture during labor, then once transition has occurred, the birth takes place quite rapidly. Quite often we need to remind the doctors that even first-timers often deliver within a half hour, and a fair number of our acupuncture babies have been delivered by residents incompletely suited up because they didn't take us at our word (a few have also been delivered by – as the nurses joke – "Dr. Sealy Posturepedic, and Nurse Percale"). If transition is complete and the pelvic floor is relaxed, then there is very little holding the baby in.

The "normal" range for second stage of labor in a US hospital is up to 3 hours. A common reason for a labor taking that long is that pushing often starts before transition is finished. Other possibilities include insufficient space in the front or back of the pelvis, inadequate contractions due to fatigue and poor quality pushing due to epidural.

Table 7.8 Main presentations and therapeutic goals for pushing

8: Main Presentations and Therapeutic Goals for Pushing		
Level	Bone	Flesh
Presentations, goals and methods for unproductive pushing	Occiput posterior – open back door: sacrotuberous ligament release, pressure or needles at UB-60, SP-6 True or functional cephalopelvic disproportion (CPD) (go to 1B)	Fatigue: • If time allows, encourage rest: Yin footrubs, Nap and Dilate protocol • If no time, activate Qi: chafe, warm moxa or needle ST-36, tapping Du-20 • Weak or irregular contractions –activate Yang: pulsing pressure at Duyin and/or LI-4; tapping at UB-67 With epidural – focus and descend Qi: pressure or needle at Du-20, pressure at GB-21

7.8.1 Evaluation of pushing productivity

As discussed in the previous section on transition, there is generally a strong spontaneous urge to push, once the head is actually in place. The argument is sometimes made that with a fully dilated cervix and a high head, pushing may in some cases speed up the descent and transition. However, pushing is also stressful and tiring for both Mom and Baby, and the extra pressure may actually impede Baby from turning. If the head is above +1 station, or if there is no rectal pressure, then in all likelihood transition is not completed; see Section 7.8 for differential assessment.

Productive pushing is easy to recognize, once the head is close to the vaginal opening. Even before it is visible, good pushes gap the labia. Then the gap gets wider and glimpses of hair become visible during pushes, but only then, as the head retreats again between pushes. At that point it becomes possible to see incremental movement forward with good pushes, or to note the lack of it.

Pushing that is strong but unproductive, due to incomplete transition or other bony obstruction, has several hallmarks. First, the scalp begins to swell (caput succedaneum). This may be mistaken for progress by an inexperienced examiner, but actually indicates that the head is jammed against a bone. When the swelling is mild, there can be hope that the soft bones will mold and the head will come through in time. However as time passes and the swelling gets worse, the likelihood of vaginal birth diminishes. A second sign of unproductive pushing is that the labia and vaginal tissues swell extraordinarily. Blood is pushed into them with the force of the push, but it is prevented from leaving by the pressure of the baby head.

Of all the difficult sights in old-fashioned hospitals, this static, "purple" pushing (so named for the color of Mom's face) is one of the hardest. If a person eats too much salty food and their fingers swell trapping a ring on their finger, is a strong hard pull the best strategy? Or does one pull on the ring gently while angling your finger back and forth? Similarly, smaller pushes with free movement of the hips work much better when the baby is a tight squeeze. If the scalp and labia swell even with gentle pushing and wiggling (as well as the more targeted approaches described below), then there is likely a bony obstruction.

Another iatrogenic form of unproductive pushing is "bad epidural pushing." While providing pain relief that is indispensable for some patients, epidural analgesia breaks the feedback loop of movement and sensation within Mom's body, leaving her unable to feel where she is pushing, and therefore less able to push effectively than without meds. Gloved birth professionals can help to reinstate the feedback loop by pressing on the vaginal wall, encouraging Mom to push into that sensation. They can also feel from inside where the force of the push is going. For acupuncturists and doulas, even without the direct touch it is often possible to see whether the push is focused and effective by looking at whether the head (once visible) moves toward the vaginal opening, and also by looking at whether the perineum bulges.

7.8.2 Differential analysis and assistance of unproductive pushing

If the head is low and there is a strong urge to push, yet pushing becomes unproductive, then there is a bony obstruction. If it is a functional CPD due to asynclitism or malpresentation, then a knee–chest reset followed by movements as for stalled transition (Section 7.8.3) may resolve the situation. If there is actual CPD, then the acupuncture treatments below may potentially purchase a few much-needed millimeters of space, in consultation with an experienced birth practitioner. However these therapeutic methods should not be undertaken lightly, or without practice.[8]

- For persistent or late-onset OP, "open the back door" manually or with needles.

- For a narrow pubic arch, needling GB-34 may help to soften the pubic symphysis, together with three needles in arrow formation at Du-24 (similar to the treatment for pubic symphysis pain). If Mom is willing to be needled at Ren-2, threading that point downward together with one or two scalp points and just Du-26 may help to create a little more flex in the cartilage.

- For bad epidural pushing, an ear needle or acupressure at Du-20 can focus the body's attention on the perineum. Bilateral pressure straight downward at GB-21 also seems to help the pushing effort focus downward and outwards.

It sometimes happens, toward the end of a long labor, that the contractions space out. In this instance, the situational treatments described in Chapter 5 include the following ways to jump-start contractions, one at a time:

- pulsing pressure at Duyin and/or LI-4

- small circles with moderate pressure at bilateral Zigong

- tapping at UB-67.

---

8 See the notes on shoulder dystocia below and in Chapter 8.

7.9 Third Stage of Labor

From an EAM perspective there are two main disorders of the third stage of labor: placenta not detaching (or falling apart with pieces still attached), and postpartum hemorrhage. Neither of these requires differential analysis, but the approaches for helping are given below.

Table 7.9 Challenge 9, third-stage emergencies.

9: Adjunctive Measures for Third Stage Emergencies	
Retained placenta	Maternal hemorrhage
Descend Qi – LV-14 pressure (in and downward), or needle LV-3 toward KD-1	Reduce blood flow: SP-1 (strong pressure with fingernail) Promote contractions: pulsing pressure at Duyin, LI-4, or UB-67, and/or nipple stimulation

7.9.1 Retained placenta

Acupressure at LV-14, pressing strongly into the intercostal space below the nipple and then downward, is quite uncomfortable. However, in my experience it has not yet failed to induce the placenta to be released and expelled. Debra Betts uses needling LV-3 through to KD-1 for the same purpose and apparently also with excellent results.

7.9.2 Maternal hemorrhage

Maternal hemorrhage is a leading cause of morbidity and mortality. It is a particular danger after long births, when muscle fatigue prevents the uterus from contracting strongly enough to close off the (greatly enlarged) uterine blood vessels under the area of the placenta. Bleeding may also result from a piece of retained placenta stuck near the opening of an artery, preventing its closure. In either case, stimulating contractions is of the essence. As the medical personnel run for their oxytocin and other meds, we can be doing our work. Indeed, with a Qi-deficient patient in a long labor, the smart money would be to start chafing the Stomach line to supplement Qi as soon as possible after delivery, while also stimulating contractions with whichever of these points is closest to hand:

- pulsing pressure at Duyin and/or LI-4

- tapping at UB-67.

A nurse or midwife will already be massaging the uterine area to restore tone, so Zigong is not an option.

Chapter 8

PREPARATION AND PRACTICE

Chapter Outline

— 8.1 Patient Safety: First, do no harm

— 8.2 Ethical Practice in Pregnancy

— 8.3 Getting Solid on the Material

— 8.4 What to Bring to a Birth

— 8.5 The Birth Team

— 8.6 Practice Structure

This chapter considers the logistics, practicalities and ethics of our work as birth professionals. It looks at the actual practice of acupuncture and acupressure during birth, implementing the concepts, techniques and differential analysis introduced in previous chapters. It is mainly for acupuncturists who have not previously attended births, but individual sections may be of interest to other care practitioners.

Section 1, "Patient Safety: First, Do No Harm," introduces concepts of safe practice in this vulnerable population. These include red flags that should trigger immediate escalation of care, as well as various ways in which acupuncturists caring for pregnant patients need to interface with Western medical providers.

Section 2, "Ethical Practice in Pregnancy," examines principles of ethical practice in light of the particular physical and emotional vulnerabilities of pregnant patients. This discussion includes the unfortunate interface between adverse events, malpractice insurance and the lapses in patient relationship that most commonly precede legal action. Advice is given for cultivating habits of practice and attention to patient experience that serve two purposes: reducing actual breaches of connection and quickly bringing subtle disruptions to a provider's attention before trouble can brew.

Section 3, "Getting Solid on the Material," provides a brief overview of the key knowledge sets that need to be in place before attending births. Beyond just reading this book, those new to birth or to acupressure will benefit from more education and preparation – marking key pages with sticky tabs, photocopying tables for reference and/or reading some suggested additional texts. For anyone who has not previously attended births and is serious about doing so now, I also strongly recommend completing a doula training program.

Section 4, "What to Bring to a Birth," overviews the paraphernalia specific to our work. A travel needle kit is nothing new for acupuncturists, but there are birth-specific items that are important to have. For those unaccustomed to attending births, other elements of a "Birth Bag" are briefly introduced, along with a checklist of what's described in this book.

Section 5, "The Birth Team," discusses the various functions that need to be carried out to support a home or hospital birth. Acupuncturists need to consider where they want to fit on the spectrum, from playing a facilitation role only during the home/hospital birth to providing ongoing support before, during and after birth.

Section 6, "Practice Structure," looks at the macro-scale, in which the temporal and financial logistics of birth work may need to be balanced with clinical practice. For most acupuncturists, this means finding a team to work with – as midwives and obstetricians generally do.

8.1 Patient Safety: First, Do No Harm

Medical safety is the prevention of harm to patients. This includes harm incurred through mistreatment, as well through treatment not given. In general, acupuncture is quite safe, though there are a few special considerations due to the specific vulnerabilities of pregnant patients. Of most concern to acupuncturists newly practicing in pregnancy should be the number of red flags that require urgent referral to primary obstetrical or emergency care. There are also situations such as breech and labor induction where an informed consent for acupuncture requires that the patient understand that Western treatments are available.

8.1.1 Direct harm from acupuncture treatment

Acupuncture is quite safe in the general population,[1] with a low number of adverse events, and those that do occur mostly quite mild, such as transient bleeding, bruising or dizziness. In 2006, I reviewed the studies of birth-related acupuncture available at that time (2000+ patients) and found no adverse events reported at all, other than one temporary drop foot. I am not aware of any pregnancy- or birth-related adverse events in literature since then, and I have been looking for them. I am also reliably informed by risk management personnel at a main insurer of acupuncturists in the United States that there have been no claims against acupuncturists for mishaps specific to pregnancy. This should be immensely reassuring to anybody worried about the actual risk of being sued for a problem occurring during pregnancy or birth.

With that understanding, it is still a statistical inevitability that as more patients are treated with acupuncture during pregnancy, some cases of pregnancy loss, stillbirth and suboptimal birth outcomes will occur within 24 hours of acupuncture treatments. In such cases, it is only human nature for patients and other practitioners to question every decision they made during the period, including whether the acupuncture could have been a factor. It is therefore the responsibility of practitioners to document treatments carefully, and stay within accepted parameters such as avoiding so-called "forbidden points" before 37 weeks' gestation. There are also a few additional risks of "wrong" treatment to be considered.

8.1.1.1 "Forbidden points"

"Forbidden points" is a general term for the points most consistently flagged in classical and recent Chinese sources for avoidance during pregnancy. These include LI-4, SP-6, GB-21, UB-32, CV-4, UB-60 and UB-67.[2] A 2015 article,[3] advocating the use of acupuncture alongside physiotherapy during pregnancy, suggested that traditional concerns regarding these points are unfounded. Although the article argued for the safety of the points in question, one of the studies cited for that purpose reported a number of withdrawals from its acupuncture group (and not the placebo group) due

---

1   Witt, C. M., Pach, D., Brinkhaus, B., Wruck, K., Tag, B., Mank, S., & Willich, S. N. (2009). Safety of acupuncture: Results of a prospective observational study with 229, 230 patients and introduction of a medical information and consent form. *Complementary Medicine Research, 16*(2), 91–97.

2   Betts, D. & Budd, S. (2011). Forbidden points in pregnancy: Historical wisdom?. *Acupuncture in Medicine, 29*(2), 137–139.

3   Carr, D. J. (2015). The safety of obstetric acupuncture: Forbidden points revisited. *Acupuncture in Medicine, 33*(5), 413–419.

to onset of early contractions. No adverse events occurred, but the example is cautionary. I recommend avoiding the above-listed points, as well as the lower abdomen and pelvic region generally, unless there is an important reason to override the contraindication. One example of such a reason is needling ST-31 for refractory vomiting; the point is often effective where gentler measures are not, and, in early pregnancy, the risk of labor initiation due to slackening of the pelvic floor is quite low.

8.1.1.2 Pneumothorax

Puncture of the lung is never a desirable outcome, but is particularly to be avoided during pregnancy. Needling GB-21 is generally best avoided during the chaos and movement of labor, and should be undertaken with care during pregnancy.

8.1.1.3 Seizure

Seizure has not been definitively established as a risk of acupuncture, but a few possible instances have been reported.[4] It has been suggested that these events may have been more benign vasovagal responses, which are a known, minor adverse event. However, given the disastrous effects of seizure during pregnancy (which may include pregnancy loss and/or fetal hypoxia) a wide margin of safety is warranted. My criteria for avoiding this risk are as follows:

- Acupuncture-naïve patients with a history of seizure, and those with a history of migraines triggered by acupuncture treatment, should not be treated during pregnancy.

- Patients who have a history of seizure but who have previously received acupuncture treatment, without event, can be treated. Treatments should be gentle, with care taken that they have eaten.

Over-treatment is a clinical phenomenon well known to acupuncturists, though acupuncture "dosage" in general is poorly studied. Use of too many needles, too large a gauge or retention for too long can cause severe post-treatment fatigue, particularly for Qi-deficient patients. During labor, excessive treatment may drain Qi and exacerbate fatigue late in labor.

---

4   White, A., Hayhoe, S., Hart, A., Ernst, E., & Volunteers from BMAS and AACP. (2001). Survey of adverse events following acupuncture (SAFA): A prospective study of 32,000 consultations. *Acupuncture in Medicine, 19*(2), 84–92.

8.1.2 Missed opportunity for Western treatment

In a small number of cases, acupuncturists have been successfully sued because patients felt that they were not adequately informed about conventional options. Potentially relevant situations include prenatal treatment for breech and labor preparation, intrapartum augmentation and use of epidural, and also the use of acupuncture to avoid Cesarean section in large babies who may be at risk for shoulder dystocia.

8.1.2.1 Breech moxa

Use of moxibustion in breech pregnancies is described in Appendix B. Obstetrical acupuncturists consider it optimally effective at weeks 33 or 34, when there is still plenty of room for Baby to turn herself. However, patients tend to hope for spontaneous resolution, and in general, contact acupuncturists as late as week 36 or even 38, when space is limited. The more aggressive Western treatment approach, manual version, is generally not performed until late in week 34, because that procedure carries a meaningful risk of membrane rupture and/or labor initiation. Altogether, this means that patients frequently request acupuncture treatment at a time when they are already eligible for manual version, and time is not on their side as Baby grows. Anecdotally, colleagues and I find that in cases where the baby has not turned with moxibustion, manual version still proceeds more easily and with a higher success rate than average. However, it is entirely understandable that parents who elected to try the moxa from week 35 to late week 36, then had no success with either approach, might then second-guess their choice. It is therefore prudent to document that patients have made their decision with awareness of the pros and cons of both approaches – I suggest use of a written information sheet to memorialize this conversation.

8.1.2.2 Labor "induction," preparation or encouragement

The phrase "acupuncture induction" is relatively common among acupuncturists, though I wish it weren't. As discussed extensively in Chapters 4, 5 and 6, acupuncture therapy can be extremely useful before and during the latent phase to assist with cervical ripening, pelvic floor relaxation and initiation of contractions. As a medical term, "induction" denotes the Western medical procedure in which Mom is "led" from latent to active phase via use of oxytocin to initiate contractions. This definition may technically be accurate to describe treatments given to Qi- or Yang-deficient patients who present with ripe cervix and relaxed pelvic floor, needing only electrical stimulation at the sacral foramina to start their contractions. However, those moms represent only perhaps 10 percent of labor preparation treatments given. Overall, the term "induction" is so strongly associated with its orthodox medical definition, that when the service is offered to patients, they may have inappropriate expectations of immediate labor onset.

It is for this reason that at least one malpractice insurance company has specifically excluded "acupuncture induction" from its general acupuncture coverage. Patients who chose "acupuncture induction" while expecting results within a tight Western time frame could experience considerable disappointment if the labor took a week or more to start – as well it might, if they started with a low Bishop Score – and then ended with a less-than-optimal birth. This is particularly a concern in light of research suggesting (though by no means proving) that induction at 39 weeks is associated with better birth outcomes. As with breech moxa, acupuncturists in litigious areas may choose to memorialize their conversation regarding "induction" with an information sheet clarifying that acupuncture treatment works to optimize maternal conditions for going into labor, but is not a substitute for Western induction.

8.1.2.3 "Acupuncture anesthesia" versus epidural

As with labor induction and breech, use of acupuncture as an exciting and mysterious substitute for a known Western entity may result in inappropriate expectations and subsequent disappointment. A quick web search will show that epidural analgesia has meaningful known risks and side effects, while acupuncture has few. However, a straight substitution should not be considered, as normal, non-medicated birth requires physical, emotional and team-building preparation. I had not anticipated this issue in planning the 2006 study my colleagues and I conducted, and indeed the acupuncture group had a somewhat higher rate of epidural usage than the non-acupuncture group. I attribute this to the misconceptions of patients who chose acupuncture for pain management, then found that – particularly in the bedridden hospital environment of that time – acupuncture alone did not provide the "painless birth" often attributed to epidural. Just as acupuncture powerfully supports smoking cessation but does not magically replace the act of quitting, acupuncture can be of enormous help in reducing pain and helping birth to go more smoothly, but works best as part of a considered plan.

8.1.2.4 Avoidance of Cesarean section

What could possibly be the downside of avoiding necessary surgery? In one case, a patient with a persistent occiput posterior (OP) baby pushed for a solid 3 hours with heroic assistance from the Acuteam; she eventually delivered vaginally, but experienced numbness down her left leg that persisted for a day or two. The numbness could have been due to the combined epidural/spinal analgesia she had received, but it could also have been from the time spent with the head wedged into the left side of her pelvis. On balance, she was better off avoiding the surgery, but had the nerve damage been permanent, she might not have been.

Even more concerning is the possibility that a labor that stalled and got moving again with acupuncture then results in a shoulder dystocia with a bad outcome. In that situation, there would be medical bills to pay, and a convincing argument could be made that without the acupuncture, the baby would have been safely removed surgically. As incidence of shoulder dystocia has risen epidemically with gestational diabetes, I have become more cautious in my treatment planning with babies over 4000 g. I support the labor enthusiastically as long as it is moving well. However, if progress should stall without an obvious constitutional or emotional reason, I am less aggressive in urging it on.

8.1.3 Red flags for escalation of care

A thorough discussion of red flags is outside the scope of this book, but a brief introduction is critical. Responsible practice as an adjunct care provider for a vulnerable population requires knowing which symptoms are potentially concerning and require urgent referral, either to primary care or to the emergency department. Resources for further study include an excellent video presentation by British midwife/acupuncturist Sarah Budd.[5] The main red flags include:

8.1.3.1 Premature prelabor rupture of membranes (PPROM)

When membranes rupture at or close to term, the wash of prostaglandins in the amniotic fluid commonly leads to cervical ripening and labor initiation. When this occurs before the fetus is well developed, it is a medical emergency. Tocolytics are administered to quiet the uterus, and treatment with steroids is given to accelerate fetal lung maturation. Acupuncture can be a powerful adjunct therapy during hospital care for PPROM, but cannot safely be used as a substitute.

8.1.3.2 Premature labor

Mild crampy sensations before term are not uncommon, particularly in summer when dehydration increases the irritability of the uterus. However, if the cramps occur at regular intervals, if they are accompanied by discharge of

---

5   https://www.healthyseminars.com/product/safety-issues-pregnancy-red-flags-acupuncturists

fluid or if the cervix shortens, then immediate medical attention is required. As with PPROM, acupuncture can work powerfully to help patients relax and seems also to quiet the uterus, but it must be used in conjunction with appropriate medical care.

8.1.3.3 Placental abruption

This is an extremely dangerous development before or during labor, in which the placenta begins to separate from the uterine wall before birth. Patients with preeclampsia or small-for-dates babies, older mothers and postdates are at elevated risk. Two main signs of placental abruption are intrapartum bleeding (which may or may not be visible) and uterine tenderness on palpation. On a contraction monitor, uterine tone may be seen to be elevated, and the fetal heart may decelerate. At home, bleeding during labor (or signs of shock suggesting internal blood loss) is an immediate trigger to call an ambulance.

8.1.3.4 Uterine rupture

Uterine rupture is rare in unmedicated, low-risk births. Risk is much higher after Cesarean section, and also with use of misoprostol for cervical ripening. For this reason, cervical ripening agents are contraindicated during vaginal birth after Cesarean (VBAC, sometimes also called TOLAC, or "trial of labor after Cesarean"). These moms are therefore excellent candidates for prenatal and intrapartum acupressure/acupuncture to help ripen the cervix, reducing the amount of force that contractions need to exert. During labor, the majority of uterine rupture incidents are preceded by sharp pain; however, in some cases there is no pain until the moment the scar opens up. Another warning sign to look out for is increased uterine tone between contractions, by palpation or on the tocometer.

8.1.3.5 Chorioamnionitis

The two key signs of chorioamnionitis, or infection in the membranes, are elevated temperature and malodorous amniotic fluid. Intrapartum fever does not always indicate infection: labor itself is an inflammatory process that may elevate body temperature. As discussed in Chapters 5 and 6, acupuncture/ acupressure can be extremely helpful as an adjunct therapy in managing a labor with fever. However, as a warning sign, it should always be brought to medical attention.

8.1.3.6 Preeclampsia/HELLP

Preeclampsia is most commonly seen in the third trimester, but may present as early as 20 weeks and as late as several weeks postpartum. Its main presentation is elevated blood pressure, usually accompanied by swelling of the hands and feet as well as protein in the urine. A related and more severe syndrome is that of HELLP, or "hemolysis, raised liver enzymes, low platelets." It is the responsibility of the primary care provider to screen regularly for preeclampsia, but everyone caring for a pregnant person should be on the lookout for sudden appearance of edema, hypertension and associated symptoms. (Acupuncturists unaccustomed to treating pregnant patients should make sure to have a large enough blood pressure cuff on hand, as a tight fit invalidates the reading.) From a Chinese perspective, the patients most at risk for preeclampsia are those with marked signs of Yin deficiency, severe Qi deficiency or Blood stasis, particularly those who have suffered severe morning sickness or previous preeclampsia. Preeclampsia is outside the scope of this book, but EAM can be extremely effective in reducing symptoms and keeping the pregnancy viable, and can be a powerful preventative for moms known to be at risk. Among American acupuncturists, Sharon Weizenbaum is expert in EAM diagnosis and herbal treatment of preeclampsia, and offers live and online training.[6] Preliminary data from the work of Zena Kocher at Allina Health Systems in Minneapolis also suggest that high-risk preeclampsia patients who receive acupuncture treatment in the antepartum unit may be able to maintain the pregnancies as much as a week longer.

8.1.3.7 Decreased fetal movements

Fetal demise after 20 weeks occurs in between 0.5 percent and 1 percent of US births. In most cases, its only sign is that movements are not felt. Acupuncturists may thus be in the position of hearing that their patients have not felt movements within the last few hours. In these cases, it's important to get the patient to her primary obstetrical provider urgently, but without inducing panic. Before jumping to conclusions, I always tap sharply on UB-67 a few times, then do the Handwich inviting Mom to breathe deeply, as both of these techniques often induce movement in babies who are merely sleeping.

8.1.3.8 Perinatal depression and psychosis

Feelings of emotional fragility and/or lability are extremely common due to fluctuating hormone levels, particularly during the first trimester and the first week after birth. A small number of the moms who experience these symptoms will develop severe depression or psychosis that may result in harm to self or baby, requiring hospitalization. However, for a surprisingly

---

6   https://www.healthyseminars.com/product/sharon-weizenbaum%E2%80%99s-complete-pregnancy-course-using-chinese-herbs

high proportion of expecting or new mothers – some 10–15 percent of new mothers – the symptoms become disabling or persistent. Symptoms normally used to screen for depression – fatigue, difficulty concentrating, disrupted sleep cycle – are so common postpartum that they lose diagnostic significance. The Edinburgh Postpartum Depression Scale[7] focuses more strongly on feelings such as self-blame, difficulty finding pleasure and humor in life, with special emphasis on thoughts of self-harm. Even without formally administering the scale, perinatal care providers such as acupuncturists should be familiar with the screening and prepared to use it as a probe into any reported low feelings or "baby blues." It is particularly important to note that perinatal depression has a 90 percent recurrence rate. Patients with a previous history of depression or other significant psychological challenges are also at elevated risk, along with those who have recently suffered bereavement or other difficult life events.

Acupuncture can be of help with perinatal depression, but should always be used integratively – and the primary determination needs to be that there is adequate social support at home. In particular, if there are thoughts of harm to self or others, then as care providers we have a responsibility to ensure the new mom and baby are not left at home alone until psychological help has been enlisted.

8.2 Ethical Practice in Pregnancy

The generalities of ethical practice are outside the scope of this book. However, two ethical issues are specific to pregnancy and important to take into account when practicing. The first of these concerns is the particular physical and emotional vulnerabilities of pregnant patients – the precious fragility of the fetal life, and the emotional intensity of labor and delivery. The second – not unrelated – is the high incidence of malpractice litigation around birth, particularly in the United States. Regarding physical vulnerability, the best that can be done is scrupulous adherence to the principles of patient safety described above. Patients' emotional vulnerability is discussed in the following section, along with providers' vulnerability to legal action.

8.2.1 Emotional vulnerability

In general, acupuncturists and birth professionals are exceptionally capable at recognizing and working with emotional intensity. I consider two principles as key.

---

7   https://psychology-tools.com/epds

8.2.1.1 First, listen carefully – what is going on?

As an experienced care provider, it is easy to fall into the trap of identifying a problem and taking steps to fix it as quickly as possible, without fully understanding the patient's preferences and priorities. Early on in my birth work, I was so strongly attached to my role of supporting normal unmedicated birth that in some cases I believe I missed cues that, staying clear and present, turned out to be a higher priority for the mom than executing the original no-epidural birth plan. The labor journey is extraordinarily complicated emotionally, often involving loss of control, alternately exciting and disappointing news, and fear based on an unknown future or traumatic past. Not uncommonly, low-grade difficulties between the patient and family may flare up in ways that you will never fully understand, but can nevertheless gently mediate by providing space, listening carefully and seeing the very best in everyone.

Sometimes during a difficult birth, Mom may need someone to be angry at, and that somebody may be you. As discussed in Chapter 2, the emotional experience of stuck Qi includes both frustration and anger. Particularly when there is a hard interface between baby and bone, the physical experience of stagnation – plus frustration, anger, and adrenaline from the challenging situation – may need to vent themselves by being directed at somebody. In the hospital this is usually nurses, techs or unskillful residents. However, at an intimate home birth, it may be you, the partner or the midwife – and in this situation you are likely the best choice. If this is happening, your best bet is to aerate the situation by creating excuses to step out and let the emotion discharge. It may also be that you are not the target of any discharge, but can help by recognizing when other members of the birth team need a break.

8.2.1.2 Ongoing informed consent per procedure

My main approach to keeping a clear emotional interface with Mom is to consider that I need a mini-informed consent – verbal, visual or tactile – for every new action I take. Without seeming insecure, it's still possible to take a moment at each new point of contact either to explain what I'm about to do, or to physically preview it and make eye contact with a silent request for approval. In this way, Mom retains a clear sense of control over my actions – I bring expertise to what I recommend, but she gets to make the call as to what I actually do. I find that in this way if any ambivalence develops about my actions – or anything else in the labor process – it will surface quite quickly, giving me a cue that I need to understand better what is going on and consider what's best to do about it.

8.2.2 Legal vulnerability

Bad outcomes occur sometimes, even if nobody is at fault. And, mistakes do also get made even with the best of intentions. As care providers it is our responsibility to cultivate behaviors of practice that minimize the risk of error, as well as habits of documentation that will provide evidence, if needed, as to whether any error was committed when a bad outcome has occurred. It is also our responsibility to maintain malpractice insurance appropriate to the degree of harm that might be incurred in case of error.

Over the years I have done various kinds of work with malpractice insurance providers, and from my discussions with them (along with background reading), I have come to understand that for acupuncturists, doulas and other non-primary providers of care during birth, actual commission of error by the provider is not the main driver of lawsuits. There are two main instances in which legal action is taken against care providers. The first is when the patient feels poorly treated by a specific provider or institution, with a sense that disrespect has been shown, an apology is owed or distressing news was delivered in a dismissive or callous manner. The second motivating factor for many lawsuits is that large medical bills are owed or a grievous loss has been sustained, so that every provider affiliated with the case is sued with little regard for her particular role in the event.

In both of these instances, the lawsuit will be defended and covered by the malpractice insurance company, even if medical error has occurred. The danger of personal exposure only arises when providers treat outside their official scope of practice, or outside of the specific provisions of the malpractice insurance. Importantly, one major provider of general malpractice insurance for acupuncturists has historically excluded moxabustion for breech, labor "induction," and also treatment during labor and delivery. It should be noted that while the term "in labor" colloquially refers to the onset of active labor, a patient who presents for an office visit with mild contractions is technically in the latent phase of labor. If an adverse event occurred with such a patient, it is a debatable point whether the insurance company would be compelled by the terms of the policy to cover any resulting litigation.

Given that some adverse outcomes and their associated legal exposure is not entirely preventable, a few tips for minimization are given below. There are a few patient situations that should be considered as "pink sticky notes." These are not full red flags requiring specific action, but rather reminders to ourselves to treat well within our zone of confidence, and to stay attentive to the emotional vulnerabilities described above.

8.2.2.1 Pink sticky notes

At the time in New York City when my practice was at its busiest, I did indeed put a pink Post-it™ note on some patient folders as a reminder to slow down and be extra attentive. The trigger for the sticky note might have been a complex medical condition, or a patient with extra emotional needs. To be honest, the most common reason I affixed one was that a previous appointment had gone less than optimally – a long wait, an extra-painful needle insertion or in one case, an herb formula that had made them spectacularly gassy. There was no sense of judgment against the patient, just a reminder to bring my very best self into the room.

Over time, the "sticky note" system has become somewhat codified in my practice and teaching work.[8] "Sticky notes" fall into two main categories: high risk of adverse outcome and high risk of relationship breakdown. In both instances, it's important to:

- keep excellent treatment notes

- pay close attention to the patient relationship

- restrict treatment methods to those with which we are familiar and comfortable.

8.2.2.2 The zone of confidence

Every practice can be seen as a bull's-eye. In the center are conditions we see commonly with excellent results, and treatment methods we enjoy doing and could do in our sleep. (Mine is the core repertory.) In successive rings outward are the patient situations we see less commonly and treatment methods that we use less frequently, and those circumstances and methods where our results have not always been optimal. The outermost ring consists of situations and treatment methods with which we have little independent experience, though we understand them based on previous instruction or reading. It feels challenging to work in this outer ring, but if we were to avoid it entirely, we would sharply reduce the number of patients we could help. One of Chinese medicine's most extraordinary and useful properties is that a majority of patient presentations, whether their Western nomenclature is familiar or not, can be assessed and assisted through the powerful lenses of Qi and Blood, Yin and Yang.

The critical "however" to this statement is that I prefer to stay out of the outer ring with "sticky note" patients. If the stakes are extra high, or if there

---

8   My online course about "Acupuncture during Pregnancy: Safe and Ethical Practice" is available on the continuing education website Healthy Seminars https://www. healthyseminars.com/product/acupuncture-during-pregnancy-safe-and-ethical-practice

has already been some disruption of patient–practitioner relationship, it's best to stay toward the center of the bulls-eye. If referral to a more experienced provider is an option, it should be taken with sticky note patients in the outer ring. If there is no option for referral, or if the patient relationship is strong and that's an important factor in the patient's care, then be confident that you are the best provider available, but stay as close as possible to the "zone of confidence" in your treatment choices.

8.2.2.3 Situations requiring extra vigilance

In several of the "red flag" situations described earlier (Section 8.1.3), acupuncture may be of great help as an adjunct therapy. These conditions include premature labor, PPROM, mild preeclampsia and perinatal depression. Those presentations, as well as TOLAC, small-for-dates babies and other births identified for any reason as high risk, should also be given "sticky note" designations. The medical and other situations below should also be considered for heightened vigilance.

THE "WINDOW OF WORST OUTCOMES"

On the population level, pregnancy loss is a sad inevitability, occurring in 10–15 percent of pregnancies. Losses occurring in the first trimester are sad, but generally accepted by society as a rough patch on the road to parenthood. The later in the pregnancy that loss occurs, the more heartbreaking the event, and the more likely that medical error will be explored as a possible cause. However, as a malpractice insurance lawyer once explained to me, the lawsuits most to be feared are those where the baby is delivered live in the early weeks of viability – these days from 19 to 32 weeks, but getting earlier all the time. In these cases, there are large hospital bills to be paid, and in some cases, the need for ongoing special care as well. Parents in this situation have no option but to pursue litigation, regardless of how much they might love their acupuncturist.

The main reason to treat second- and early third-trimester patients with caution is not the fear of litigation, of course, but the desire to do everything we can to keep Baby safe and healthy at this critical time. There is no reason to think that appropriate acupuncture treatment will dislodge a healthy pregnancy at any point. However, patients in general come to us when they are not fully healthy. Knowing that Qi- and Yin-deficient patients in particular are vulnerable to premature labor or membrane rupture, I use conservative treatments such as ear seeds, bodywork and exercises when possible. If needling, I include Qi-raising points such as Du-20 and ST-13 (unless there are already signs of Qi rising). Treating during pregnancy is out of the scope of this book, though many of the assessment and treatment approaches in it will lend themselves to doing so. I do urge practitioners to seek additional training or mentorship in the particular needs of pregnant patients, or else to refer to more experienced practitioners.

Large babies
As discussed in Section 3.3.2.3, shoulder dystocia is a not insignificant risk with babies over 4000 g. I therefore consider the size alone to warrant a sticky note, particularly if Mom is not large.

Non-medical sticky notes
In her book on acupuncture during pregnancy and birth, Zita West describes a situation in which she was preparing to apply moxabustion to a patient with breech presentation and then was overcome with anxiety at the door to the patient room. Listening to her inner voice, she managed the situation without giving any actual treatment, and was very glad that she had done so – as the patient later suffered a severe hemorrhage.

One of the most important reasons to treat a patient conservatively (or not at all) is simply that you have a bad feeling. Even laying aside the possibility of prescience, our emotions are based on a powerful human capability to register and assimilate a huge number of subconscious cues. Knowing as we do now that dogs can sense incipient epilepsy as well as undiagnosed cancer, we should respect our own capability to warn ourselves when a situation is more complex than it appears.

Another important reason to treat conservatively or consider referring a patient is if it is clear that one of you annoys the other. Awkward pauses, humor falling flat, severe or persistent verbal misunderstandings and (these days) severe disjunction of political views all constitute sticky notes. In the vast majority of cases, these issues get smoothed over with no further ramifications. However, they are an indication to stay within one's comfort zone, and to treat conservatively if there are also medical concerns.

8.2.3 Disagreement with primary care
One of the most difficult ethical dilemmas in birth work is how to handle situations where we feel that the current plan of care is not in the best interest of the patient. Ethically speaking, openly questioning the provider's choices is almost never the right choice. A patient's relationship with the primary care provider and faith in their judgment is the main safe space of the birth. Tearing that open with a conflicting action plan will in most cases only exacerbate the situation at hand. However, there are occasional

situations where medical error can be prevented by timely intervention. Steps for thinking the situation through and finding the best course of action are presented below. Needless to say, in emergent situations, there may not be time for a full workup, which is all the more reason to practice the process with less urgent disagreements, so that it will be fluid and quick when needed.

8.2.3.1 Identify the level of disagreement

Actual lapses in judgment by primary providers do happen. However, they are much less common than first-principle disagreements over how – and to what extent – birth should be managed. Anytime you find yourself questioning a medical decision, press yourself to identify more closely the nature of your disagreement. Some possibilities include:

- philosophical disagreement with the provider

- philosophical disagreement with the institution's care in general

- frank medical error by the provider

- understanding of the situation that is different than the provider's

- thinking the provider might actually see things your way if they had more information.

For many doulas and acupuncturists in the United States, philosophical disagreement with institutions and/or providers is all too common. And quite often, apparent bad calls by practitioners are in response to institutional or the American College of Obstetricians and Gynecologists (ACOG) guidelines over which they have no control. However, if the practitioner is showing poor judgment, particularly at a home birth where there are no other medical staff members assessing safety, you should at least consider speaking up. This is best done in private communication with the provider. I once thought through a nuclear option in detail – thinking I would text a midwife and then show it to her on my phone, "If you don't transport now I'm calling 911." A whispered question, "Are you going to transport?" was a much better choice.

Speaking up need not be confrontational. At the hospital, I have made a practice of politely inquiring into the reasoning behind provider choices that seem off to me, and have very often either learned something or, after listening carefully, found the opportunity to share my view. In some of these cases, they have at least delayed oxytocin or C-section orders so as to give my approach a try. My beloved colleague Tzivya finds the best success with a three-step approach:

- Articulate clearly that your aim is to make their work go better (i.e. safe, healthy, happy patient and baby).

- Make a specific, time-bounded request with an anticipated goal, e.g. "For the next three contractions can I try stimulating these toe points?"

- If things improve, you are then in a position to negotiate for more time without them losing face.

Also consider back channels: is there a nurse, midwife, resident or other practitioner who sees things your way and is in a better position to ask for change? Your patient may be in a position to ask for a change of staff as well, although be careful with this option, as it may earn the patient a reputation for being "difficult."

8.2.3.2 What's at stake?

Briefly ask yourself: What's the worst possible downside of what's happening? Preventable primary Cesarean section is bad, but postpartum hemorrhage at home is worse.

Then consider the best- and worst-case scenarios of possible intervention. If you think there's a chance the provider will change course in relation to a question and discussion from you, that's worth considering. However, if you don't have a sense of someone both empowered to make the decision and also willing to listen to you, there's just no point going there.

8.2.3.3 Where do you think the patient stands?

As discussed above, undermining the patient's faith in their primary provider is not an option. However, if the patient is already questioning the provider, or a new proposed intervention is in direct conflict with Mom's birth plan, then you can be a strong ally in supporting the patient's request for private time to consider any new intervention. (Debra Pascali-Bonaro, legendary doula trainer, birth activist, blogger and filmmaker,[9] suggests that the two best ways to create space in a birth room are asking for time to "pray on it," and pulling out a vibrator for "natural stimulation.")

Often if I have been using acupressure only in deference to a patient's fear of needles, I will propose trying acupuncture and E-stim at this juncture to see whether change can be effected using our strongest non-pharmaceutical tools. If it cannot, then this can provide Mom with better peace of mind that the team tried everything first, rather than jumping into a procedure.

---

9   https://www.debrapascalibonaro.com

8.2.3.4 How sure are you? Get a second opinion

If on consideration of the issues above, you feel that it's important to at least try to effect change in the plan of care, one last step is useful. This is to text or call a knowledgeable colleague for a quick check-in. Emotions run high in birth, and particularly if you are new at it, the egregiousness of the perceived error may diminish somewhat once you've gotten it off your chest. Conversely, talking to a colleague may provide the chance to rehearse your talking points and strengthen your confidence in speaking up.

8.3 Getting Solid on the Material

Putting this book's material into practice will require different types of prep work, depending on your current practice situation. Those who are already practicing acupressure, bodywork and/or acupuncture during birth can of course hit the ground running, just incorporating the parts they find useful. For the rest, this section considers the subjects of practicing birth bodywork and other techniques, building a personal practice resource, charting and background reading.

8.3.1 Bodywork practice

Even if you are an experienced bodyworker, it is critically important that you practice the hand techniques described here before using them in a clinical setting. Ideally, find a partner who will practice them on you as well, so you have a sense of how the techniques work from both sides.

For acupuncturists in clinical practice, many of the techniques are well suited to pregnancy, women's health and even the general population. It is particularly important to practice the sacrotuberous and sacrospinous ligament releases, as these are tricky to get at first. Beyond their role as terrific additions to prelabor treatments, they can sometimes be quite useful in treating sciatica or coccyx pain.

8.3.2 Personal practice resource

In my PhD work on acupuncture during stroke rehabilitation, I investigated the balance of competing imperatives: consistent, evidence-based practice versus meeting the individual needs of patients as they unfold in the course of treatment. I concluded that the best practice would be to have practitioners decide on their treatments individually and freely, as they always have, but to provide written support for the decision-making process. This book's structure roughly follows the approach I developed for providing written support, though with less overt emphasis on the clinical research. My years in the clinics of seasoned practitioners led me to think of treatment planning as an algorithm, briefly summarized here:

- Is this a commonly seen presentation? If so, do what you always do for that (this is the core repertory, situational treatments and common constitutional approaches).

  - Did it work? If not, try the same treatment principle with stronger stimulation (or with a stronger modality).

- If those approaches still didn't help, take a step back and reassess your understanding of the situation (this is the text in Chapter 6).

  - If no new insight emerges from this reassessment, start with the best treatment plan you can think of based on what you *are* certain of about the case (e.g. acupressure at SP-6 in a Blood-deficient patient who is not dilating), then:

- Consult the research literature, and/or reach out to expert colleagues or mentors for advice.

  - *Please note that online social media is not an appropriate venue for medical consultation.* Practitioner groups are excellent for discussing cases after the fact, but any consultation with colleagues needs to be private and specific.

  - You will also find that when you are in the midst of a difficult case, that is not the best time to scan through research papers looking for something. Instead, build yourself a personal practice resource.

The personal practice resource can be on paper or electronic, for higher capacity and rapid searching. Evernote, Dropbox and Google Drive are all convenient places to make a folder and populate it with useful research and articles to read during down time. Some items will likely need to be on paper, including:

- acupressure guides for other birth team members (these may be copies of Debra Betts' handouts or something you made individually)

- other information sheets including care package handouts

- consent and charting materials (see below).

8.3.3 Consent and charting materials

Practicing acupuncturists do not normally need additional consent forms for labor and delivery. However, if using a malpractice insurance company that does not cover labor, you will want to draw up an agreement that for the duration of the labor you are in a doula–client relationship, not an acupuncturist–patient relationship. In your charting materials, you should refrain from explicit references to diagnosis and treatment. Analysis and assistance are fine.

I strongly recommend use of a timeline-based record of every birth encounter, even for doulas who do not normally chart. Examples are available at Citkovitz.com. If you choose to make your own, the following information should be included:

- Maternal name, age, gender identification and other demographic information if relevant.

- Other members of the birth team, clearly identifying primary provider.

- Gestational age (weeks/days).

- Parity – how many times pregnant and how many times delivered.

- Most recent cervical exam and time (record each subsequent exam and time as well). Include dilatation, head station, effacement, cervical quality and cervical position (anterior, mid, posterior).

- Notes on course of any previous labors (this is extremely important!).

- Notes on course of pregnancy – in particular:

    - Vomiting (this gives some indication of constitution and may be a flag for deficiency).

    - How much sleep over the last days and weeks (this affects Yin and Qi reserves).

    - Ankle swelling? (None at all suggests Yin deficiency; lots and early onset suggest Qi and Yang deficiency, as well as damp waiting to obstruct the labor.)

    - Does Baby have a favorite place to hang out? Is he there now, and can you check, too? (This gives you a chance to palpate and connect.)

- Notes on her menstrual and other health history:

  – Were periods regular? Painful? (And if so, relieved by warmth?) Scanty or heavy?

  – Any other health issues you should know about?

- Current presentation:

  – Any pain? (Always ask this first, and if Mom does have pain, ask all your other questions while starting work to relieve the pain.)

  – Location of pain? Fixed or changing? Frequency and intensity of contractions?

  – Time and circumstances of labor onset (gradual contractions building, water breaking, induction, etc.)

- Notes on EAM analysis if relevant – complexion, manner, pulse, tongue, possible constitutional factors based on signs and symptoms.

After the pages for this background information, you will want plenty of structured space (and multiple two-sided backup sheets) on which to make your birth timeline. Use a margin at the left, for noting the time. (Use the 24-hour format – I can state from experience that it makes life much easier.) Then, in the rest of the space, record all observations and interventions made by you and any other practitioners, noting their names carefully. Also record anything else of note – patient vomited, change of position, contractions increased or reduced in intensity, change of nurses, etc. This can seem excessively detailed in an uneventful labor, as for example when you find yourself alternating the same two or three activities for hours at a time. However, it is remarkable how difficult it is to remember the events of a labor with any precision as to time, so often the timeline proves invaluable in pulling together a coherent narrative.

Acupuncturists will need to add two columns, one for each needle (i.e. SP-6 left, SP-6 right) and one indicating that it has been removed and appropriately disposed of. Ear seeds do not need to be so listed, but magnets and tacks should be. On the chart we use at the hospital, a separate line at the bottom of each page requires the current acupuncturist in the case to visually inspect each needle site listed and sign that all of the points are needle-free before starting a new chart page. This is critically important in preventing inadvertent souvenirs (we learned this lesson the hard way once, in 2008).

8.3.4 Background reading

Below are a few favorites, sorted by type. This should be considered a beginning, not a comprehensive reading list.

8.3.4.1 Acupuncture practice

1. Betts, D. (2006). *The Essential Guide to Acupuncture in Pregnancy and Childbirth*. Hove, UK: Journal of Chinese Medicine. This text by a beloved mentor and colleague is essential. The section on birth is not large but all of her information is clear and solid, light on theory and very strong on experience.

2. West, Z. (2001). *Acupuncture in Pregnancy and Childbirth*. Edinburgh, UK: Churchill Livingstone. I find this book by a British midwife/acupuncturist less useful clinically than the Betts, but there are interesting segments, stories and tidbits of information. In particular, a section on use of E-stim advises mimicking brain wave frequencies, a practice I still use (hence the 2 Hz for calming).

8.3.4.2 Acupuncture integration

1. Roemer, A. (2005). *Medical Acupuncture in Pregnancy: A Textbook*. Stuttgart, Germany: Thieme. I disagree with the author's fundamental premise that the Spleen governs the cervix. However, the book is well organized and offers useful integrative explanations and illustrations.

2. David, S. S., & Blakeway J. (2009). *Making Babies*. New York: Little, Brown. This book beautifully exemplifies how to talk to moms and Western providers about Chinese medicine concepts, without either dumbing them down or sounding mystical.

8.3.4.3 Conventional Western medicine

1. Oxorn, H. (1986). *Human Labor and Birth*. New York: McGraw-Hill (Fifth Edition). This edition of the book has long been superseded, but I love its illustrations and deep detail; for example, there's nearly a whole chapter on ROP position. It's also quite a bit cheaper than the current edition.

2. Cabaniss, M. L., & Ross, M. G. (2010). *Fetal Monitoring Interpretation*. Philadelphia, PA: Wolters Kluwer/Lippincott Williams & Wilkins. This is an expensive, authoritative and dizzyingly thorough guide to interpreting fetal monitor tracings. It's worth borrowing from the library if you spend a lot of time in hospitals.

3. Buckley, S. J. (2015). Executive summary of hormonal physiology of childbearing: Evidence and implications for women, babies, and maternity care. *The Journal of Perinatal Education*, 24(3), 145. Although dense, this book is essential reading for understanding the interrelated physical and emotional terrain in which we work.

8.3.4.4 Mother-friendly Western medicine

1. Simkin, P., Hanson, L., & Ancheta, R. (2017). *The Labor Progress Handbook: Early Interventions to Prevent and Treat Dystocia*. Hoboken, NJ: John Wiley & Sons. Penny Simkin is a physical therapist and one of the founders of the doula movement. This book is a classic for doulas and extremely useful in understanding the progress and bottlenecks of labor.

2. Davis, E., & Pascali-Bonaro, D. (2010). *Orgasmic birth: Your Guide to a Safe, Satisfying, and Pleasurable Birth Experience*. Emmaus, PA: Rodale.

3. Simkin, P., & Klaus, P. (2004). When Survivors Give Birth. Seattle, WA: Classic Day.

8.3.4.5 Chinese medical history and practice

1. Wu, Y. L. (2010). *Reproducing Women: Medicine, Metaphor, and Childbirth in Late Imperial China*. Berkeley, CA: University of California Press. This beautifully written book chronicles a fascinating shift in Chinese medical practice around pregnancy and birth from the Ming to the Qing dynasties.

8.3.4.6 Web resources
The following online resources are also useful.

- **https://healthyseminars.com** The leading provider of online continuing education in acupuncture, Healthy Seminars has a strong focus on women's health. My online classes are available there, along with those of a number of my beloved mentors and colleagues, including Debra Betts from New Zealand, the wonderful British midwife-acupuncturist Sarah Budd and Sharon Weizenbaum in the United States.

- **Whitepinehealingarts.org** Sharon Weizenbaum is an extraordinary herbalist and acupuncturist with particular expertise in women's health. She blogs with extremely valuable clinical pearls, and her online graduate mentorship program has improved the diagnostic and herbal medicine skills of hundreds of acupuncturists. Her blog on carp and daikon soup is the best Chinese medical discussion of polyhydramnios I have seen.

- **Ravenlang.com** Raven Lang is a legend. She founded the first two birthing centers in North America, as well as the first non-medical midwifery school, before apprenticing with groundbreaking acupuncturist Miriam Lee in the 1980s. Her website contains links to her books and recorded teachings.

- **DONA.org** Doulas of North America is one of the largest and best-known organizations training and certifying doulas. Its program is not the longest or most demanding, but for women's health acupuncturists, it can be a great start. Debra Pascali-Bonaro (see orgasmic birth reference earlier and next) offers trainings at least once per year in Brooklyn, NY.

- **Orgasmicbirth.com** This inspiring film and ongoing blog community is the work of Debra Pascali-Bonaro, one of the earliest doulas in North America. She began her work by photographing births, and has gone on to become one of the most articulate voices showing why mother-friendly birth is not a luxury but a cultural and global necessity.

- **https://www.magamama.com** This is the site for Kimberly Ann Johnson, who does wonderful work exploring and healing the pelvic floor. Her book *The Fourth Trimester: A Postpartum Guide to Healing Your Body, Balancing Your Emotions, and Restoring Your Vitality* ((2017) Shambhala Publications) is an excellent resource, as is her podcast, available on the website.

- **Spinningbabies.com** The "belly mapping" handout – one of many resources generously offered on this website – has been helping breech and occipital posterier moms to find and fix their babies' positions since 2004.

- **Milescircuit.org** The Miles Circuit is another phenomenal resource generously offered to the public. It is a series of positions and movements that together take about 90 minutes and gently but powerfully encourage optimal fetal positioning before or during early labor.

8.4 What to Bring to a Birth

As with one's purse, backpack or travel toiletry bag, a well-stocked birth bag will have a number of obvious necessaries, and also a number of personal preferences that will be filled in over time. Here are some suggestions.

The basics:

- practice resource, consent and charting materials

- spare pens and paper

- vibrating massager

- warming packs

- hand-held fan (manual and/or battery-operated)

- small spray bottle for misting

- peanut ball

- small comb for gripping.

Special practice tools:

- needle kit including plenty of ear needles and 1 in. needles thin enough to bend and tape, also 1.5 in., 2 in. and 3 in. needles, hand sanitizer, Q-tips for closing the hole and a compact sharps container

- moxa poles, lighter, jar for ashes and aluminum foil for extinguishing[10]

- small, light E-stim machine (the ES-130 is compact and reliable)

- tape for securing needles

- ear seeds

- aromatherapy oils.

Great additions:

- extra hair clips and ties

- breath mints

- honey sticks (these are little straws filled with honey that you suck out) https://www.gorawhoney.com/raw-honey-sticks

---

10 Stick-on moxa may be more convenient for traveling, and can be ordered from Kamwo. com or other EAM suppliers.

For you:

- full overnight kit including spare fleece, change of clothes, toothpaste/ toothbrush, deodorant, etc.

- extra cash

- granola bars, etc.

- feminine hygiene stuff

- water bottle

- small first aid kit (band-aids, etc.).

8.5 The Birth Team

In Chinese herbal medicine, ancient convention analyzes formulae in terms of four main functions, as follows:

- The *Emperor* is the main herb, given in the largest dosage, which therefore dictates the basic treatment principle of the formula – warming and activating, cooling, etc.

- The *Minister* is an herb with similar properties to the Emperor, which simply serves to strengthen its function.

- *Assistant* herbs have properties markedly different from those of the Emperor, sometimes even diametrically opposed. They may reduce side effects or moderate harsh properties of the Emperor, or they may serve a distinct but related function, such as an herb that calms the spirit in a formula to treat menstrual cramps.

- *Courier* herbs may guide the formula's effects to a specific area of the body, or they may "harmonize" the formula, helping the strong flavors of the other herbs to blend for better taste as well as function.

This framework has a parallel in the labor and delivery process: a birth team works best when all of these roles are capably filled, though casting schemes may vary, with one person filling more than one role or multiple people sharing.

The Emperor provides leadership to the birth, holding the positive vision of its joyous outcome and making final decisions on all intermediate steps. This function may be held by the person having the baby – or by Mom and partner together, with the latter functioning as Minister. In some cultures or situations, the role of Minister may be held by the baby's father, or the birthing person's mother. It may also be abdicated to medical personnel, due to fear or intimidating circumstances. One of the most important team functions of an East Asian medicine (EAM)-informed birth practitioner can be to gently return leadership to Mom by functioning as an effective Minister, showing unconditional warmth and respect for Mom's well-being and preferences.

In some cases, an Assistant is urgently needed: Mom may be experiencing fear or frustration that seeks resolution, or the Emperor may be a less-than-optimal medical practitioner. At other times, friends or family members may be in the Assistant role, and what is needed is a Courier to harmonize their potentially chaotic good intentions, often by directing them into acupressure.

Many of us naturally gravitate to one role or another. Reading the room, and shifting roles as needed, is a critical element of attending births. A colleague of mine jokes about the "doula booby prize," where at the end of a birth Mom can't thank you enough and swears she couldn't have done it without you, while her partner sits stone-faced on the sidelines, waiting for you to leave. This is a clear indication of a doula holding onto the Minister role too long, rather than harmoniously supporting the partner to perform it.

8.6 Practice Structure

Birth is not a sport for lone wolves. Even solo doulas need considerable backup, as two clients per month is not nearly enough to live on, and three patients due in the same month can easily go into labor on the same day (or a day when one is sick or injured). For acupuncturists with a clinical practice, it's even worse: the time-commitment needs of acupuncture and birth treatments are diametrically opposed. Acupuncture patients need you to be in a pre-agreed spot for hours at a time, while births require complete flexibility.

8.6.1 Group practice

The logical solution to this problem, used by most obstetricians and midwives, is group practice. This allows acupuncturists to have reliable clinic days and birth days, as well as days off. An optimal practice size, in my view, consists of three to five senior practitioners and three to five junior practitioners, who follow and assist the senior providers and grow into providing backup or taking on additional clients as demand allows. A full discussion of practice logistics and finances is outside the scope of this book. However, some suggestions follow.

A joint venture need not involve creation of a big new business with associated overhead. With only a website and a Google Voice number, prospective clients could be directed to whoever is on backup duty that day. Initial visits would then be equitably distributed by the calendar, as would birth encounters.

Labor preparation treatments would optimally be included in a package with the birth, and divided between practitioners so that nobody is a stranger by the day of the birth. Although state regulations need to be checked carefully regarding bundling of treatments, it can be useful to bundle other services as well. For example, a Cesarean section recovery package could include a hospital visit for pain and swelling, a home visit to moxa the scar and teach mother warming, then a series of office visits 8 weeks hence for scar therapy. A postpartum home visit is also a most-welcome addition to a birth package, as most patients can benefit greatly from treatment, but are too overwhelmed to make the journey out.

8.6.2 Mixed-discipline practice

Most births can benefit greatly from constitutionally appropriate acupressure and other non-invasive techniques described in this book. That said, by no means does every birth require the full range of an acupuncturist's skills for the whole duration of the birth – nor would that be financially feasible for many. The problem is, it's not clear in advance which births will be smooth and easy and which will require every trick in the book. In a mixed-discipline practice, acupuncturists could provide labor preparation and other pregnancy services, as well as constitutionally appropriate recommendations for intrapartum acupressure and other approaches. Doulas could perform their usual prenatal, intrapartum and postpartum roles, with on-call availability of acupuncturists for difficult births and/or postpartum house calls. (If the doula has also read this book, then a phone call providing advice on differential assessment might be sufficient.)

Acupuncturists might also consider the practice structure of following midwives in order to gain birth experience. While this might not be sustainable long-term, the benefits to both of a time-bounded mentorship would be considerable.

8.7 Then and Now

Earlier this month my colleagues Debra Betts, Sarah Budd, Zena Kocher, Sabine Wilms and I gave a series of talks at the famous traditional Chinese medicine congress in Rothenburg, Germany, on the obstetrical herb formulas of revered 17th-century gynecologist Fu Qing-zhu. I spoke about his prescriptions for labor and delivery, and their relevance to contemporary birth acupuncture practice in the United States. In discussing his formulas for difficult birth due to blood deficiency, bony obstruction and Qi stagnation, Fu Qing-zhu complains about practitioners who begin the mother pushing too early, "before the head is at the birth gate" – a complaint I hear commonly from my colleagues about obstetricians today. In discussing management of stillbirth, he warns that initiating contractions before the fetus has dropped into the pelvis can exhaust the baby – a common presentation in contemporary "failed inductions" that lead to C-section.

Yi-Li Wu's excellent book, *Reproducing Women*, describes the evolution of medical discourse on labor and delivery from the Ming to the Qing dynasties and beyond. She quotes Chinese medical doctor Feng Shaoqu in 1934[11] lamenting the rise of Western birth practices, in a passage that sounds equally familiar to modern readers:

Western-style childbirth medicine has refined and excellent instruments and adroit surgical skills. I deeply admire them. But often they do not understand what the illnesses of pregnancy and postpartum consist of. Some are dazzled by money, while others cherish their time, and before the time for "the melon to ripen and drop" arrives [i.e. the proper time of birth], they have already recklessly used surgical methods to make [the baby] come out. Women in childbirth who have undergone Western surgical techniques must then have surgery the next time they give birth. The result of this is that humankind's original ability to give birth will be reduced day by day.

Today, Raven Lang, the trailblazing midwife who founded the first two birth centers in North America, describes multiple waves of infatuation with new interventions at the expense of natural birth rhythms.

In the first 60–70 years of the 20th century, science and technology had taken over the practice of medicine. Birth had been relegated to hospital care, and during that time it lost something essential, its humanity. When technology became the template for all women and babies during childbirth, much of the old-fashioned support and guidance that women once received got lost and the birthing woman lost authority over her own experience. Instead, her body became a battleground between her instincts and hospital protocols, and birth

---

11 Siming Songshi jiachuan chance quanshu miben (The complete secret book of childbearing transmitted by the Song family of Siming), compl. and suppl. By Feng Shaoqu (Shanghai: Zhongxi shuju, 1934), translated by Yi-Li Wu, *Reproducing Women*, Berkeley, University of California Press, 2010

became a heroic industry of extraction in the name of safety, rather than a rite of passage that involved the sacred.

Just as my curiosity and study on childbirth arose, it simultaneously rose throughout all of North America. Childbearing women no longer wanted to acquiesce to the institutional practice of birth and in the 1970's a mere 10% of them began to have their babies at home. Midwifery, a profession that had been outlawed in most states made a needed comeback. It did this because of a desperate desire women had to have it. With a great deal of effort and a few decades to get midwives licensure, a huge body of silenced knowledge was regained by midwives and birthing women.

Due to these changes, childbearing women were now listened to in ways they had not been for decades.

Since the 1970's to the end of the 1990's, terrific positive changes were made in hospitals. Women were no longer separated from their mates during labor and delivery, the leather straps were discarded, hospitals developed rooming-in for mothers and babies, and lactation consultants were available in the first day or two of a hospital stay. This makeover looked good, and it was. But, in the process of these positive changes, the Cesarean rate jumped from 5.5% in 1970 to 15.2% by 1978, and by the year 2015, according to the American Congress of Obstetricians and Gynecologists (ACOG) the national average of Cesareans jumped to 32% in one mere generation! Despite the good that was being accomplished, something still remained quite wrong in the industry of birth.

Science and technology continued to rise exponentially during these years of rising Cesareans. It brought us widespread use of antibiotics and surgery. It enabled us to collect data and monitor the health and well being of mothers and babies as pregnancy progressed. These additions to our health care are important and are tools that save lives. However, we must be aware that only a few women and babies need them, because when birth is left to itself it is normally a safe process. Today obstetrical decisions are made because of numbers, graphs, and pictures that scientific data provide. Due dates determine destiny. Rules and regulations of hospitals and of ACOG are all too often absolute and do not allow individual considerations or treatment plans. Great strides in childbirth have been made, no question, but we are still in big trouble.

From three experts 300 years apart, responding to the pressures of their own time and place, it is possible to draw some general conclusions:

1. Certain social systems, reimbursement structures and frailties of human nature may favor excess intervention, including surgery.

2. Those forces are remarkably persistent over time, and across cultures.

3. As surgical birth becomes safer and more accepted, curiosity and expertise as to the nature and conduct of vaginal birth diminish.

For those of us who work to develop and foster such expertise, it is tempting to think in terms of a crusade – a Yin army – fighting to turn the cultural tide from birth-as-surgery back to birth-as-sacred-life journey (with high-tech interventions available as needed). But a battle needs an enemy. This might be individual care providers and institutions making decisions we disagree with, or the systemic forces that can incentivize unhealthy decisions. Either way, we are fighting against reality itself: the very definition of stagnation. Stagnation happens, it's a part of life – but it's not a working strategy for success.

What's most needed is to nourish the flow of culture in a positive direction – which happens through positive interactions accumulated steadily over time. My colleague Zena Kocher had been a fixture in the antenatal unit of her hospital for years, and everyone knew that the patients were happier and more relaxed when her team was there – but it was only recently when they ran the numbers on high-risk preeclampsia that they realized that patients were staying pregnant for many days longer. Australian acupuncturist and researcher Kate Levett's PhD project was a combination of six simple, evidence-based techniques, including acupressure, taught to moms and partners for use before and during labor. The techniques were well known and commonly used in birth: they included simple acupressure, yoga and breathing exercises. Moms who took the course not only had fewer C-sections, they also had fewer epidurals, labor augmentation interventions and neonatal resuscitations, second stage of labor was shorter and perineal trauma was milder. And just yesterday I was encouraged to receive an email from a younger colleague who is currently starting a new acupuncture program at a hospital on the West Coast, with advice from Debra, Zena and several others. She wrote:

Our first patient that we saw at the hospital was headed in on Tuesday for an induction due to low amniotic fluid and the week prior, Natalie sent her home with strict homework for pre-birth acupressure and moxa on ST36 and she got to the hospital on Tuesday with increased fluids and 8 cm dilated!

Interventions like antenatal acupuncture, intrapartum acupressure and home care homework can be normalized, slowly but surely – it just takes as many of us as possible, showing up and making ancient wisdom as available as possible in our modern world. Over the past 15 years I have tried to do my part by teaching this material to patients, families and practitioners, as well as consulting and mentoring for new hospital programs. I encourage others to do the same; information on these courses, as well as mentorship for practitioners and new programs, is available at my website, Citkovitz.com.

Of all the Yang forces eternally pushing for unnecessary intervention, perhaps most basic is the earnest wish to do something, in the face of birth's emotional and physical intensity. This urgency to act is particularly understandable in people who are action-oriented to begin with, and those whose anxieties have been stoked by the culture around them –whether those people are birth partners or health care providers.

One recent approach to reduction of excessive Yang has been through reason, with observational and clinical research demonstrating that outcomes are not improved by excessive surgical, pharmaceutical and monitoring interventions. Less direct but perhaps equally important is the nourishing Yin, by providing something to do in birth that is not surgical or pharmaceutical. This work is already underway by a giant, peaceful Yin army of birth educators, midwives, doulas, nurses, physicians, acupuncturists and massage therapists using a magnificent spectrum of preparation and comfort measures that give moms and their birth teams a sense of orientation to the events of birth, as well as specific measures to take. I have found EAM exceptionally useful for both these purposes, and hope that readers will, too.

Acupressure Point Locations and Names

Table A1 contains the names and locations of all acupressure points used in this book. Illustrations of point locations can be found below (Figures A1 to A10) and in Chapter 2 (Figures 2.4 and 2.5). Names and locations are not provided for points used for needling only, as those trained in acupuncture will either know the information or have their own, more precise reference resources. For convenience and ease of use during birth, the app version of "A Manual of Acupuncture"[1] is highly recommended; it provides both line drawings and video of point locations. Point locations can also easily be found in Google and Google Images.

Table A1 Point names and locations (acupressure points only).

Point	Chinese name	English translation	Figure	Location
Clavicle points			A4	Along underside of clavicle
Du-14	Dazhui	Big hammer	A5	In the depression below the (very prominent) spinous process of the seventh cervical vertebra
Du-20	Baihui	Hundred Meetings	A8	At the highest point of the head, on the line connecting the tops of the ears
Duyin		Solitary Yin	A9	Under the second toe, at the center of the distal crease

---

1   Deadman, P., Al-Khafaji, M., & Baker, K. (1998). *A Manual of Acupuncture* (pp. 256–325). Hove, UK: Journal of Chinese Medicine Publications.

Ear Apex			A10	At the highest point of the ear Alternate: find and prick venules near the top of the ear
Ear Cingulate Gyrus			A10	On the surface of the earlobe, anterior and inferior to the deepest point of the intertragic notch
Ear Endocrine			A10	On the superior aspect of the bottom of the intertragic notch, slightly posterior and medial to its deepest point
Ear Liver			A10	Posterior and slightly superior to Point Zero, where the floor of the ear begins to rise toward the antehelix
Ear Point Zero			A10	At the center of the ear, on the superior aspect of the antihelix where it merges with the floor of the ear
Ear Shenmen			A10	In the superior aspect of the triangular fossa, ¼ to ⅓ of the way from its apex to its base
Ear Sympathetic			A10	On the wall of the ear, at the anterior inferior corner of the triangular fossa
Ear Thalamus			A10	At the midpoint of the base of the antitragus, following a ridge from the tip of the antitragus down to where it meets the floor of the ear
Ear Uterus			A10	At the midpoint of the base of the triangular fossa, where the floor and wall of the ear meet
GB-21	Jianjing	Shoulder well	A5	Tender point in the middle of the trapezius muscle, approximately midway between Du-14 and the acromion of the shoulder
GB-30	Huantiao	Jumping circle	2.5	Tender point in a depression in the buttock, ⅓ of the distance between the greater trochanter and the top of the coccyx
GB-31	Fengshi	Wind market	2.5	Tender point in the iliotibial band on the lateral thigh, slightly more than ⅓ of the say from the knee to the greater trochanter

GB-34	Yanglingquan	Yang hill spring	2.5	Tender point in the depression approximately 1 in. (2.5 cm) anterior and inferior to the head of the fibula
GB-41	Zulinqi	Foot container of tears	2.5	Distal to the junction of the fourth and fifth metacarpal bones, in a depression just lateral to a large tendon
Hand points			A1	Along the distal palmar crease, including HT-8
HT-8	Shaofu	Lesser mansion	A1	In the depression between the fourth and fifth metacarpal bones, slightly below the distal palmar crease, where the tip of the little finger falls when fully flexed
Inner thigh points			2.4	Along the Liver and Kidney channels, approximately midway up the inner thigh
KD-1	Yongquan	Bubbling spring	A9	On the sole of the foot, in the depression formed when the toes are flexed
LI-4	Hegu	Adjoining valley	A2	Tender point in the flesh between thumb and forefinger, at the midpoint of the metacarpal bone. Note: for obstetrical use, the most tender and useful point is usually found much closer to the wrist, near where the metacarpal bones meet
Liver Gummies			A6	Tender nodules along the posterior edge of the tibia, from above the ankle bone to below the knee
LV-2	Xingjian	Movement between	A3	Just proximal to the webbing between the first and second toes
LV-3	Taichong	Great rushing	A3	Tender depression distal to the junction of the first and second metatarsal bones
LV-8	Ququan	Spring at the bend	2.4	Tender point at the inner knee, just superior to the medial end of the popliteal crease in a depression between two large tendons

LV-14	Qimen	Cycle gate	A4	Directly below the nipple (or where it would be on a flat chest); in the sixth intercostal space at approximately the level of a bra strap
PC-6	Neiguan	Inner gate	A1	On the inner forearm, approximately 2 in. (5 cm) above the wrist crease in a depression between the two largest tendons, slightly to the thumb side of the midline
PC-8	Laogong	Palace of work	A1	On the transverse palm crease, in the depression between the second and third metacarpal bones
SI-11	Tianzong	Heavenly gathering	A5	Tender point in the center of the scapula
Soojok uterus			A9	Depression in the fleshy area underneath the bases of the toes, between the distal heads of the third and fourth metatarsal bones
SP-1	Yinbai	Hidden white	A3	On the flesh just proximal and medial to the corner of the great toenail
SP-6	Sanyinjiao	Three Yin crossing	A4, A6	In a tender depression a hand's breadth above the inner ankle, just behind the tibia
SP-9	Yinlingquan	Yin mound spring	A4	In a tender depression below and behind the medial condyle of the tibia
ST-31	Biguan	Thigh gate	A4	At the juncture of the torso and upper thigh, at the junction of lines drawn down from the hipbone and across from the pubic bone, in a depression that deepens when the leg is lifted
ST-36	Zusanli	Leg three miles	A4	A hand's breadth below the outer eye of the knee, in a depression one finger width lateral to the crest of the tibia
ST-44	Neiting	Inner court	A3	Just proximal to the webbing between the second and third toes

TH-5	Waiguan	Outer gate	A2	On the outer forearm, approximately 2 in. (5 cm) above the wrist crease in the hollow between the ulna and radius, directly opposite PC-6
UB-31–34 (sacral points)	Ba Liao	Eight bone-holes	A5	Tender spots at and around the holes in the sacrum
UB-17	Geshu	Diaphragm transporting point	A5	Between the spine and the lower corner of the scapula, approximately 1.5 in. (3.8 cm) lateral to the spinous process of T7, at the highest point on the paraspinal muscle
UB-60	Kunlun	Kunlun mountains	A7	In the depression between the outer ankle bone and the Achilles tendon
UB-67	Zhiyin	Reaching Yin	A3, A7	On the flesh just proximal and lateral to the corner of the fifth toenail
Waist points			A5	Tender points on the side, approximately 1 in. (2.5 cm) above the crest of the hipbone

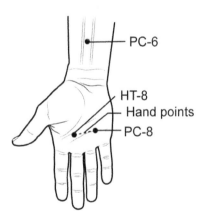

Figure A1 Points of the inner forearm and palm.

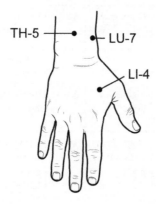

Figure A2 Points of the outer forearm and hand.

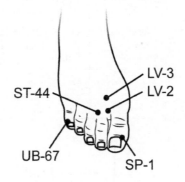

Figure A3 Points of the dorsum of the foot.

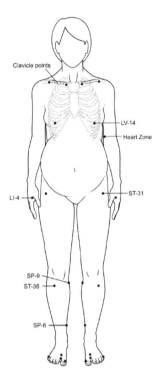

Figure A4 Points of the frontal torso and legs.

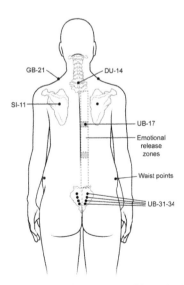

Figure A5 Points of the upper and lower back.

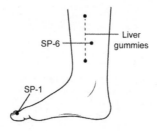

Figure A6 Points of the medial leg and foot.

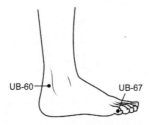

Figure A7 Points of the lateral leg and foot.

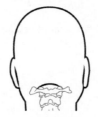

Figure A8 Points of the head.

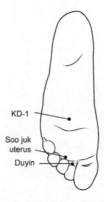

Figure A9 Points of the sole of the foot.

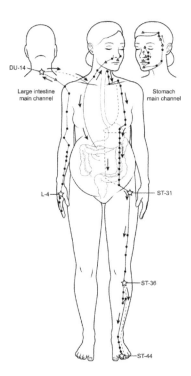

Figure A10 Points of the Large Intestine, Stomach and Du channels.

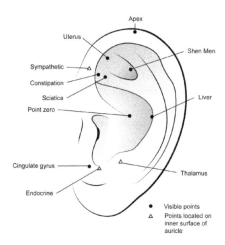

Figure A11 Points of the ear.

Moxibustion for Breech Presentation

Moxibustion at UB-67 for breech presentation is a simple, safe procedure that can be done at home. It can also be used for transverse or oblique lie. When performed correctly, it is seen to increase the frequency of fetal movements, and the likelihood of babies turning head down. It is important to follow guidelines for correct timing, application and "dosage."

Timing

The Western method for addressing breech presentation is external cephalic version, an uncomfortable procedure in which a midwife or doctor manually encourages the fetus to turn. The procedure carries a significant risk of initiating labor, and is therefore usually performed after the middle of the 34th week, when fetal development is sufficient that a preterm birth would not be terribly dangerous.

The optimal time for breech moxa to be performed is between 33 and 35 weeks, when Baby still has plenty of room to move. Another advantage of this early time frame is that if the fetus does not turn with moxa alone, external version is still an option. Of course, moms typically wait until 36 or even 38 weeks to call, when there is less available space. Cautions and modifications of the procedure for that situation are discussed below.

Method

Basic use of moxibustion is described in Section 5.4. For UB-67, the challenge is to apply sufficient heat to the small point without overheating it or the surrounding area, or making it so much trouble that parents won't do it. Experience has shown that a highly efficient method is to secure the moxa poles in a stable holder; for example, a canister of "play-doh" or other child's modeling clay. I have also seen the moxa pole secured by closing a hardcover book on it, but of course close attention must be paid to keep the burning end of the stick far from the flammable pages. Once two sticks have been stably located, 2–3 ft (60–90 cm) apart and facing each other, Mom can then position her feet between them, either seated or on hands and knees. She can then regulate distance and temperature simply by moving her feet.

Some East Asian medicine (EAM) traditions – notably the Japanese – use "direct" moxa, in which a very pure form of the herb is rolled into tiny threads and burned directly on the acupuncture point. Others use small manufactured "stick-on" poles, which are applied directly to the point and make less smoke. There are also "smokeless" moxa poles, which are more concentrated and burn hotter with less smoke, and even a topically applied "liquid" moxa that contains warming herbs. Other than the liquid moxa, which I am quite certain is useless for this purpose, I do not have strong recommendations for or against the others. To my knowledge nothing other than the large moxa poles has been evaluated in clinical trials. I personally have tried direct moxa with what appeared to be inferior results (though my sample is small and my direct moxa skills are not the best).

Dosage

It is important that moxibustion be done daily, and for a long enough period each day. The clinical trials showing most effectiveness of the method have in general had daily treatments of at least 15 minutes, performed for at least a week. I recommend to my patients that they do the procedure 20 minutes per day for 10 days. The extra 5 minutes and 3 days are safety buffers to ensure that even if they cheat a little, they get an adequate dose. I also recommend finishing out the course whether or not Baby turns, as it is my belief (based on EAM principles plus experience) that the extra Yang pushed into the body by the moxa helps keep Baby well positioned.

If moms have completed one course and Baby has not turned, I do not advocate repeating the course, though I am not against it if they are still before 37 weeks. Debra Bettts, who has seen a higher volume of these patients than I over more years, reports feedback from midwives she works with that for moms who undergo external cephalic version, having done the moxibustion, the version is easier and less uncomfortable than for those who have not.

After 34 Weeks

The methods below can be used to optimize fluid volume and position for maximum maneuverability after the ideal time window has passed. The methods are effective in my experience, but time-consuming and labor intensive. The larger Baby is, the more room she needs to turn and the more important it is to include them.

Hydration should start 6 or more hours before treatment, with at least 8 oz (227 g) per hour. Miso soup, coconut water and pear juice seem to be most potent for increasing amniotic fluid, but anything will do other than caffeine (which is a diuretic) and water alone (which in high quantities can alter Mom's electrolyte balance).

To further increase amniotic fluid, moxa on ST-36 should be performed for 10–15 minutes each side, or both together. The technique can be sparrow peck (see Chapter 5) or steady heat. This should be done after at least 3 hours of hydration, and at least 3 hours before the UB-67 moxa.

To increase space, Mom can take a supported knee–chest position during the UB-67 moxa. This is done by starting on hands and knees, then adding pillows under the chest and bump until it is reasonably comfortable to fold the arms and relax the upper body downwards, turning the head and relaxing the cheek on another pillow. This position has the benefit of lifting the uterus away from the sacrum and pelvis, which optimizes fetal maneuverability. However Mom may feel uncomfortable pressure on the lungs and liver; this can be alleviated somewhat with more support under the chest. In this position, it is easiest for a partner or helper to do the UB-67 moxa from behind.

If possible, this treatment should be followed by a session of swimming or relaxing in the water, belly-down as much as possible. With the bump supported by the water, Baby has maximum freedom to move.

Cautions and Modifications

Important cautions for this procedure include:

- Neuropathy or severe pedal edema. These moms are at high risk for burns or infections, and should not casually self-regulate the temperature. Instead, a partner should apply the moxa one toe at a time, keeping their own fingers right near the point to objectively assess temperature.

- Fibroids, previous Cesarean birth, bicornuate uterus or other known uterine anomaly. It is my sense, based on experience, that babies held in place by physical constraints of the uterus such as fibroids will not turn with moxibustion alone. However I don't see any harm in trying the procedure at 33–36 weeks. I would be conservative about suggesting moxa after that time.

- Twins. In general I do not advocate the use of moxibustion for multiple pregnancies. It should be avoided when the twins share an amniotic sac, as the cords may become tangled. It is unnecessary if Baby A (the lower one, who will deliver first) is head down. In cases where Baby A is breech and the sacs are separate, I would consider whether there still seems to be adequate room for Baby A to turn. In no case would I encourage use of moxa without agreement from the primary care provider.

Written Instructions

I strongly advocate providing patients with written instructions for performing the procedure, rather than relying on verbal transmission. I also suggest that the written instructions should clearly indicate that patients are responsible for discussing the plan of care thoroughly with their primary providers. In particular, moms should be explicitly aware that external cephalic version is an option, and is not to be confused with moxibustion.

Moxibustion for Threatened Miscarriage

This moxibustion and visualization technique comes originally from the the great Chinese medical practitioner and martial artist Ken Ark Fu Gong. I learned it as a treatment for threatened miscarriage, and in the decades since have also used it successfully for other kinds of vaginal bleeding and premature shortening of the cervix during pregnancy. The point used for this technique is Du-20; located at the very top of the head, it is frequently used to raise Qi. The method is an advanced variation of sparrow peck moxa (see Chapter 5).

Sparrow peck moxa is quite meditative. It takes a little while to really get the feel of it, developing a sense that you are pushing Qi into a point that is happily receiving it, and then, after a number of repetitions, feeling something change once the body is done – an increased sense of resistance to your push, or something along those lines. For those who feel quite solid on the regular sparrow peck technique, a more advanced method is to reverse direction, using the moxa to pull the Qi upward. Steps are as follows:

1. With a moxa pole lit and fingers near the point checking for warmth, bring the pole in to warm the point.

2. Have a feeling of connecting with the point, and imagine the warmth of the moxa filling and strengthening Mom's spine down to the perineum (the other end of the Du channel).

3. Once you feel a sense of connection (this may take a few seconds, especially at first) pull the moxa pole away from the point very slowly, as though you are tugging hard on a rope to raise the muscles around the perineum and hold Baby in.

Repeat this action for approximately 15 minutes, every other day if possible, depending on the severity of the situation. Be reasonable about logistics though – if a house call is not possible, then Mom staying at home in bed may be more important than coming to your office. Not every partner will be confident and mindful enough to learn this technique, but it may be worth a try. I don't think the technique can possibly cause harm, other than a sore spot on the scalp.

Labor Preparation

As a medical term, "labor induction" means leading the patient into labor, by initiating contractile activity. I avoid the phrase, not because acupuncture can't initiate contractions – it can, as we have seen – but because in most cases where contractions haven't started spontaneously there's a reason why. Challenges of position, hormonal activity, cervical ripening and/or emotional preparedness cause delayed labor onset more often than simple lack of contractions. Accordingly, most moms benefit more from preparatory work based on their personal situation, than from generic stimulation of contractions. Also, as discussed in Chapter 8, use of a Western term for an East Asian medicine (EAM) procedure can be problematic if Mom is not entirely clear in her expectations.

The approach described below is to systematically assess and assist Mom's progress toward active labor. The landmarks along the way are the same as those discussed in Chapter 7 – engagement, cervical ripening and initiation of contractile activity. However, there are some differences in approach, because for labor preparation there is more time for homework and self-care to promote the important hormonal and emotional shifts toward readiness. The steps below summarize the main components of a labor preparation visit, with needles or with targeted acupressure, bodywork and home care. There is no need to use the specific methods I describe, particularly for those who have their own acupuncture or bodywork practice, but I do suggest sticking to the overall architecture of the session, as follows:

- initial information gathering; choose position for session

- relax body and spirit

- sequentially assess and support labor preparation goals, one main goal per session. These are:

- – engagement

- – hormonal changes and tissue softening

- – cervical ripening

- – initiation of contractions.

- • teach labor preparation homework as appropriate.

Tight for time, or overwhelmed by all the choices below? Acupuncture or pressure at the standard "labor induction" points, LI-4, SP-6 and UB-32, can provide a push in the right direction for many moms after week 37 – as long as occiput posterior (OP) has been ruled out. SP-6 nourishes Yin and Blood and promotes dilatation, while LI-4 can either nourish or move Qi depending on whether it's stimulated gently or strongly. All three points have also been shown to have some effects promoting hormonal and/or contractile activity, so they're safe bets for a generic first session where Mom seems healthy and balanced, or time has been taken up by initial intake and checking for red flags. However, if there are any actual problems to solve, it's better to address them specifically using the information in the sections to follow.

D1 Initial Information Gathering

It would be possible to spend half the session with Mom in a chair opposite us, asking questions in order to get a better idea of what exactly is going on and how we can best help. However, every minute spent talking is one not spent doing bodywork or acupuncture. This section details the essential points of information that really do need to be gathered before the session starts. These include:

- • What is the timing of the pregnancy and any anticipated intervention, e.g. induction at 39 weeks, or 42?

- • Visual assessment and brief palpation of the belly: Is Mom's back excessively curved? Has Baby dropped yet? Is the occiput posterior (OP) or anterior (OA)?

- • Any clues as to constitutional challenges?

- • Red flags – is there anything going on that requires urgent medical referral?

D1.1 Time parameters and associated therapeutic goals

Therapeutic goals are set in relation to time parameters. Usually, Baby will begin to engage at 36–38 weeks for first-time moms, but will stay higher longer in multiparas. Hormones should also be getting in gear at this time, with signs such as feeling emotional or chatty, lower back pain, or even nausea or diarrhea. Loss of the mucus plug is a sign of early cervical ripening. If these signs are not seen, or if a vaginal exam indicates that Baby is still high or cervix is still firm at or after 38 weeks, then therapeutic principles of softening the pelvic floor and/or promoting hormonal activity are in order. Differential assessments and therapeutic methods for each of these sequential goals are discussed below. The approximate expected time frame is as follows, but each individual's progress will differ. Every section should be consulted until its associated goal is reached:

- Week 36, initial information gathering; assess and address bony obstacles to engagement.

- Weeks 37, support hormonal shift and tissue softening.

- Weeks 38, promote cervical ripening.

- Week 39, if Baby is still high, strongly promote engagement and tissue softening; if engaged, promote cervical ripening.

- Week 40, if engaged with ripe cervix, promote contractions; otherwise strongly address cervical ripening or previous goals as appropriate.

Situations that affect therapeutic goal setting are as follows:

- If an early induction is planned for medical reasons, strongly promote hormonal shift and tissue softening (or other goals based on Mom's progress); also address any constitutional imbalances identified.

- If there has been premature rupture of membranes (PROM), assess and address occiput posterior position (OP) as the most likely cause; if OP is ruled out, then use sequential goals plus hip rocking, etc. to stretch tissues.

- If Mom is planning a vaginal birth after Cesarean section (VBAC), then use the same time parameters, but with closer attention to staying on schedule, increasing frequency and/or intensity of sessions and home care, or referring to an experienced women's health acupuncturist.

D1.2 Visual assessment and palpation

Just as bodyguards automatically size up everyone in the room, we can use the initial moments of an encounter to process important visual information about Mom and her likely labor journey. Specifically:

Has Baby dropped yet? With a little practice, the eye can trace a shift from apple to pear shape in the torso. There is also a marked change in gait as Mom's center of gravity shifts both downward and backward as Baby enters the pelvis. Baby weight that has been out in front of her, rotating the pelvis forward, now moves backward and downward, tilting the pelvis backward as it goes. Moms will usually notice and report this shift; heartburn and shortness of breath also improve, while urinary urgency worsens. If in doubt, it is possible to gently palpate the head in the lower abdomen, checking whether it is free to move and how many finger widths are palpable above the pubic symphysis (see Figure 3.6).

Once Mom is on the table, it is also useful to measure with a tape, from the top of the pubic symphysis to the top of the bump. This will help to track progress from session to session, and can also be used at the end of a session if it looks or feels as though significant change has taken place.

Is the back excessively arched? One common form of bony obstruction is that as Baby's weight pulls the pelvis forward, a back that is already weak or tight may arch excessively, sending Baby's weight further out in front, which only increases the pull on the strained muscles. This swayback posture is a leading cause of back pain in pregnancy; acupuncturists also see it in men; my colleagues call it "beer belly back pain." When the pelvis is tilted forward, engagement is more difficult, as gravity is not working at a favorable angle to bring Baby's head into the pelvis. Cervical ripening may also be delayed, as more of Baby's weight rests forward against the pubic bone and stomach muscles, meaning less pressure on the cervix and pelvic floor.

Is Baby OP? Visual assessment and palpation are described in Section 7.1.2; a typical OP bump is high in the center, above the navel, with a slight dip around the navel area where there should be a smooth outward curve. OP is not always easy to identify visually, particularly if Mom has a heavy build. If palpating along the bump does not resolve the question, the OP approach outlined in Section D3.1 should still be used any time there is prelabor rupture of membranes (commonly caused by OP), or if there is back or sacral pain; the approach is quite gentle and will not cause harm.

In addition to these bony considerations, observation of Mom's flesh and spirit is helpful to understanding what may delay labor onset.

- Look for signs that Mom's spirit is either stuck or checked out. How is her affect as she walks in? Does she meet your eyes and interact in an ordinary way? Is there a sense of frustration or other emotional heaviness? Or any delay or disconnect? Usually there is not, but it is important to inquire further if something doesn't seem right.

- Is Mom's flesh far to the Yin or Yang end of the spectrum – pale, soft and moist, or excessively slender and ropy? Does she hold herself tightly upright, or more slack? Are her movements rapid and restless, or slow and heavy? If an imbalance is severe enough to hold back labor inside the body, it usually shows itself outwardly as well.

D1.3 Basic medical history and red flags for referral to primary care

Ask about Mom's age and medical history, including any previous pregnancies. Older patients are more prone to Yin or Blood insufficiency even if they look great, while medical history can give clues to possible constitutional challenges. Previous pregnancies and labors provide the most important cues about what to look for and help with this time around, particularly if there were losses or other emotional difficulties. Also, remember multiparas tend not to engage before 39–40 weeks, so Baby not dropping before this time is not necessarily a problem.

- Are vaginal exam findings available? See Chapter 7 for discussion of significance.

- Ask about menses. Extra-painful cramps suggest stagnation – often cold that should be warmed before labor. Regularity, duration and consistency are also clues to constitution (see Chapter 2).

- Course of this pregnancy. Was there severe morning sickness or fatigue? These suggest insufficiency or obstruction of Qi or Yin. Were Braxton–Hicks contractions on schedule? This is not necessarily a problem, but may signal emotional or experiential disconnect with the pregnancy.

Also ask about any other current symptoms; check ankle swelling, musculoskeletal pain, heartburn or constipation, insomnia, etc. *These are cues to imbalance and obstruction, and respond well to acupuncture or acupressure.*

Any of the "red flag" symptoms below should be referred to primary care for evaluation. They are discussed more thoroughly in Chapter 8.

- Vaginal bleeding: other than a few streaks of blood with the mucus plug, any bleeding requires urgent referral.

- Unusual itching: cholestasis needs to be ruled out.

- Excessive swelling of the ankles or (especially) of the hands, headaches, dizziness, sudden weight gain, abdominal pain or feeling generally unwell can be warning signs for preeclampsia.

- Decreased fetal movements.

- Feelings of sadness, guilt, worthlessness, anxiety or lack of interest in activities can all suggest prenatal depression, particularly if appetite or sleep are affected.

D1.4 Choose positioning for the session

I usually suggest seating Mom on a sturdy stool, or a chair with a small back that allows you to work on her back. Support the head and shoulders well with pillows as Mom leans forward onto a table or treatment bench. It is usually most comfortable to fold the arms cradling the head. This position naturally opens the back and helps Baby drop into the pelvis.

The side-lying position is better for addressing OP position, or lower-body complaints such as sciatica or severe swollen ankles. It may also be preferred for various reasons, including fatigue. Have plenty of pillows on hand to support Mom's head, upper leg and possibly the baby bump. If time allows, it's best to address both sides by starting the session with the non-problem side up for the relaxation sequence, then have Mom turn by coming up on hands and knees, then down on the other side.

Other positions are fine, too. The main constraints are that pregnant people should not lie flat on their backs for more than 30 seconds, and that fluid loss from ruptured membranes should be minimized by keeping Mom mostly horizontal.

D2 Relax Body and Spirit

Whatever the specific therapeutic goals, labor preparation works best when mind and body have settled down onto the table together. Downward movement along the large muscles of the back – the "emotional release areas" – is an EAM staple for letting go of sticky emotions and physical tightness. Those already trained in bodywork can make their own choices about technique; the acupressure sequence described below has proven highly effective over the years, particularly in the seated position. If Mom is seated, you will likely want to start out standing and finish sitting on a chair behind her; make sure to have this set up in advance for a graceful transition.

Acupuncturists may choose do to an abbreviated version of the acupressure sequence below, by simply palpating downward along the inner and outer Bladder channels of the back, releasing any tight areas with acupressure and/or needles. Treatment may also include:

- birth basics points for relaxation and hormones: Sympathetic, Uterus, Shenmen, Liver, Endocrine

- other ear or body points by presentation or symptom – Constipation or Sciatica points, Bladder point for OP, Kidney point for Yin or Yang deficiency, points along the antihelix for back pain, etc.

The acupressure sequence begins with helping the head, neck and shoulders to relax. This is similar whether in side-lying or forward-leaning position:

- Open the channels of the back by gently chafing down along the paraspinal muscles from the neck to the top of the pelvis.

- Use the fingertips to dredge along the muscles and channels of the scalp.

- Use the thumb and middle finger to grasp downward along the neck from the occiput to the base, two or three times. The final pass should be slower, pausing to press comfortably into the muscles of the neck for 5–10 seconds each, or longer if desired.

- Gently grasp the trapezius muscles of the shoulders, both sides simultaneously, until they soften and relax – usually a minute or two.

Once neck and shoulders have relaxed, address the back and emotional release areas. Start with round rubbing or gentle chafing, downward along the large muscles of the back, to warm and soften the muscles.

Then, to open the emotional release areas more deeply, the thumbs will move downward along the large muscles of the back, making gentle contact with redirecting pressure to move Qi downward through the emotional release zones, as follows:.

- With both hands gently resting on the shoulders, let the thumbs make contact at the top of the paraspinal muscles, the large ridges 1–2 in. (2.5–5 cm) outside the spine. This will be slightly below the level of the large prominent vertebrae at the top of the back.

- As Mom inhales, leave the thumbs where they are, so that they press slightly into the muscle rather than rising with Mom's breath and staying at skin level. As she exhales, you should have a feeling of downward movement (this technique is actually redirecting pressure; see Section 5.2.2.1).

- Stay with this point for another in- and out-breath, letting Mom's body catch on that it can trust your thumbs not to make any sudden moves, and using your thumbs to press against and release the tight muscles. Then move your thumbs downward one rib space per breath. If you can't feel the ribs under your fingers, it's fine to guesstimate about an inch per two breaths.

- Most important is to be relaxed and present yourself, keeping your hand movements steady and moving the thumbs right on schedule with every breath. If you notice tight areas, you can return to them with gentle thumb circles starting above the tight place and working downwards.

- When you reach the hipbones in the back, you will need to move your thumbs inward along the pelvis until you reach the top of the sacrum. Keeping the pace at 1 in. (2.5 cm) per breath, descend along the sacrum to either side of the coccyx.

- Conclude the releasing sequence with slow, deliberate thumb circles along the top of the pelvis, from the sides all the way down to the sacrum again, followed (optionally) by thumb circles at any areas that were tight on the first pass.

- Finally, stand up, ask Mom how she is doing and repeat the initial round rubbing or gentle chafing downward along the muscles to close the sequence.

For side-lying sessions, hip rocking and round rubbing or chafing down the back should be followed by round rubbing on the muscles of the hip and buttock area. Then, dredge down the Gallbladder channel, and perform grasping and thumb circles on any tight areas identified. For OP, particular attention should be paid to loosening up the sacroiliac joint, hip and buttock.

D3 Address Bony Challenges to Engagement – Week 36 and After

Assessing engagement has already been discussed above under "Visual assessment and palpation." First babies often drop between 36 and 38 weeks, and can be considered behind schedule if still high after 38 weeks. Subsequent babies usually drop later, and labor usually starts shortly thereafter (unless Mom is Yang deficient or damp, in which case she may need help with initiation of contractions).

A common reason for late engagement is bony obstruction – most commonly OP or swayback posture, discussed below. *If found, they should be addressed as soon as possible* – the therapeutic methods suggested are gentle and safe before 37 weeks. Table D1 summarizes the assessments and approaches.

Table D1 Assessing and addressing challenges to bony engagement.

Assessment/ goal	Therapeutic methods in session	Homework
Swayback? Open the lower back	Seated relaxation sequence, plus: • Warm the lower back • Repeat relaxation sequence for lower back • Coach Mom on flattening the back	• Repeat back flattening exercise two or three times a day (provide instructions) • Add Hula Hips and daily foot soaks as time allows
Occiput posterior? Open space and encourage rotation	• With right* side up, 5 minutes relaxation sequence • Turn right side down, rock hips 20–30 minutes plus acupressure or acupuncture to open space • Reassess position *Most OP is ROP; if no change in session, palpate for possible LOP or ask primary provider	• If no change during session, teach UB-67 moxa (provide instructions) and Miles Circuit • Cat/Cow on hands and knees, 3–5 minutes, three to five times a day • Avoid sitting leaned back or knees above hips • Foot soaks or moxa if Yang or Qi deficient

D3.1 OP (plus or minus PROM)

OP position at or before engagement is extremely common. In many cases it is a simple matter of habit due to Mom's relationship with gravity, and one or two sessions of hip rocking and homework will lead Baby to engage in a better position. OP can also be caused by a pelvis narrow in front, in which case it will persist for three or more sessions. Therapeutic goals should then shift to softening the pelvic floor, particularly the sacrotuberous ligament release, which can increase space at the pelvic outlet for posterior delivery (see Section 6.2.1). When Baby is engaged OP, cervical ripening and initiation of contractions may also be slow, as the head is not well situated to press on the cervix.

OP is a common cause of PROM, where membranes rupture but labor does not start within 4 hours. This is because the membranes can easily tear by catching between Baby's occiput and Mom's bony sacrum. Amniotic fluid is a rich soup of hormones and prostaglandins; if the head is placing appropriate pressure on the cervix, and Yin and Yang are functioning adequately, then the steady drip of amniotic fluid should normally be enough to ripen the cervix and start contractions. However in OP, the head is pressing back into the sacrum and not down onto the cervix, so contractions don't start. Although PROM can happen in other situations – infection or inflammation, often with underlying Yin deficiency; or QI stagnation – OP is by far the most common. Whether or not OP has been confirmed, the gentle hip rocking is beneficial for PROM, as it stretches the tissues to encourage cervical ripening.

The therapeutic goals for OP are to open space and help Baby turn. Specific methods are as follows:

- Start with the right side up[1] for the relaxation sequence described above, approximately 5 minutes.

- Turn to right side down, place pillows for comfort and find a rocking movement that will be comfortable and sustainable for 20–30 minutes.

- Open space in the pelvis and Dai/Belt channel, and encourage repositioning.

  - Acupressure: strong pressure for 1 minute each on bilateral LV-7, Waist points, and GB-31; optional moxa or ear seed at UB-67.

  - Acupuncture: constitutional treatment plus moxa on UB-67; at 37 weeks or more, add Dai opening points, SP-6 and UB-60, can substitute needles or ear tacks for moxa.

- Rock the hips very gently for 20–30 minutes (making sure not to disturb needles if they are in).

---

1   It can be difficult to distinguish which side an OP baby is on from external palpation. However, it is safe to assume they are on the right, as this is quite a bit more common and there is little downside to getting it wrong at this early stage. If there is no change at all after the first session, or if there is any back pain during or after the session, then simply reverse sides.

- Reassess position: it is rare that Baby will not turn with this treatment, especially before engagement. If there has been no change, teach UB-67 moxa, plus either the homework below, or the Miles Circuit (easily found on their website, www.milescircuit.com).

Homework to discourage return to OP:

- Cat/Cow on hands and knees, 3–5 minutes three to five times per day.

- Avoid sitting in a leaned-back position, or with knees higher than hips (e.g. bucket car seats; put a pillow in them).

- Consider adding constitutional homework, particularly hot foot soaks or moxa for Yang- or Qi-deficient moms.

D3.2 Swayback posture

As discussed in Chapter 2, the swayback posture is a form of functional cephalopelvic disproportion (CPD) where Baby has trouble engaging properly because Mom's pelvis is tilted forward. This situation generally presents with a tight, sore, excessively arched lower back, and is often compounded by some combination of cold and deficiency. If the skin of the back, sacrum or upper buttocks is cool to the touch, or Mom reports commonly feeling cold anywhere else, then warming the back and body will be important to resolving the situation.

A labor preparation session for this presentation follows directly from the relaxation sequence, and has three parts:

- Thoroughly warm the muscles of the lower back, using a heating pad, heat lamp or round rubbing for 5–10 minutes (I don't use moxa for this, as it only heats one point at a time). If cold is pronounced and it's convenient, soak the feet in hot water during the treatment.

- Repeat the latter part of the relaxation sequence, with thumb pressure down the back starting just below the bottom rib, followed by thumb circles in the tight lumbar area and along the top of the sacrum and the sacroiliac joint.

- Coach Mom on consciously flattening the back. This will be a modified version of Cat/Cow, rebalancing Yin and Yang movements within the lower back.

  - Supporting Mom's lower back with your hand, invite her to sit mostly upright, leaning forward into the table slightly and supporting some weight with her arms.

– Ask her to arch her back very slightly away from your hand, while inhaling – only until she feels the back muscles engage comfortably. In this position there will usually be resistance as the bump presses against her legs.

– On the exhale, invite her not to actively curve the back, but merely to relax whatever muscles she has been engaging in order to arch – in the back and all the way to her neck. Repeat this once or twice.

– Once she has felt a sense of truly relaxing out of the arch, invite her to inhale in the neutral relaxed position, then exhale and curve the back outwards, pressing into your hand and relaxing the head forward to make a "C" shape, still supported by her arms on the table.

– Finish in the neutral position, by chafing the right and left sides of the lower back separately, using enough pressure with the root of your palm that the muscles and pelvis jiggle with the movement. This should take 3–5 minutes:

Homework to alleviate swayback

• Ask Mom to repeat the exercise two or three times per day, leaning forward on a table or desk (make sure to provide written or video instructions).

• As time allows, add Hula Hips and daily foot soaks (hot if she is cold or temperature neutral; warm at bedtime if she is Yin or Blood deficient).

D4 Hormonal Shifts and Support Tissue Softening – Weeks 36–38 and After

Engagement occurs in conjunction with initial softening of the pelvic floor and cervix. This softening takes place over the last month of pregnancy, due to a combination of high relaxin levels, increased baby weight and the cervical ripening cycle in which tissue stretch increases secretion of prostaglandins, which in turn make the tissue stretchier (see Figure 3.14). When the hormones are appropriately online, moms will often notice the shift, feeling more emotional. The hormonal cycle is easily disrupted: by insufficiency of either Yin or Yang, by strong or stagnant Qi that will not allow Baby to drop and the pelvic floor to soften, or by a spirit that is emotionally stuck or not ready for labor. Supporting the process thus requires some additional information gathering regarding possible constitutional imbalances. Addressing imbalances and promoting a hormonal shift is the essence of labor preparation – whether it takes place with a baby that is still high at 41 weeks, or at week 37 before any problems are apparent. Constitutional assistance can begin at week 36, while methods to soften the pelvic floor should usually wait until week 38. Relevant therapeutic goals and methods are summarized in Table D2.

Table D2 Supporting hormonal shifts and tissue softening.

Assessment/ goal	Therapeutic Methods in Session	Homework
Deficient Yin? Nourish Yin	• Footrubs, press SP-6, gentle chafing inner ankle • Needling KD-6, SP-6, PC-6, etc.	Encourage hormones: • Pressure LI-4, SP-6, thumb circles at sacral points • Baby pictures, cute animal videos, romantic movies, nipple stimulation, orgasm, semen (oral, or vaginal only if membranes are intact) • Ear birth basics seeds or needles
Deficient Yang? Warm Yang	• Heating pads, Handwich • Moxa inner ankle, lower back • Hot foot soaks, Cat/Cow	
Trauma/Fear/Heart Qi locked up? Open and descend Heart Qi	• Side-lying, have Mom warm heart center, top of fundus with hands; press KD-1 • Needle RN-17 & 15, HT-3, KD-1	
Urgent encouragement (any presentation)	• E-stim, Ear Endocrine to Uterus • Du-26	

The lines of questioning below address the most important constitutional challenges to address before birth. If session time is short, they can often be asked during the physical set-up of the session, or during other steps of the session as occasion arises:

- Identify any gross Yin/Yang imbalances – is Mom markedly hot or cold, dry or damp, restless or lethargic?

- Qi/Blood sufficiency and flow – ask about energy, sleep, appetite, constipation, heartburn or hemorrhoids, body sensations.

- Spirit or emotional challenges – look for visible emotion, tension; ask leading questions such as "Are you feeling ready for the birth?", "What are your main stressors at this point?", "Are you getting any down time?"

- Final open question – "Is there anything else you'd like me to know?"

Yin and Blood deficiency can be addressed through footrubs, pressure on SP-6 and gentle chafing of the inner ankle. Acupuncturists can needle KD-6 and PC-6, adding SP-6 after 37 weeks.

Yang deficiency can be warmed with heating pads, the Handwich or moxa on the inner ankle and/or lower back; lifestyle homework can include hot foot soaks and Cat/Cow.

If fear or other emotions appear to be a factor, pressure at KD-1 can be useful to calm and root the spirit, as well as working with the emotional release points. Invite Mom to breathe deeply into the points to press your thumbs against them, and ask about any associated issues or feelings that may arise. If the treatment is helpful, it can be taught to a partner or birth team member. Ear seeds are useful, and acupuncturists are encouraged to use their full range of diagnostics for emotional challenges.

Occasionally, Mom will appear ambivalent, mildly dissociated or "checked out." In these situations, it can be very useful to physically and ritually reconnect the heart and uterus. Mom can lay one hand at the chest center and one at the top of the fundus, while the acupuncturist may choose to needle points such as Ren-17 and 15, HT-3 and KD-1.

Home activities that encourage the labor hormones include romantic movies, babies and cute animals (live or video), nipple stimulation, orgasm and acupressure at LI-4 and SP-6, along with thumb circles at sacral points (these should wait until week 37). It should be noted that semen is rich in prostaglandins, and is helpful both systemically and locally to facilitate tissue stretch.[2] The birth basics ear seeds can help these to work, particularly Endocrine and Uterus.

Home activities that encourage the labor hormones include:

- oxytocin-promoting activities including babies and cute animals (live and video), romantic movies, kissing and physical contact, and orgasm

- semen, vaginally (unless membranes are ruptured) or orally

- acupressure at LI-4 and SP-6, and thumb circles at sacral points (these should wait until week 37).

If Baby has not engaged by 38 weeks, and there is no sign of bony obstruction, then it is time to begin helping the pelvic floor to relax and directing Qi downward. Suggested methods include strong bilateral pressure on the Waist points, LV-7 and GB-21, along with dredging downward along the GB channel (iliotibial band) on the thigh. Acupuncturists may needle points such as ST-31, UB-60 toward KD-3 and Du-20. Useful homework includes the Sumo Walk and Squat, dancing, and gentle bouncing.

---

2   If membranes are ruptured, vaginal sex should be avoided; however, oral intake of prostaglandins also helps to ripen the cervix.

The sacrotuberous ligament release (Section 6.2.1) is a direct and powerful way to soften the pelvic floor. It should be done on any first-time Mom who has not dropped after 38 weeks, and any time induction is imminent. It can also be done lightly to get an idea of the pelvic size and shape, at the initial visit or anytime there is any concern or question regarding pelvic shape; for example, with persistent OP, which may be caused by a narrow pelvis. I strongly encourage practitioners to use this technique as often as possible at first, in order to improve technique and thumb strength, as well as learning the normal range of pelvic shapes – wide and narrow, long and short.

Acupuncturists can needle UB-60 and 67 downward to strongly descend Qi, but only if the head is still unengaged; otherwise the sudden increase in pressure on the cervix may lead to swelling.[3] If induction is imminent, or if Mom is behind schedule and her pulse is not yet floating, then LU-7 can be needled to circulate the Qi and encourage descent. Electrical stimulation between Ear Endocrine and Sympathetic can also help to initiate hormonal activity that is missing in action; it is particularly useful when moms are being induced early for medical reasons. For robust patients and those with Qi stagnation, useful empirical points for pelvic floor release may include ST-31, Du-26 and any tight areas around GB-27 and GB-28.

Homework for strongly promoting hormonal activity includes acupressure, with 5 minutes each every 4 hours on SP-6, LI-4, GB-21 and thumb circles on the sacral points. Strong nipple stimulation (e.g. with a breast pump) may also be useful.

D5 Support Cervical Ripening and Early Dilatation – Week 38 and After

As hormones soften the pelvic floor and Baby engages, the cervix should begin to respond to the increased stretch by softening further, shortening and dilating to 3–4 cm. Some US providers monitor this progress with weekly vaginal exams; otherwise loss of the mucus plug between 37 and 39 weeks is an important signal that cervical ripening is occurring on schedule. Relevant assessments and therapeutic goals are summarized in Table D3.

---

3 I learned this technique from Canadian obstetrical acupuncturist Jean Levesque – along with the urgent caution that it should be used only when the head was still high or the cervix was fully dilated.

Table D3 Promoting cervical ripening.

Assessment/ goal	Therapeutic Methods in Session	Homework
Cold? Warm lower abdomen	• Heating pads, Handwich • Moxa inner ankle, lower back	• Hot foot soaks, Cat/Cow
Deficient Yin or Blood? Nourish Yin/ Blood, gently move Qi	• Gentle Liver Gummies, hip rocking, footrubs, press SP-6, LV-8 • Handwich with Belly Breathing (if anxiety) • Needling KD-6, SP-6, PC-6, LV-8, etc.	• Warm foot soaks at bedtime, can add magnesium • Dancing or gentle bouncing, Belly Breathing • Gentle Liver Gummies or footrubs, press LV-8
Qi stagnation? Move stuck QI, soften Liver channel	• Side-lying relaxation sequence: hip rocking, dredge GB channel, loosen tight points in hip/buttock area • Liver Gummies	• Sumo Walk, dancing or gentle bouncing • Pressure at Waist points, GB-21, LI-4 • Needling LV-3, LI-4, SP-6, etc.
Trauma? Open/descend Heart QI	• Side-lying, have Mom warm heart center, top of fundus with hands; press KD-1 • Needle RN-17 & 15, HT-3, KD-1	Repeat heart/fundus warming daily, adding Belly Breathing and partner acupressure at KD-1
Urgent encouragement (any presentation)	• Strong Liver Gummies • E-stim, SP-6 to SP-6 or LV-2 to LV-5 (bilateral)	Also address Hormones/Tissue Softening

The main obstacle to cervical effacement and dilatation is Qi stagnation, plus or minus underlying factors such as cold or Yin deficiency. Take a moment and imagine that you have a very full bladder, but the facility is far away; notice a clenching in the pelvic floor, lower abdomen and inner thighs, as the body clenches itself against downward release. Points along the Liver channel can be very effective in softening this tightness, as can warmth, deep breathing, and movements, large and small. Helping a mom to find what works best for her is not only important for cervical ripening, but will also give her and her birth team valuable tools to use in active labor. If constitutional imbalances have been identified, they provide the most important cues as to what will help.

Qi stagnation is common among strong, energetic moms who are used to more vigorous exercise than they get in late pregnancy. It is also common with work stress or emotions such as anger and frustration (fear and grief usually need a more delicate approach; see the paragraph below). Vigorous movement is usually best for moving Qi and softening the Liver channel. Useful methods to teach for labor preparation and birth include the Sumo Walk, dancing or gentle bouncing, as well as hip rocking, Liver Gummies, and pressure on GB-21 and the Waist points. Acupuncturists may needle points such as LV-3, LI-4 and SP-6 (after 37 weeks). If the pulse is not yet floating, LU-7 may be added. If induction is imminent, the homework methods can be performed every 4 hours. E-stim can be added to acupuncture sessions, connecting SP-6 to opposite SP-6, or connecting same-side LV-2 and LV-5 points, as preferred.

Cold easily stagnates Qi, and is therefore a common and important impediment to cervical ripening. Anyone who feels cold, or suffers painful menstrual cramps that improve with warmth, can benefit from warming therapies during labor preparation and birth. Methods include heating pads, the Handwich, moxibustion at the inner ankles or lower back and abdomen, hot foot soaks and vigorous Cat/Cow.

In a number of cases, slow dilatation reflects Qi stagnation with underlying deficiency of Yin or Blood, or vulnerable emotions such as fear, anxiety, unresolved grief or past trauma. These moms generally do not respond well to vigorous movement, strong pressure or aggressive needling – the strong stimulus is painful or overstimulating and causes further clenching or emotional withdrawal. If the issue seems primarily traumatic or emotional, the methods described above to descend the Heart Qi for engagement and initial tissue softening should be used, along with methods that nourish Yin and Blood. These include the Handwich with Belly Breathing, footrubs, gentle chafing of the Liver Gummy area, and acupressure on SP-6 and LV-8. Gentle hip rocking, dancing or bouncing are also beneficial to softly move QI. Acupuncturists may needle points such as SP-6, LV-8 and HT-3.

D6 Promote Contractions – 40 Weeks, or 1 Week Before Scheduled Induction (Assuming Engagement and Cervical Ripening)

In general, it is better to accomplish as much cervical ripening and dilatation as possible through relaxation and gravity, sparing contractile activity for active labor. It is almost never appropriate to promote contractions before at least the beginning of engagement: when the head is in place, the shape of the pelvis funnels contractile force down toward the cervix. When the head is out of the pelvis, the uterus's strength will be dissipated due to lack of downward focus, in some cases even reducing Baby's freedom to find his best angle of approach. Considerations and methods for promoting contractions are summarized in Table D4.

Table D4 Promoting contractions.

Assessment/ goal	Therapeutic methods in session	Homework
Some contractions: Contraction wrangling	Chafe ankle 3 minutes, tap UB-67 for 30 seconds; repeat for 20 minutes then reassess contraction regularity, intensity, duration	Warm Yang, encourage hormones: see above under Hormones/ Tissue Softening
No contractions: Promote contractions	• Needle Ear birth basics, LI-4, SP-6 • Strong manual or electrical stimulation at UB-32 (not crossing midline)	

Initiation of contractions is Yang's responsibility: if Baby's head is engaged but contractions have not started, usually Mom has some combination of Yang/Qi deficiency and damp. Occasionally, there is indeterminate obstruction – a short cord, or true CPD – and in other cases the spirit is just holding back. The same methods used to warm Yang and address spiritual challenges at engagement should be used as appropriate, while also promoting contractions. All of the methods for encouraging hormones should also be used: ear birth basics, pressure at LI-4, SP-6, and thumb circles at sacral points; as well as romantic movies, nipple stimulation and (especially) orgasm.

If Baby is engaged, the cervix is ripe and there is already some irregular contractile activity, then contraction wrangling (Section 6.5.1) almost always succeeds in nudging Mom into labor within hours. It has four steps, and is easily taught to doulas or clever family members:

- With a relaxed hand, vigorously chafe and warm the inner ankles (KD-1 to KD-7 area) for 4 minutes, while Mom keeps you posted of any contractile activity.

- If a contraction starts before 4 minutes is up, time it and let it run its course, then restart the 4 minutes of chafing (the goal is regular contractions every 5 minutes or less, each lasting about a minute).

- If no contraction arises during the 4 minutes of chafing, then tap or press smartly at UB-67 for 30 seconds, or until a contraction starts. A short fingernail can be just the right amount of stimulus; it can also work to place an ear seed on the point and press or tap sharply with the fingertip. I find it's actually important that the pressure has a brisk, Yang quality to it, perhaps three or four taps per second.

  - If contractions do not start immediately, experiment with the intensity and regularity of the tapping – sometimes irregular tapping seems more effective than a regular rhythm, and softer pressure works better for some sensitive or Yin/Blood-deficient moms.

- – For birth professionals, this same tapping usually produces an acceleration in the fetal heart rate of a sleeping baby, which can be handy in interpreting a tracing that looks a little flat.

- After 20–30 minutes of this, step back and reassess what the contractions do on their own. If induction is imminent, as with prelabor rupture of membranes, the method can be repeated hourly or alternated with the acupressure below until the rhythm continues independently.

If the tapping does not reliably start contractions, or if there is no contractile activity to begin with, then stronger methods are needed. Together with careful differential diagnosis of bone, flesh and spirit challenges, strong manual or electrical stimulation at the sacral points is very effective for initiating contractions.

Manual stimulation tends to work best in the seated position. After some relaxing bodywork, Ear birth basics seeds or needles can be placed, along with LI-4, SP-6 and constitutional points as appropriate. Palpate the sacral points carefully, noting which seems most reactive and pressing it at various angles until one feels as though it will let the needle in. Then needle carefully with a 3 in. needle, or longer if Mom is large. If you hit bone, withdraw to skin level and redirect until you can feel clearly that the needle is inside the hole.

- Once both needles are in place, stimulate both simultaneously with small, rapid back-and-forth or lift-and-thrust movements – whatever you usually use is fine, as long as you can keep it up with gusto for a full minute (this may take some practice).

- If you're new at this or Mom's sacrum is tricky, and you keep bumping up against the bone rather than sliding smoothly into the sacral foramen, then consider adding a second set of needles in the hole above or below. This gives you a second chance to get needles into the holes, and if that fails, then you can consider adding E-stim (if it is not your first session with this patient, and you feel comfortable that she will not faint). I find needles inserted over but not in the holes to be ineffective at initiating labor with manual stimulation alone.

- Rest for 4 minutes between stimulation, and repeat five times for a 30-minute treatment, stimulating the other needles as appropriate. If contractions initiate before the 4-minute mark, time their duration and ask Mom to rate their intensity from 1 to 10 for reference.

For electrical stimulation, I prefer a side-lying position so that Mom can relax more deeply, and to prevent possible fainting with the strong stimulation. If the sacral points are tricky, you can ask Mom to curl forward. Start with Ear birth basics, SP-6, LI-4 and constitutional points as appropriate.

- Find the two sacral points on each side that seem the most active and needle them, trying to get all the way into the holes if possible.

- Connect E-stim leads from the top to the bottom point on each side – do not cross the midline. Most machines do not actually differentiate positive and negative poles; if yours does, then run the current down the channel.

- Set frequency and intensity according to Mom's constitution as well as your own experience and preference, increasing intensity every 5 minutes or so as tolerance builds:

  - If there is Yin or Blood deficiency, or anxiety, start with very mild intensity, increasing only as it's truly comfortable.

  - If anxiety is a factor, use 1–2 Hz for the first 10 minutes; once Mom feels more relaxed, begin alternating with 50 Hz.

  - For Yang and Qi deficiency, alternate 10 Hz with 100 Hz.

Homework for promoting contractions includes:

- Acupressure at LI-4, SP-6 and thumb circles at sacral points, 5 minutes every few hours while awake.

- Oxytocin-promoting activities including babies and cute animals (live and video), kissing and physical contact, and orgasm; also semen, vaginally (unless membranes are ruptured) or orally.

D7 Summary Table and Final Note
The time frames and associated therapeutic goals for labor preparation are summarized in Table D5.

Table D5 Therapeutic goals according to timing or situation.

Gestational age	Key items	36 weeks	37 weeks	38 weeks	39 weeks	40 weeks	41 weeks or after	Early medical induction	Prelabor rupture of membranes
1. Information gathering	Baby high or low? Swayback or occiput posterior (OP)?	?	?	?	?	?	???	?	???
	Obvious imbalances?	?	?	?	?	?	???	???	?
	Red flags?	?	?	?	?	?	?	?	?
	Other complaints?	?	?	?	?	?	?	?	?
	Choose position	✓	✓	✓	✓	✓	✓	✓	✓
2. Relaxation	Get settled	✓	✓	✓	✓	✓	✓	✓	✓✓✓
	Open back	✓	✓	✓	✓	✓	✓	✓✓✓	✓
3. Bony engagement	Swayback?	✓	✓	(✓?)	(✓?)	(✓?)	???	✓	✓
	OP?	✓	✓	(✓?)	(✓?)	(✓?)	???	✓	???
4. Hormones and tissue softening	Deficient Yin or Yang?		?	(✓?)	(✓?)	(✓?)	?	?	?
	Trauma/ Heart Qi locked up?		?	(✓?)	(✓?)	(✓?)	?	?	?
	Encourage hormones	✓		(✓?)	(✓?)	(✓?)	✓	✓✓✓	✓✓✓
5. Cervical ripening and dilatation	Cold?			?	?	(✓?)	?	?	?
	Deficient Yin or Blood?			?	?	(✓?)	?	?	?
	Qi stagnation?			?	?	(✓?)	?	?	???
	Trauma?			?	?	(✓?)	?		?
6. Promote contractions	Some contractions					?	???		???
	No contractions					?	???		???

?	Assess this now
✓	Do this now (unless there's a reason not to)
??? or ✓✓✓	Most important to assess or do for this situation
(✓?)	This should be in order by now, if it's not, then stay back and keep working on it before moving on to this week's goal

Any discussion of labor preparation written after 2016 is remiss if it does not discuss the Complementary Therapies in Labor and Birth protocol developed by Australian acupuncturist and women's health researcher Kate Levett.[4] This is a combination of six simple, evidence-based techniques taught to moms and partners for use before and during labor. These were originally taught in a weekend course, but can be adapted to other formats. The techniques include acupressure (from Debra Betts' handout), visualization and relaxation, breathing, massage, yoga techniques and facilitated partner support. Results were extraordinary, with the group who took the course showing significantly fewer instances of Cesarean sections, epidural use, labor augmentation, perineal trauma and resuscitation of the newborn; duration of second stage was also shorter.

If any drug achieved all of those improvements in clinical outcome with no adverse events, it would be hailed as miraculous and would quickly become the standard of care. However, as an educational program, it has not yet been widely adapted. It is incumbent on those of us who understand the value of birth preparation to till the ground, demonstrating the usefulness of acupressure and other techniques for labor preparation and support. Levett's techniques can easily be mixed and matched with the homework described above, for use both before and during labor.

---

4   Levett, K. M., Smith, C. A., Bensoussan, A., & Dahlen, H. G. (2016). Complementary therapies for labour and birth study: A randomised controlled trial of antenatal integrative medicine for pain management in labour. *BMJ Open*, 6(7), e010691.

Appendix E

Postpartum Care

East Asian medicine (EAM) can be extraordinarily helpful during the postpartum period, helping Mom to rebuild her Qi and Blood while accommodating a newborn's schedule and nutritional needs. A thorough discussion of postpartum care is outside the scope of this book: in particular, acupuncture can help to quickly resolve musculoskeletal pain including back and pelvic pain and rectus or symphysis diastasis. Postpartum vulvar pain, varicosities and urinary incontinence also respond extremely well to timely acupuncture treatment.

A few key techniques for early postpartum recovery are presented below, for use under the dual safety net of Mom's primary care provider, and/or mentorship by experienced EAM practitioners. The constitutional care packages from Chapter 4 can also be used for self-care – though time is always a challenge. The key is to pick one intervention that also provides some pleasure and much-needed recharge time, and to make it a ritual of whole-family care.

Postpartum "Mother Roasting"

Raven Lang may be the most important living progenitor of the acupuncture and birth community in North America. As a midwife in the 1970s, she founded the first free-standing birth centers in the US and Canada, delivering innumerable babies, publishing a seminal book on home birth,[1] and training midwives. In the 1980s Raven also attended acupuncture school and assisted in the clinic of Miriam Lee, an acupuncturist in San Francisco who (legend has it) had her busy clinic shut down by the police until scores of passionate patients showed up at the courthouse, leading to the legalization of

---

1   Raven, L. (1972). *Birth Book*. Chicago, IL.

acupuncture in the United States. Raven's self-published booklet on "Mother Roasting" (available on her website) is based on her research into traditional postpartum practices worldwide, which very often include both protecting mothers from the cold and also proactively warming their lower back and abdominal areas. Raven's recommendations, which I follow enthusiastically, are as follows:

- Warming sessions of 40–60 minutes per day should begin as soon as convenient after birth, and continue until 5–10 total sessions have been completed, or they stop feeling good to Mom.

- Warming may be done with pole moxa, a moxa pot or box (sold in Chinese medical supply stores) or other equipment such as heating pads, rice bags or hot rocks.

- The back and front should be warmed on alternate days. The areas to be warmed are:

  – the lower back, from about L-2 to S-2, from the midline out over the sacroiliac joint

  – the lower abdomen, from above the pubic bone to below the navel.

- The treatment should feel good at all times, and should be modified or discontinued if the heat becomes uncomfortable.

- While providing adequate ventilation, make sure that Mom is well covered and not exposed to direct drafts.

Post-Cesarean Section Care

Cesarean section is now the most common surgery in the United States, and numbers are high in other countries as well. Its high prevalence seems to have engendered widespread amnesia regarding the seriousness of this abdominal surgery. When acupuncturists come to the hospital to train, I have them watch at least one of the surgeries in order to understand experientially what a shock to the system it is – including the extreme cold of the operating room, many degrees below anything the uterus ever expected to encounter.

I practice and teach post-C-section care in three distinct stages:

- acute recovery, within a week after surgery

- scar therapy, any time after 10 weeks (even years later)

- labor preparation for the next labor.

Acute recovery

After C-section, it is particularly important to do mother warming – carefully – as soon as possible after the sutures are removed. In addition to warming the whole area, the scar should be thoroughly warmed – it's critically important to monitor the heat level with clean fingers resting near but not touching the scar, as there may some numbness or hypersensitivity. This may feel strange for acupuncturists, who are trained not to moxa anything that looks swollen or inflamed. However, during C-section the uterus and fascia are exposed to cold drafts unlike anything that nature could ever have imagined, and moms tend to report that the scar loves and craves the heat, at least for the first several days. Once it stops feeling great, it is time to stop the treatment. Also, it does sometimes happen that after moxa a small pustule forms, as though the scar is extruding some hidden bacteria. This is a positive outcome of the treatment, not a negative one – without the heat increasing local immune response, the bacteria might have lingered.

Acupuncturists should also think in terms of reinstating channel flow across the cut area. Those good with their hands may want to try redirecting pressure on Leg, Arm and Upper Torso points, with the aim of helping Qi to move through the areas where the fascia has been cut and twisted. I work with distal points on the first treatment, e.g. SP-4, PC-6, LU-7, KD-6, ST-36, plus ear seeds for pain as needed. Then over the next two or three treatments I move closer to the area (Mom will be quite appropriately protective of the whole abdomen at first). I look for tender points moving inward along the course of the Stomach channel and extra vessels, such as ST-32, GB-31, LV-8 and the inner thigh points, with points like Ren-9 (there is usually retained fluid) and GB-26. ST-25 and 31, and KD-16 are usually the closest I get before 6 weeks.

Scar therapy

Up to about 6 weeks, the body builds the scar up, adding scar tissue like a sculptor piling on clay, not sure yet what she will decide in the moment. After that time, the tissue that is pulled on frequently stays, and tissue that is not used gets reabsorbed. I don't feel that it's at all appropriate to interfere in the building-up phase, so I usually wait until I am quite sure it is completed – about 10 weeks. At that point (or whenever Mom comes in, which may be years later) I begin scar therapy.

With acupuncture, "surround the dragon" by placing 1 in. needles in a circle 1–1.5 in. (2–4 cm) away from the scar, inserted about ½ cun at about a 45° angle pointing inward (for the bottom of the circle, you may need to adjust technique and angle to accommodate the top of the pubic hair). Over the next two to five treatments (depending on the age and severity of the scar) move the needles progressively closer and begin needling directly into the tough parts; I often use ½ in. needles for this as they penetrate better. The whole scar will soften and lighten in color, but parts will remain tough; begin surrounding these until they let go. The manual work described below will also help to break them up.

This manual stretching of the scar works with or without acupuncture, though of course the combination is faster and more complete. With Mom lying comfortably on her back, knees supported, have your hips at about the level of her mid-thighs and face toward her. Lay your eight fingertips (not counting the thumbs) across the length of the scar, and equalize the pressure between fingers by bending the middle fingers more. Then, ever so slowly, let your fingers sink into the flesh of the scar – only as fast as Mom's body invites you in. This usually feels like sinking downward as she exhales, then holding steady as she inhales so that the tissues stretch themselves against your quiet, curious fingers. Over about 5 minutes (longer if you have time and Mom feels it's helpful) let your fingers drop constantly inward, never backing off a millimeter, but instead gently exploring any resistance. You may find your hands twisting away from each other to increase torsion on a particularly tight place; if in doubt as to what to do, simply hold steady and check in frequently with Mom. As with mother warming, this manual scar therapy usually feels quite pleasant, like scratching an itch she didn't know she had. Make sure to take before and after pictures, as the scar often becomes markedly flatter and paler after each session. Occasionally the color darkens temporarily as circulation increases, but this always subsides. It's quite hard to predict how many sessions will be needed to "finish" the work – as there will never be no scar. Better to suggest starting with three and then making a plan after that.

Labor preparation

A small but significant number of vaginal births after Cesarean result in "scar dehiscence" – tearing open under the force of the contractions. The third phase of post-C-section care is therefore to provide treatments to ripen and soften the cervix and pelvic floor as much as possible, so that the uterus does not have to work as hard. Within the time parameters given in Appendix D, stay on the early side, aiming for a ripe cervix with contractions during week 39 rather than week 40.

Other Postpartum Challenges

EAM treatment and self-care can be very helpful in helping the body to heal from the birth, as well as managing the challenges of lactation and sleep deprivation. It can also be helpful in the prevention and treatment of postpartum depression, though of course coordination with Mom's primary care and support network is critical. Common postpartum issues that respond well to EAM therapeutic methods include:

- afterpains

- constipation, hemorrhoids and tears

- insufficient lactation and mastitis

- fatigue and mild depression.

Afterpains

During the days and weeks after birth, the uterus contracts itself back from its expanded pregnant state to the size of a pear. Those contractions may be below the pain threshold, like the prenatal Braxton–Hicks contractions, or they may be quite uncomfortable, like severe menstrual cramps. Whatever comfort measures were most useful during birth should also help to relieve these afterpains, particularly warming therapies for cold moms and Liver Gummies if there is stagnation involved. Pressure or needling at SP-6 may also be helpful, along with any tender points above it, particularly in the belly of the calf muscle (SP-8 area). If persistent, a single office visit to an acupuncturist for a full treatment can usually resolve them.

Constipation, tears and hemorrhoids

Constipation is extremely common after birth, as the metabolism accommodates to the fluid loss of birth and the need to send much of its fluid intake back out again as breast milk. This is particularly for Yin- and Blood-deficient types. Tears and hemorrhoids only complicate matters: the first few bowel movements can be quite uncomfortable, and there is a natural urge to postpone them as long as possible. Unfortunately, the large intestine is a drying chamber, so the longer a stool remains in it, the harder and sharper it gets. Three basic principles make it possible to heal as quickly as possible.

First, keep bowels as soft as possible with ample hydration, fiber and slippery, Yin- and Blood-nourishing food and drinks. These include:

- coconut water, smoothies, green juices and fruit juices, especially prune or pear

- healthy fats, which are also needed for producing breast milk: avocados are particularly good, as is coconut oil

- cooked vegetables, particularly okra; fresh, cooked or dried fruit

- nuts and seeds, only if the area is not too raw.

Second, keep the perineum clean and dry. I recommend the Yin care wash, which has a balanced combination of cooling and flesh healing herbs. It can be mixed with water and sprayed on with a mister or squirt bottle, then patted dry.

Third, keep Qi moving in the right direction. Round rubbing on the abdomen can be done as self-care for 1–2 minutes every time Mom lies down to sleep, or by a partner or helper in 5–7-minute sessions. Stack the hands one atop the other and rub in a large circle, clockwise from the right hip up below the right ribs, across to the upper left, down to the left hip, then across to start again. This is the trajectory of the large intestine, and rubbing it like this both physically encourages movement, and also strengthens the Qi of the abdomen generally. The pace should be steady and deliberate, perhaps 2–3 seconds per direction, with as much pressure as is comfortable.

If there are tears or hemorrhoids, then acupressure, moxa or needling at Du-20 can help to raise Qi and take pressure off the area. Acupuncturists may also want to palpate for tender points around UB-57.

Milk production

Insufficient lactation has two basic presentations: Qi stagnation and Blood deficiency. If milk has not come in at all, or if there are possible signs of both, then the methods below can be combined. Make sure to keep pressure within Mom's comfort zone.

With Qi stagnation, relaxation and let-down are inhibited by muscular tension in the shoulders, as well as the back and shoulder blade. Strong pressure downward at GB-21 almost always breaks up the tension and increases milk flow instantly. It's also extremely useful to teach family members a simple regimen of prefeeding massage: neck, traps, between the shoulder blades, then coming around on each side from the shoulder blade (with special emphasis on a tender point in the middle, Small Intestine-11) around the shoulder and upper arm to the pectorals.

Inhibited lactation due to Blood deficiency takes more work to resolve, including a nourishing diet high in protein and fat, and moxa or round rubbing for several days or even weeks. As a rule of thumb, if someone had scanty periods or other Blood deficiency signs pre-pregnancy, then some nourishing work will be needed on the back end to get lactation up to speed. The preferred method is Moxa at UB-17, both sides, 15 minutes daily or as close as possible – at least for the first week, after which it can be weekly or as needed. Debra Betts hears from midwives to whom she has taught this method, that the milk actually appears creamier after a week of treatment, as well as more abundant. If digestion is poor or appetite is low, also moxa ST-36 for 5 minutes.

If moxa is impossible, substitute round rubbing at the mid-back, as well as chafing down the outer shin from ST-36 and gentle shoulder rubs as described above. Other items from the Qi and Blood deficiency care packages in Chapter 4 can also be useful if time allows.

Mastitis

When breast tissue becomes inflamed and infected, acupuncture's ability to clear heat and flush out stuck Qi in a particular body area is extremely valuable. The same heat-clearing points on the foot used in labor work well to clear heat and reduce fever – LV-2, plus its neighbors ST-44 and GB-43. Local points Ren-17 (in the chest center) and ST-18 (at the base of the breast directly below the nipple, one rib space above LV-14) move Qi where it is stuck in the breast. Debra reports hearing from one of her midwife students that a patient's fever reduced a full degree and her breast became less swollen within an hour of treatment. Antibiotics for mastitis are widely regarded as a necessary evil, but in many cases acupuncture treatment is enough to help the body mount its own successful immune defense, along with hot compresses and other home remedies.

Fatigue and postpartum depression

Fatigue and postpartum depression are distinct but related challenges. They differ in frequency and severity, with fatigue due to interrupted sleep nearly universal in contemporary households, while clinical depression affects an estimated 10–15 percent of mothers in the West. It is not known how many suffer mild or moderate subclinical symptoms not rising to the level of diagnosis. While postpartum depression is complex, multifactorial and poorly understood by Western medicine, the link between sleep and mood regulation is clear experientially, and is increasingly strengthened by basic and clinical research. Of all the ways in which to help the world, it's hard to imagine a point of higher leverage than preventing or mitigating even one case of postpartum depression, given its potential severity and critical impact on the entire trajectory of two lives.

From an EAM perspective, the problems are closely related manifestations of insufficiency and/or stagnation. Fatigue represents a mild to moderate disruption of one's ability and interest to engage in life, while depression is more severe, affecting the emotions and, at worst, the spirit's willingness to remain tied to the body. As with birth, each type responds differently to the challenges of sleep deprivation and new motherhood. In addition to the care package interventions, a few methods may be key.

Yin- and/or Blood-deficient moms tend to be hardest hit, as their sleep and capacity for self-soothing is often less than optimal at baseline. The experiential quality of Yin deficiency fatigue can be a sort of low-grade agitation, like a cranky child – life is overstimulating and every stimulus is noxious, but lying down in a quiet bedroom only provides an empty stage for anxious thoughts to dance on. The therapeutic goal is to soothe the agitated spirit and nervous system, so that sleep can be both deeper and easier to achieve within an unstable schedule. Key methods include:

- belly Breathing, with exhale twice the length of inhale

- footrubs, pressure on KD-1 or gently chafing on the inner ankle

- relaxing self-acupressure on points such as Yintang (at the "third eye" between the brows); any tender points along the occiput; SP-6, PC-6 or LV-3. These can be done for three deep breaths' duration any time there is a spare 30 seconds

- downtime away from home and baby, e.g. yoga class or even just a walk around the block.

Blood-deficient moms may have similar challenges with sleep and overstimulation, but the emotional quality differs from Yin deficiency. Baby crying and dirty diapers lead less to anger and frustration, and more to feeling scattered, overwhelmed or even dissociated. Mom may have difficulty emotionally connecting to her new life and feel like a stranger, hovering purposelessly although there is work to do. In this case the therapeutic goal is rooting the spirit in the body while also building more Blood to keep it there. Key methods include:

- Moxa or rubbing/chafing on UB-17 and ST-36; moxa is particularly important if appetite is not good or milk supply is low.

- Moderate, regular cardiovascular exercise, e.g. at least two walks per day of at least 15 minutes' duration.

- If at all possible, consider familiar social activities, e.g. yoga or tea with old friends.

Yang- and Qi-deficient moms tend to experience fatigue frequently and easily, but in the more familiar, physical sense of lassitude and weakness. There is often also a sense of overwhelm, but it is more at the infinite volume of household work to be done, rather than sensory stimulation. When severely affected, Yang-deficient moms may experience joylessness – not dissociated, particularly, but more aware of the emptiness rather than the fullness of any particular glass. Key methods include:

- sunshine and air as early as possible in the day, even if only for a quick turn around the block

- as much regular cardiovascular activity as possible, ideally four sessions per week

- moxa at ST-36, especially if appetite is not good

- hot foot soaks or ankle chafing.

Moms with Qi stagnation, like those with Yin deficiency, tend to feel an angry or agitated edge within their fatigue – an itch that will not be scratched by sleep. This is particularly a challenge for strong women accustomed to plenty of exercise and/or control over their lives. Most important for these moms is to move their Qi, as often and as much as possible.

- If financially feasible, jogging strollers and/or child care for daily exercise breaks are optimal.

- Otherwise, creativity can be exercised in finding ways to move throughout the day – one martial artist colleague with a colicky baby simply walked in circles holding him all day.

The self-care and lifestyle methods described above can be very helpful in managing fatigue, but should not be considered as cure-alls for severe fatigue or depression. Experienced perinatal acupuncturists and herbalists can be a powerful resource, but should always be consulted alongside one's primary care provider.

Glossary of Medical Terms

This Glossary includes terms used in the text, as well as a few terms or abbreviations that are commonly used in birth settings and may be confusing to acupuncturists.

Active phase of labor: the period when labor progresses most rapidly, previously considered to begin at 3–4 cm based on data from the 1950s; current assessments suggest that 5 cm (Europe) or 6 cm (US) is more appropriate.

Amniotic Fluid Index (AFI): an estimate of the amount of amniotic fluid in the uterus, based on ultrasound findings.

Android: pelvic shape with less space and larger ischial spines than gynecoid pelvis, tends toward longer labor.

Anthropoid: pelvic shape with a very narrow pubic arch, tends toward occiput posterior delivery.

AROM: artificial rupture of membranes; used for labor augmentation.

Asynclitism: when the fetal head enters the pelvis at an oblique angle forward or backward.

Attitude: the relationship of the fetal parts to each other, e.g. head tilted (asynclitism) or not flexed (military attitude).

Augmentation of labor: the use of membrane rupture or pharmaceutical agents such as oxytocin to increase contractions.

Bishop Score: 0–13 scale of cervical factors, used to assess likely induction outcome; score <6 indicates need for cervical ripening.

Cephalic: indicates that the fetal presenting part is the head (versus the buttocks or feet in breech presentation).

Cervical edema: swelling of the cervix under pressure when pushing begins too soon.

Cervical ripening: softening, effacement and dilatation of the cervix before and during early labor.

Cervidil: see Dinoprostone.

CPD: cephalopelvic disproportion – the fetal head is too big to fit through the pelvis.

Crowning: during second stage of labor, when the fetal head passes through the cervix.

Cytotec: see Misoprostol.

Descent: descent is the movement of the fetal head (or other presenting part) down into the pelvis and through the vaginal canal.

Dinoprostone: a synthetic preparation of prostaglandin E1: a pharmaceutical agent used for cervical ripening, usually in a removable ring or tampon; more expensive than Cytotec (misoprostol).

EAM: East Asian Medicine is a general term for all of the styles of practice derived from the initial Chinese texts of the Han dynasty (200 BCE to 200 CE). These spread across the various nationalities of East Asia, including China, Korea, Japan, Vietnam and others. The term is used in preference to the now-outdated 'Oriental Medicine'. The related term 'Traditional Chinese Medicine' (TCM) specifies a distinct practice style codified in China during the 20th century.

EDD: estimated due date; 280 days from last menstrual period (LMP) (40/0) = 10 menstrual cycles.

Effacement: measurement (0–100%) of cervical thinning.

EFW: estimated fetal weight; normal range 3000–4000 g (6.6–8.8 lb).

Engagement: the point when the widest part of the fetal head (or buttocks, if breech) enters the pelvis.

Epidural analgesia: a procedure where a large hypodermic needle is used to place a thin, wire-like catheter just outside the membranes surrounding the spinal cord, delivering small amounts of analgesic agents as needed. For labor, it is placed in between the third and fourth lumbar vertebrae.

Erb's palsy: a temporary or permanent paralysis of the arm due to nerve damage sustained during delivery with shoulder dystocia, when the shoulder is pushed down away from the head with excessive force.

FD: fully dilated.

First stage of labor: the events of labor from first perceived contractions to full dilatation of the cervix.

FT: fingertip, term used to indicate some cervical dilatation but less than 1 cm.

Gestational diabetes mellitus (GDM): new onset high blood sugar or glucose tolerance test readings during pregnancy. Type A2 requires medication and may be induced at 39 weeks as babies tend to be large. The milder type A1 is controlled with diet and managed as a normal pregnancy. Types B through H indicate that the disorder predates the pregnancy.

Gravida: number of pregnancies, within the GPA (gravida, para) system of reporting; G2P1 indicates a woman who is currently pregnant with her second child. The TPAL system (term, preterm, abortus, living) includes more complete obstetrical information.

Hematocrit: indicates the ratio of red blood cell volume to total blood volume, which is normally about 38–46 percent pre-pregnancy and which should drop during pregnancy as fluid in the blood increases. Anything below 33 is considered anemic. The assessment may also be made in terms of hemoglobin levels, with anemia defined as below 11 g/dl in the first and third trimesters, and 10.5 in the second trimester.

Hypoxic brain injury: damage that occurs to brain cells with reduced oxygen supply for over 8 minutes. If severe, long-term complications can include cerebral palsy, seizures, or cognitive, motor or sensory disabilities.

Induction of labor: the stimulation of uterine contractions before they begin on their own; if the cervix is not yet ripe, stimulation of contractions will usually be preceded by a cervical ripening agent such as misoprostol or dinoprostone.

Latent phase: consensus on an exact clinical definition is poor, but generally understood as the time during which contractions are relatively regular and painful, but not yet rapidly progressive (i.e. active phase).

Lie: refers to the direction of Baby's position; longitudinal (could be head up or down), transverse (horizontal across the belly) or oblique; both of the latter are incompatible with vaginal birth but appropriate for moxibustion as with breech.

Lithotomy position: Lithotomy (removal of stones from the bladder or internal organs) is one of the oldest-known surgeries. It was performed with the patient supine, legs spread and raised in stirrups. A reclining version of this position is still used for birth in some institutions.

LMP: last menstrual period.

Misoprostol: a synthetic preparation of prostaglandin E2, indicated for prevention of non-steroidal anti-inflammatory drug (NSAID)-induced gastric ulcers but used off-label as a cervical ripening agent; it is orders of magnitude less expensive than dinoprostone.

Molding: slight reshaping of the soft fetal skull under pressure during delivery; usually resolves within 1–3 days.

Multipara: a person who has given birth more than once.

Nullipara: a person who has never given birth.

OA: occiput anterior; preferred birthing position; may be ROA or LOA (right/left).

Occiput: medical term for the back of the head, which is especially large and protuberant in neonates.

OP: occiput posterior; often results in painful "back labor" (pain); may be ROP or LOP but more commonly ROP.

OT: occiput transverse; distinguish from transverse lie; may be ROT or LOT (right/left). Both are normal at engagement, though LOT is more common.

Oxytocin: an important signaling molecule with many functions. As a hormone, it binds to uterine tissue and produces contractions; as a neurotransmitter it mediates experiences of love, trust and bonding.

Parity: the number of times a mom has delivered a fetus of potentially viable age (over 20 weeks).

Pitocin: US commercial name for synthetic oxytocin, used to induce or augment labor, and postpartum to expel the placenta and prevent hemorrhage (see also Syntocinon).

Platypelloid: flat pelvis shape tending toward slow engagement and/or transverse delivery.

Position: the rotational position of the fetus on its longitudinal axis, described by the orientation of the occiput (or sacrum, in breech); e.g. OP, LOA, etc.

Primipara: term commonly used to describe a person pregnant for the first time; it can also indicate a person who has given birth once, creating potential for confusion. The term "Nullipara" is clearer.

PPROM: premature prelabor rupture of membranes.

Preeclampsia/HELLP: See Section 8.1.3.6.

Presentation: refers to the part that first "presents" to the outside world; i.e. cephalic (head), breech (buttocks), footling (foot), shoulder; compound presentation indicates multiple parts, e.g. head and hand.

Preterm: indicates a fetus of gestational age less than 37 weeks (see also Term).

PROM: prelabor rupture of membranes; indicates that the amniotic sac has ruptured with fluid loss, but labor has not started within 4 hours (see also PPROM, SROM, AROM).

Prostaglandins: local inflammatory signaling molecules (eicosanoids) secreted when tissue is stretched; in labor they soften tissue and open oxytocin binding sites.

Second stage of labor: delivery of the fetus.

SROM: spontaneous rupture of membranes; indicates that the amniotic sac has ruptured spontaneously, either during labor or with subsequent spontaneous labor onset.

Station: measured from the ischial spines; range of −5 (head above the pelvis) to +5 (head at the vaginal opening).

Syntocinon: commercial name for synthetic oxytocin, used to induce or augment labor, and postpartum to expel the placenta and prevent hemorrhage (see also Pitocin).

Tachysystole: designates more than five contractions in 10 minutes; commonly seen during induction with topical application of misoprostol in Yin-deficient moms.

Term: previously used to indicate any fetus past 37 weeks of gestational age, the designation has now been more closely specified: early term (37–38 weeks); full term (39–40 weeks) and late term (41–42 weeks)

Third stage of labor: delivery of placenta and management of any postpartum bleeding.

TOLAC: trial of labor after Cesarean section (see also VBAC).

TPAL: See Gravida.

Transition: the final, intense phase of the first stage of labor, when the fetus descends the final distance from mid-pelvis to pelvic outlet, usually turning its head to do so.

VBAC: vaginal birth after Cesarean section.

Subject Index

Author Index